Handbook of Stereotactic and Functional Neurosurgery

NEUROLOGICAL DISEASE AND THERAPY

Advisory Board

Handbook of Stereotactic and Functional Neurosurgery

edited by
Michael Schulder
New Jersey Medical School
Newark, New Jersey, U.S.A.

associate editor
Chirag D. Gandhi
Mt. Sinai School of Medicine
New York, New York, U.S.A.

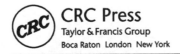

CRC Press
Taylor & Francis Group
Boca Raton London New York

CRC Press is an imprint of the
Taylor & Francis Group, an **informa** business

First published 2003 by Marcel Dekker, Inc.
This edition published 2011 by Informa Healthcare

Published 2019 by CRC Press
Taylor & Francis Group
6000 Broken Sound Parkway NW, Suite 300
Boca Raton, FL 33487-2742

© 2011 by Taylor & Francis Group, LLC
CRC Press is an imprint of Taylor & Francis Group, an Informa business

First issued in paperback 2019

No claim to original U.S. Government works

ISBN 13: 978-0-367-44681-9 (pbk)
ISBN 13: 978-0-8247-0720-0 (hbk)

**Visit the Taylor & Francis Web site at
http://www.taylorandfrancis.com**

**and the CRC Press Web site at
http://www.crcpress.com**

A CIP record for this book is available from the British Library.

Library of Congress Cataloging-in-Publication Data available on application

Series Introduction

The *Handbook of Stereotactic Neurosurgery* provides comprehensive information regarding the use of this important therapeutic maneuver in the treatment of neurological disease. Technical aspects are discussed in stereotactic with frames, frameless stereotactic, and stereotactic radiosurgery. Localization techniques are described in detail. The clinical use of stereotactic neurosurgery in movement disorders, particularly Parkinson's disease, is thoroughly discussed. There are many important advances in this area. The various surgical approaches are discussed by the leading authorities in the field.

Stereotactic neurosurgery is outlined for other indications as well, such as chronic pain, spasticity, and epilepsy. Indications, approaches, and techniques are covered. This book provides a comprehensive approach to stereotactic neurosurgery, both for the neurosurgeon who needs technical details and for the neurologist who must refer patients to the neurosurgeon and evaluate the results of neurosurgical intervention. For all those involved in the care of patients who undergo functional stereotactic neurosurgery, this handbook will provide detailed information to which they can refer. This is indeed a landmark book for functional neurosurgery, which clearly has gained importance in the treatment of a variety of neurological diseases in recent years.

William C. Koller

Foreword

This is an exciting time to be in stereotactic surgery. In a little more than 50 years, it has developed from a concept used in the animal laboratory to a technique that promises to permeate all of neurosurgery.

Before human stereotactic surgery was born, functional neurosurgery consisted of a few adventurous procedures confined to interrupting pathways that were conveniently located superficially and were not overlain by other eloquent tracts. The only functional operations that were generally practiced were open anterolateral cordotomy and pain procedures involving cutting of peripheral or cranial nerves. Interrupting pain pathways within the brainstem was practiced by a relatively small group of neurosurgeons. Surgery for movement disorders often was directed to ablation of the motor cortex or pyramidal tracts, with acceptance of paralysis as a necessary trade in exchange for involuntary movements. The few neurosurgeons who attacked the extrapyramidal system recognized the great morbidity and mortality of their operations. Perhaps the most common functional procedure was prefrontal lobotomy, which involved separating the anterior frontal lobe pathways with a back-and-forth motion of a knife, spatula, or icepick.

It was the abhorrence of prefrontal lobotomy as it was then practiced that motivated Ernest A. Spiegel, a Jewish neurologist born in Vienna who had fled to Philadelphia, to adapt to patients a technique developed for use in laboratory animals half a century before by neurosurgeon Sir Victor Horsley and engineer Robert Clarke. Spiegel recruited Henry T. Wycis, a former student and neurosurgical colleague at Temple Medical School, to develop with him techniques to allow stereotactic targeting to be used in patients. They developed a procedure that used intracerebral landmarks visualized by intraoperative X-ray, rather than skull landmarks as had been used in animals.

Human stereotactic surgery was born in 1946, when Spiegel and Wycis injected alcohol stereotactically into the globus pallidus and dorsomedial thalamic nucleus of a patient for treatment of Huntington's chorea. During the next decade, other eminent neurosurgeons entered the field, including Lars Leksell, Traugott Riechert, Jean Talairach, Gerard Guiot, Hirotaro Narabayashi, Blaine Nashold, Sixto Obrador, B. Ramamurthi, Georges Schaltenbrand, Keiji Sano, Sir John Gillingham, and Manuel Velasco Suarez. That decade saw the most exciting and productive development of new surgical indications that has ever been seen. The field was launched with a series of empirically determined targets for almost all the indications we still use. One pervading philosophy was that every insertion of an electrode into the human brain was a unique opportunity to study human neurophysiology and pathophysiology. That led to better understanding of the human brain and, in turn, to better targets for more indications.

By the 1960s, stereotactic surgery was commonly used, mainly as the major treatment for Parkinson's disease. When L-dopa became available in 1968, activity in the field almost ceased, and it was only the dedication of a handful of neurosurgeons that kept the field of stereotactic surgery alive.

During the 1960s and 1970s, stereotactic techniques expanded significantly. Leksell had experimented with using stereotaxis to focus radiation to small targets within the brain, and introduced the Gamma Knife in 1968. The field of stereotactic radiosurgery was practiced at only a few centers with the Gamma Knife or proton beam technology until the 1990s, when computers made it possible to administer the focused radiation with a commonly available linear accelerator. Meanwhile, the Gamma Knife became available commercially and has proliferated, so that stereotactic radiosurgery is now commonly available.

In the 1980s, when there was a dearth of surgery for Parkinson's disease, fetal or adrenal tissue was transplanted into the caudate nucleus, with limited success. It was not until 1992 that Lauri Laitinen reawakened stereotactic surgery by resurrecting Leksell's technique for pallidotomy. As interest reawakened in stereotactic surgery, the use of thalamotomy for tremor also increased.

Also in the 1980s, implantable stimulators were developed for long-term stimulation of various sites for pain management, but this activity waned as difficulties with patient selection and establishing benefit became apparent. However, when Alim Benabid and Jean Siegfried reported that the use of those same stimulators in the same pallidotomy target provides a benefit similar to that of pallidotomy with perhaps less risk, the door opened to the use of implanted stimulators for other indications at other sites. Long-term stimulation of the thalamus for treatment of tremor has emerged as well, such as stimulation of the subthalamic nucleus for Parkinson's disease.

It was also in the 1980s that computed tomographic scanning was introduced. A marriage between imaging modalities and stereotactic surgery was only natural, as both were based on spatial orientation of specific targets within the brain. The first image-guided procedures involved biopsy or aspiration of abscesses. As imaging improved and magnetic resonance imaging became widespread, the use of stereotactic guidance for tumor resection developed. The use of a three-dimensional volumetric target depended on the availability of adequate computer power, and was pioneered by Pat Kelly. Tumor resection became more accurate, and injury to surrounding areas was avoided. Such volumetric display of a tumor volume also made brachytherapy more efficient and practical, although it was subsequently largely supplanted by stereotactic focused external beam radiation. Such image-guided neurosurgery is an immediate outgrowth of computer science. The revolution in computers has had more impact on stereotactic surgery than on any other branch of neurosurgery, and perhaps any other surgical field. Because computer science will undoubtedly continue to mature at an ever more rapid pace, stereotactic surgery promises to follow that same pattern.

We have crossed the threshold of a new millennium. Stereotactic surgery has become the most rapidly advancing field within neurosurgery, and the future promises even more. As computer science moves ahead at a dizzying rate, new techniques in imaging and image guidance will be incorporated into image-guided surgery. Chronic stimulation techniques are becoming more widespread, and new targets and new indications are being sought. Stereotactic radiosurgery and stereotactic radiotherapy are now commonly available, and with new experience will come sophistication in the use of these modalities, particularly for treatment of tumors.

The seeds are being planted for the use of stem cells or genetically modified cultured cells for the treatment of degenerative diseases and movement disorders. For the first time we will treat the underlying disease process or neurochemical abnormality and not merely suppress the symptoms. The genetic abnormalities that allow tumors to grow are being identified, so they might be corrected to treat or prevent brain tumors. The delivery of radiation is becoming more sophisticated, so lesions might be treated more effectively with less radiation to normal tissues. The physiological abnormalities that produce seizures are being identified, so they might be corrected. Stereotactic surgery will be increasingly important to obtain tissue to study these techniques, to prepare treatment tissues, or to deliver the cells to their site of action.

The fields of functional neurosurgery and stereotactic surgery are diverging. Functional neurosurgery will, for the foreseeable future, remain a subspecialty that requires additional training in the neurological and computer sciences. Stereotactic surgical guidance will be used for every neurosurgical procedure by every neurosurgeon to make neurosurgery safer and more effective. Image guidance is rapidly becoming indispensable to every neurosurgical operation.

This is indeed an exciting time to be in stereotactic surgery! And the future promises to be even more exciting.

Philip Gildenberg, M.D., Ph.D
Houston Stereotactic Center,
Houston, Texas, U.S.A.

Preface

The Latin derivation of "stereotaxy" refers to a system in physical space; the term "stereotactic" means to touch in space. Both concepts apply well to the expanding field of stereotactic neurosurgery. The history of stereotaxis began with the development of the experimental Horsley-Clarke apparatus in 1908. The adaptation of this system by Spiegel and Wycis in the 1940s spurred the growth of functional stereotactic surgery, which was used primarily for the treatment of patients with parkinsonism. With the advent of L-dopa in the late 1960s, stereotactic surgery became a relatively obscure part of neurosurgical training and practice, limited to a few centers.

Digital sectional imaging—computed tomography and then magnetic resonance imaging—has fueled a renaissance in stereotaxis, and then some. In the last 15 years, for instance, stereotactic biopsy has gone from being a "high-tech" procedure reserved for academic institutions to a routine part of daily neurosurgery. The incorporation of frameless stereotaxy has been even more rapid. Radiosurgery, a subject that at first drew little interest (mostly negative) at major meetings, is now performed at hundreds of sites in the United States and is discussed avidly in large international forums.

Functional stereotaxy has made a comeback as well, as the limitations of chronic medical therapy for parkinsonism became apparent and the surgical technology improved. The advent of implantable stimulators has made

nonablative functional stereotactic surgery a realistic possibility for community neurosurgeons. In part, this and other technological advances have
spurred interest in surgery for patients with other movement disorders, pain,
spasticity, and epilepsy.

Several excellent textbooks now provide detailed descriptions of the
underlying theory and outcomes for the various subsets of stereotactic procedures. Perhaps because of their heft, however, they have not served as a
practical guide for neurosurgeons. This book hopes to address that need. It
is meant as an adjunct to the above-mentioned textbooks and monographs,
which contain important information that any stereotactic neurosurgeon must
thoroughly understand. A handbook such as this reflects the ongoing development of stereotaxis as part of every neurosurgeon's treatment arsenal.

Michael Schulder

Contents

Contributors

John R. Adler, Jr., M.D. Department of Neurosurgery, Stanford University School of Medicine, Stanford, California, U.S.A.

Eben Alexander III, M.D. Department of Neurosurgery, University of Massachusetts Medical School, Worcester, Massachusetts, U.S.A.

Ahmed Alkhani, M.D. Division of Neurosurgery, University of Toronto, and Toronto Western Hospital, Toronto, Ontario, Canada

Ron L. Alterman, M.D. Division of Stereotactic and Functional Neurosurgery, The Hyman-Newman Institute for Neurology and Neurosurgery, Beth Israel Medical Center–Singer Division, New York, New York, U.S.A.

Arun Paul Amar, M.D. Department of Neurological Surgery, Keck School of Medicine, University of Southern California, Los Angeles, California, U.S.A.

David W. Andrews, M.D. Department of Neurosurgery, Thomas Jefferson University, Philadelphia, Pennsylvania, U.S.A.

Michael L. J. Apuzzo, M.D.   Department of Neurological Surgery, Keck School of Medicine, University of Southern California, Los Angeles, California, U.S.A.

Hooman Azmi, M.D.   Department of Neurosurgery, New Jersey Medical School, Newark, New Jersey, U.S.A.

Roy A. E. Bakay, M.D.   Department of Neurological Surgery, Rush Medical College, Rush-Presbyterian-St. Luke's Medical Center, Chicago, Illinois, U.S.A.

Gene H. Barnett, M.D., F.A.C.S.   Brain Tumor Institute, Department of Neurological Surgery, The Cleveland Clinic, Cleveland, Ohio, U.S.A.

Francis J. Bova, Ph.D.   Department of Neurosurgery, University of Florida Brain Institute, Gainesville, Florida, U.S.A.

Jeffrey A. Brown, M.D.   Department of Neurological Surgery, Wayne State University School of Medicine, Detroit, Michigan, U.S.A.

John M. Buatti, M.D.   Department of Radiation Oncology, University of Iowa Health Care, Iowa City, Iowa, U.S.A.

Kim Burchiel, M.D., F.A.C.S.   Department of Neurological Surgery, Oregon Health and Science University, Portland, Oregon, U.S.A.

Steven D. Chang, M.D.   Department of Neurosurgery, Stanford University School of Medicine, Stanford, California, U.S.A.

Joseph C. T. Chen, M.D., Ph.D.   Division of Neurosurgery, Department of Surgery, University of California at San Diego, San Diego, California, U.S.A.

G. Rees Cosgrove, M.D., F.R.C.S.(C)   Department of Neurosurgery, Massachusetts General Hospital, and Harvard Medical School, Boston, Massachusetts, U.S.A.

Denny Demeria, B.Sc., M.D.   Division of Neurosurgery, Department of Surgery, University of Saskatchewan, and Regina General Hospital, Regina, Saskatchewan, Canada

Antonio A. F. DeSalles, M.D., Ph.D.   Department of Neurosurgery, UCLA School of Medicine, Los Angeles, California, U.S.A.

Fernando Díaz   Department of Neurosurgery, Wayne State University, Detroit, Michigan, U.S.A.

M. Beverly Downes   Thomas Jefferson University, Philadelphia, Pennsylvania, U.S.A.

Thomas L. Ellis, M.D.   Department of Neurosurgery, Wake Forest University School of Medicine, Winston-Salem, North Carolina, U.S.A.

Emad N. Eskandar, M.D.   Department of Neurosurgery, Massachusetts General Hospital, and Harvard Medical School, Boston, Massachusetts, U.S.A.

Kelly D. Foote, M.D.   Department of Neurosurgery, University of Florida, Gainesville, Florida, U.S.A.

William A. Friedman, M.D.   Department of Neurosurgery, University of Florida, Gainesville, Florida, U.S.A.

Robert E. Gross, M.D., Ph.D.   Department of Neurological Surgery, Emory University School of Medicine, Atlanta, Georgia, U.S.A.

Sagi Harnof, M.D.   Department of Neurosurgery, The Chaim Sheba Medical Center, Tel Hashomer, and The Sackler School of Medicine, Tel Aviv University, Tel Aviv, Israel

Alan C. Hartford, M.D., Ph.D.   Department of Radiation Oncology, Northeast Proton Therapy Center, Boston, Massachusetts, U.S.A.

Paul A. House, M.D.   Department of Neurosurgery, University of Utah Health Sciences Center, Salt Lake City, Utah, U.S.A.

Zvi Israel, B.Sc., M.B.B.SD.   Department of Neurosurgery, Hadassah University Hospital, Jerusalem, Israel

Yücel Kanpolat, M.D.   Department of Neurosurgery, University of Ankara School of Medicine, Ankara, Turkey

Douglas Kondziolka, M.D.   The Center for Image-Guided Neurosurgery, University of Pittsburgh School of Medicine, Pittsburgh, Pennsylvania, U.S.A.

Krishna Kumar, M.B., M.S., F.R.C.S.(C), F.A.C.S., S.O.M.   Division of Neurosurgery, Department of Surgery, University of Saskatchewan, Saskatchewan, and Regina General Hospital, Regina, Canada

Michael L. Levy, M.D.   Division of Neurosurgery, and Department of Surgery, University of California San Diego, San Diego, California, U.S.A.

Danny Liang, B.A.   Department of Neurosurgery, New Jersey Medical School, Newark, New Jersey, U.S.A.

Jay S. Loeffler, M.D.   Massachusetts General Hospital, and Harvard Medical School, Boston, Massachusetts, U.S.A.

Deon Louw, M.D.   Consultant Neurosurgeon, Foothills Medical Center, Calgary, Alberta, Canada

Andres M. Lozano, M.D., Ph.D., F.R.C.S.(C)   Department of Surgery, University of Toronto, and Toronto Western Hospital, Toronto, Ontario, Canada

L. Dade Lunsford, M.D.   The Center for Image-Guided Neurosurgery, University of Pittsburgh School of Medicine, Pittsburgh, Pennsylvania, U.S.A.

Robert J. Maciunas, M.D.   Department of Neurological Surgery, Case Western Reserve University, Cleveland, Ohio, U.S.A.

Allen H. Maniker, M.D.   Department of Neurological Surgery, New Jersey Medical School, Newark, New Jersey, U.S.A.

David A. Marks, M.D.   Department of Neurosciences, New Jersey Medical School, Newark, New Jersey, U.S.A.

David P. Martin, M.D.   Department of Neurosurgery, Stanford University School of Medicine, Stanford, California, U.S.A.

Sanford L. Meeks, Ph.D.   Department of Radiation Oncology, University of Iowa Health Care, Iowa City, Iowa, U.S.A.

G. Robert Nugent, M.D.   Department of Neurosurgery, Robert C. Byrd Health Sciences Center, Morgantown, West Virginia, U.S.A.

Bryan Rankin Payne, M.D. Department of Neurosurgery, Louisiana State University, New Orleans, Louisiana, U.S.A.

Arun Angelo Patil, M.D. Department of Neurosurgery, University of Nebraska Medical Center, Omaha, Nebraska, U.S.A.

Warwick J. Peacock, M.D., F.R.C.S. Department of Neurosurgery, University of California at San Francisco, San Francisco, California, U.S.A.

Gerhard Pendl, M.D. Department of Neurosurgery, Karl-Franzens University Graz, Graz, Austria

Edward C. Pennington, M.S. Department of Radiation Oncology, University of Iowa Health Care, Iowa City, Iowa, U.S.A.

Ramiro Pérez de la Torre Department of Neurosurgery, Wayne State University, Detroit, Michigan, U.S.A.

M. Raphael Pfeffer Department of Radiation Oncology, The Chaim Sheba Medical Center, Tel Hashomer, and The Sackler School of Medicine, Tel Aviv University, Tel Aviv, Israel

Steven N. Roper, M.D. Department of Neurological Surgery, University of Florida, and Malcolm Randall VA Medical Center, Gainesville, Florida, U.S.A.

Oskar Schröttner, M.D. Department of Neurosurgery, Karl-Franzens University Graz, Graz, Austria

Michael Schulder, M.D. Department of Neurosurgery, New Jersey Medical School, Newark, New Jersey, U.S.A.

James M. Schumacher, M.D. Department of Neurological Surgery, Center for Movement Disorders, University of Miami, Miami, Florida, and Neuroregeneration Laboratory, McLean Hospital, and Harvard Medical School, Boston, Massachusetts, U.S.A.

Theodore H. Schwartz, M.D. Department of Neurological Surgery, Weill Cornell Medical College, New York Presbyterian Hospital, New York, New York, U.S.A.

Ashwini D. Sharan, M.D. Department of Neurosurgery, Thomas Jefferson University, Philadelphia, Pennsylvania, U.S.A.

Konstantin V. Slavin, M.D. Department of Neurosurgery, University of Illinois at Chicago, Chicago, Illinois, U.S.A.

Robert Smee, M.B., B.S., F.R.A.N.Z. Department of Radiation Oncology, Prince of Wales Hospital, Randwick, New South Wales, Australia

Matthew Smyth, M.D. Department of Neurological Surgery, University of California at San Francisco, San Francisco, California, U.S.A.

Timothy Solberg, Ph.D. Department of Radiation Oncology, UCLA School of Medicine, Los Angeles, California, U.S.A.

Angelyn M. Solko, Pharm D. Harborview Medical Center and University of Washington School of Pharmacy, Seattle, Washington, U.S.A.

Deepa Soni, M.D. Department of Neurosurgery, Brigham and Women's Hospital, Children's Hospital, and Harvard Medical School, Boston, Massachusetts, U.S.A.

Roberto Spiegelmann, M.D. Department of Neurosurgery, The Chaim Sheba Medical Center, Tel Hashomer, and The Sackler School of Medicine, Tel Aviv University, Tel Aviv, Israel

Philip Starr, M.D., Ph.D. Department of Neurological Surgery, University of California at San Francisco, San Francisco, California, U.S.A.

Todd P. Thompson, M.D. Department of Neurosurgery, Straub Clinic and Hospital, Honolulu, Hawaii, U.S.A.

William D. Tobler, M.D. Department of Neurosurgery, University of Cincinnati, and Mayfield Clinic and Spine Institute, Cincinnati, Ohio, U.S.A.

Thomas H. Wagner, Ph.D. Department of Neurosurgery, University of Florida Brain Institute, Gainesville, Florida, U.S.A.

Marshall T. Watson, Jr., M.D.   Department of Neurological Surgery, University of Rochester, Rochester, New York, U.S.A.

Ronald F. Young, M.D., F.A.C.S.   Gamma Knife Center, Northwest Hospital, Seattle, Washington, U.S.A.

Randa Zakhary, M.D., Ph.D.   Department of Neurological Surgery, University of California at San Francisco, San Francisco, California, U.S.A.

Lucía Zamorano, M.D.   Departments of Neurosurgery and Radiation Oncology, Wayne State University, Detroit, Michigan, U.S.A.

Edward J. Zampella, M.D.   Chatham Neurological Associates, Summit, New Jersey, U.S.A.

1

Intracranial Stereotactic Surgery: Indications

Joseph C. T. Chen
University of California at San Diego, San Diego, California, U.S.A.

Michael L. J. Apuzzo
Keck School of Medicine, University of Southern California, Los Angeles, California, U.S.A.

1 INTRODUCTION

The indications for stereotactic neurosurgical methods have, at one point or another, encompassed all major categories of differential diagnoses. Stereotactic techniques, introduced in the early 20th century, applied instrumentation in a minimally invasive, precise, and reproducible manner for research purposes. The first report of a stereotactic device in the English language literature is the report of Horsely and Clarke, which described a device for accessing the dentate nucleus of the cerebellum in monkeys [1]. Despite this early start, stereotactic methods were not attempted in humans until nearly 40 years later when Spiegel and Wycis inaugurated the era of human stereotaxis for ablative neurosurgical procedures [2]. They developed the paradigm of contemporary stereotactic technique, combining the use of a stereotactic device, radiographic imaging, and a quantitative anatomic atlas.

Since then, stereotactic methods have been progressively refined and are now applied for a wide range of indications to accomplish both diagnostic and therapeutic goals. This chapter provides a brief outline of the wide indications for stereotaxis in both historical and contemporary neurosurgical practice.

2 NEOPLASTIC

2.1 Diagnostic

Biopsy is the most common indication for the use of stereotactic methods. Before the introduction of modern stereotactic methods, biopsies involved free-hand needle aspiration or craniotomy guided by indirect radiographic procedures, such as angiography or ventriculography. Modern imaging and frame-based stereotactic procedures rapidly obtain diagnostic material with minimal patient mortality and morbidity [3,4]. The vast majority of brain lesions visible on imaging studies can be safely biopsied with high diagnostic yield [5]. Lesions with possible vascular pathology and those with significant associated mass effect, however, should be excluded from consideration.

2.2 Radiosurgery

Perhaps no more important method of treating brain tumors has been introduced in the last 20 years than stereotactic radiosurgery. Radiosurgery uses precise delivery of energy in the form of convergent beams of high energy photon or charged particle radiation to tumor tissue on a hypofractionated basis. Devices designed to deliver radiosurgical doses include the Leksell Gamma unit and a number of linear accelerator-based devices. Radiosurgery has been found to yield survival rates comparable to open surgical intervention for metastatic tumors of the brain [6,7]. Radiosurgery may also be used as effective adjuvant or primary treatment of carefully selected extra-axial tumors, such as meningiomas of the skull base or vestibular schwannomas [8,9]. It is imperative that neurosurgeons become familiar with the techniques and indications for stereotactic radiosurgery to maintain leadership in this field.

2.3 Brachytherapy

Use of brachytherapy has gradually declined since the introduction of conformal radiation therapy and radiosurgical methods. Brachytherapy, using the stereotactic implantation of radioactive seeds into the mass of tumor tissue, has the advantages of allowing delivery of highly concentrated radiation energy with a tighter dose fall-off than radiosurgical methods [10–12]. In practice, however, brachytherapy has several disadvantages that have contributed to its disuse. These include hazards incumbent on the use of radioactive materials in the operating suite and the invasive nature of the procedure. At our center, since the advent of radiosurgical methods, brachytherapy is no longer used.

2.4 Other Indications for Neoplasms

Approximately 3% of gliomatous tumors may be associated with a significant cystic component. Cyst drainage by stereotactic techniques can provide an important means of palliation for these patients. Colloid cysts have been treated with similar techniques, although recurrence rates remain high [13]. Craniopharyngiomas have been treated with stereotactic techniques using aspiration and the instillation of radioactive isotope into the cyst cavity in selected cases [14,15].

3 STEREOTACTIC CRANIOTOMY

Recent advances in imaging coupled with the availability of high-performance computing has made possible the introduction of stereotactic-assisted craniotomy for tumor, vascular, and other mass lesions. These stereotactic methods were initially introduced by Kelly, using a frame-based stereotactic system [16,17], and have since been moved to so-called frameless systems by a number of other groups [18,19]. Frameless systems differ fundamentally from their frame-based counterparts. Frame-based systems are designed to mechanically constrain instrumentation to a direct path to tumor tissue. Frameless systems are, by design, unable to provide mechanical constrainment of an operative corridor. Frameless systems instead report back the location of a freely mobile pointing device. Such frameless systems should, therefore, not be considered as replacements for frame-based stereotactic devices, as their roles are different.

Currently, stereotactic craniotomy is used for a variety of indications and should be a part of every neurosurgeon's armamentarium. Stereotactic craniotomy is most useful for small, deep-seated lesions where reliance on surface anatomic landmarks can be misleading. Furthermore, for convexity lesions, stereotactic guidance can allow for smaller, more localized craniotomies than would be possible with the use of surface landmarks coupled with eyeball evaluation of radiographic studies.

Despite the advantages of stereotactic craniotomy, these methods are still not pervasively used. Several factors account for this. First, most devices of the present generation are complex, with poor user interfaces and cumbersome if not outright awkward set-up requirements. The complexity of these devices often necessitates additional operating room staff expressly for the use and care of this equipment. Second, the devices continue to be very expensive, making access to this technology feasible for higher volume services only. This situation, however, may only be transitory, as evolution of these products will likely remedy many of the present shortcomings.

A separate issue from the shortcomings of the devices themselves is that use of these devices demands a different style of operating to minimize the occurrence of intraoperative brain shift and subsequent loss of registration. Experienced users of these devices minimize use of diuretics and dissect tumor tissue out circumferentially rather than internally debulking the mass [17].

The future direction of stereotactic craniotomy will likely see it in combination with intraoperative imaging technologies capable of updating images during the surgical procedure, thereby rendering unnecessary the need to control brain shift [20].

4   FUNCTIONAL NEUROSURGERY

Access to small, deep-seated targets for the purpose of effecting a change in the function of the brain, whether for treatment of movement disorders, pain, or psychological disorders, represents the earliest indications for stereotaxy.

4.1   Movement Disorders

Movement disorder surgeries were widely practiced in the 1950s. Targets included thalamic nuclei as well as the pallidum. With the introduction of L-dopa, however, surgical interventions for movement disorders fell by the wayside, reaching a nadir in the late 1970s. The eventual development of dyskinesias, on-off phenomena, and other side effects in long-term patients with Parkinson's disease led to a re-exploration of surgical techniques for the treatment of movement disorders. Furthermore, the discovery of the Methyl-phenyl-tetrahydropyridine (MPTP) model of Parkinson's disease led to the development of animal models and a re-evaluation of the pathophysiology of movement disorders, allowing for a rationalized surgical approach to this set of diseases.

Ablative surgeries have been the core of stereotactic surgery for movement disorders since Spiegel and Wycis undertook their procedures. Ablation includes physical methods, such as use of a leukotome; chemical methods, such as alcohol or glycerol injection; radiofrequency coagulation; and freezing methods. Of these methods, radiofrequency ablation methods are generally safer and more reproducible.

Recently, deep brain stimulation (DBS) has revolutionized the field of movement disorders surgery. Deep brain stimulation, utilizing classic targets for movement disorders including the ventralis intermedius (VIM) nucleus of the thalamus for tremor [21,22], globus pallidus for dystonia [23,24], and the subthalamic nucleus of Luys for Parkinsonism [25] has shown significant promise in recent years. Subthalamic nucleus stimulation, in particular, results in long-term amelioration of all the cardinal signs of Parkinsonism. Deep brain stimulation has a number of advantages over ablative surgery, including the ability to adjust stimulation parameters to titrate effect and reversibility of the procedure.

Biological approaches, including gene therapy, stem cell and tissue transplant for movement disorders are a nascent technology that promises applicability to a wide range of neurologic disorders, including degenerative and demyelinating disease. Early results from these approaches, however, have been disappointing thus far. Currently tissue transplant has not yielded results comparable to either DBS or ablative procedures [26,27]. Despite these early disappointments, it is a virtual certainty that these technologies represent the near future of neurologic treatment. Many groups, in both academics and industry, have been actively involved in the development of these methods.

4.2 Psychiatric Disorders

After the introduction of classic physiologic methods to the study of the forebrain, interest turned to how the results of these studies could be applied to the clinical realm. Because of the horrid conditions within psychiatric facilities at the time and the primitive nature of nonsurgical therapies (e.g., insulin and electric shock), the advent of psychosurgery held great promise. Stereotactic variants of psychosurgical procedures have included cingulotomy [28], anterior capsulotomy [29], tractotomy [30], and others.

Evaluation of the psychosurgical literature is difficult, partly because of reporting methods, partly because diagnostic categories in psychiatry have changed greatly over the years. It appears, however, that certain categories of illness do respond to surgical intervention (e.g., obsessive compulsive disease, anxiety), whereas others do not (e.g., schizophrenia).

As with movement disorders, the introduction of effective drug therapy led to the demise of psychosurgery. Furthermore, political trends as well as the lack of a sound theoretic scientific basis for these procedures made continued widespread use of these methods untenable. Nevertheless, a few centers have continued these procedures on a limited basis. Advances in neuroscience research may, in the near future, provide a more firm basis for the re-exploration of surgical interventions for psychiatric disease.

4.3 Seizure Disorders

Stereotactic methods, as applied to seizure disorders, encompass both the diagnostic and therapeutic realm. From the standpoint of diagnosis, implantation of stereotactic depth electrodes for localization of seizure activity in mesial temporal structures is a common technique. In some centers, especially in Europe, arrays of stereotactically implanted depth electrodes are used in preference to the surface grids commonly used in North America.

Ablative stereotactic procedures have been used in the treatment of seizure disorders in highly selected patients [31,32]. It is unlikely, however, that these techniques will replace the current strategies of resective surgery, especially given high rates of success and safety with open surgery. Recently, work has been done with stimulation of deep brain structures for the treatment of seizure disorders. This work, still unpublished as of this writing, appears to be promising. The efficacy of such procedures remains to be investigated in the coming years.

4.4 Pain

The current generation of deep brain stimulation electrodes was initially conceived and devised for use in treatment of chronic pain. Currently, DBS is limited to a few specialized centers treating pain syndromes unresponsive to all other modes of therapy. Because of the subjective nature of pain and the pervasive coincidence in these patients of significant psychiatric overlays, objective analysis of the results from surgical intervention is extraordinarily difficult. Most of the published data suggest that modest improvements can be realized in highly selected patients [33]. An emerging modality is cortical stimulation, whereby primary motor cortex is chronically stimulated by implanted strip electrodes placed with stereotactic guidance and electrophysiologic localization [34]. These technologies hold hope for a late recourse for patients with chronic localized upper limb and facial pain. Other modalities used in chronic pain have included cingulotomy and thalamic ablative procedures with mixed success.

5 OTHER INDICATIONS

5.1 Hematoma

Stereotactic aspiration on intracerebral hemorrhage is a method practiced in some centers for removal of both acute and subacute lesions. It has been suggested that superior results can be obtained after aspiration of these lesions [35,36].

5.2 Abcess

Intracranial infection can, in many instances, be treated successfully by stereotactic abscess aspiration. Lunsford et al. have reported good results with overall bacteriologic identification of 97% and cure rates of 72% for patients presenting with a wide range of diagnoses and underlying illnesses [37,38].

6 CONCLUSION

In the more than 50 years during which stereotactic brain procedures have been practiced, gifted neurosurgical pioneers have applied these methods to virtually all major diagnostic categories. The reason for this is simple: stereotactic devices are the only means by which one can efficiently target and access any arbitary volume within the space occupied by the brain.

As the basic medical science of the brain yields discoveries leading to treatments for currently uncurable disorders of the brain, it is likely that stereotactic methods will be the vehicles of treatment for these therapeutic modalities. Stereotactic methods are already sufficiently powerful to be applied on a daily basis to the majority of neurosurgical practice.

REFERENCES

1. Horsley V, Clarke RH. The structure and function of the cerebellum examined by a new method. Brain 1908;31:45–124.
2. Spiegel EA, Wycis HT, Marks M, Lee AJ. Stereotaxic apparatus for operations on the human brain. Science 1947;106:349–350.
3. Heilbrun MP, Roberts TS, Apuzzo ML, Wells TH, Jr, Sabshin JK. Preliminary experience with Brown-Roberts-Wells (BRW) computerized tomography stereotaxic guidance system. J Neurosurg 1983;59(2):217–222.
4. Apuzzo ML, Chandrasoma PT, Cohen D, Zee CS, Zelman V. Computed imaging stereotaxy: Experience and perspective related to 500 procedures applied to brain masses. Neurosurgery 1987;20(6):930–937.
5. Chandrasoma PT, Smith MM, Apuzzo ML. Stereotactic biopsy in the diagnosis of brain masses: Comparison of results of biopsy and resected surgical specimen. Neurosurgery 1989;24(2):160–165.
6. Auchter RM, Lamond JP, Alexander E, Buatti JM, Chappell R, Friedman WA, Kinsella TJ, Levin AB, Noyes WR, Schultz CJ, Loeffler JS, Mehta MP. A multiinstitutional outcome and prognostic factor analysis of radiosurgery for resectable single brain metastasis [see comments]. Int J Radiat Oncol Biol Phys 1996;35(1):27–35.
7. Alexander E 3rd, Moriarty TM, Davis RB, Wen PY, Fine HA, Black PM, Kooy HM, Loeffler JS. Stereotactic radiosurgery for the definitive, noninvasive treatment of brain metastases. J Natl Cancer Inst 1995;87(1):34–40.

8. Kondziolka D, Lunsford LD, Coffey RJ, Flickinger JC. Stereotactic radiosurgery of meningiomas. J Neurosurg 1991;74(4):552–559.

9. Kondziolka D, Lunsford LD, McLaughlin MR, Flickinger JC. Long-term outcomes after radiosurgery for acoustic neuromas [see comments]. N Engl J Med 1998;339(20):1426–1433.

10. Apuzzo ML, Petrovich Z, Luxton G, Jepson JH, Cohen D, Breeze RE. Interstitial radiobrachytherapy of malignant cerebral neoplasms: Rationale, methodology, prospects. Neurol Res 1987;9(2):91–100.

11. Bernstein M, Gutin PH. Interstitial irradiation of brain tumors: A review. Neurosurgery 1981;9(6):741–750.

12. Gutin PH, Phillips TL, Wara WM, Leibel SA, Hosobuchi Y, Levin VA, Weaver KA, Lamb S. Brachytherapy of recurrent malignant brain tumors with removable high-activity iodine-125 sources. J Neurosurg 1984;60(1):61–68.

13. Kondziolka D, Lunsford LD. Stereotactic management of colloid cysts: Factors predicting success. J Neurosurg 1991;75(1):45–51.

14. Gutin PH, Klemme WM, Lagger RL, MacKay AR, Pitts LH, Hosobuchi Y. Management of the unresectable cystic craniopharyngioma by aspiration through an Ommaya reservoir drainage system. J Neurosurg 1980;52(1):36–40.

15. Lunsford LD, Pollock BE, Kondziolka DS, Levine G, Flickinger JC. Stereotactic options in the management of craniopharyngioma. Pediatr Neurosurg 1994;21(suppl 1):90–97.

16. Kelly PJ. Stereotactic craniotomy. Neurosurg Clin N Am 1990;1(4):781–799.

17. Kelly PJ. Tumor Stereotaxis. Philadelphia: WB Saunders, 1991.

18. Roberts DW, Strohbehn JW, Hatch JF, Murray W, Kettenberger H. A frameless stereotaxic integration of computerized tomographic imaging and the operating microscope. J Neurosurg 1986;65:545–549.

19. Smith KR, Frank KJH, Bucholz RD. The NeuroStation—a highly accurate, minimally invasive solution to frameless stereotactic neurosurgery. Comput Med Imaging Graph 1994;18(4):247–256.

20. Black PM, Moriarty T, Alexander E 3rd, Stieg P, Woodard EJ, Gleason PL, Martin CH, Kikinis R, Schwartz RB, Jolesz FA. Development and implementation of intraoperative magnetic resonance imaging and its neurosurgical applications. Neurosurgery 1997;41(4)831–842; discussion 842–845.

21. Tasker RR. Deep brain stimulation is preferable to thalamotomy for tremor suppression. Surg Neurol 1998;49(2):145–153; discussion 153–154.

22. Benabid AL, Pollak P, Seigneuret E, Hoffmann D, Gay E, Perret J. Chronic VIM thalamic stimulation in Parkinson's disease, essential tremor and extrapyramidal dyskinesias. Acta Neurochir Suppl 1993;58:39–44.

23. Tronnier VM, Fogel W. Pallidal stimulation for generalized dystonia. Report of three cases [in process citation]. J Neurosurg 2000;92(3):453–456.

24. Kumar R, Dagher A, Hutchison WD, Lang AE, Lozano AM, Globus pallidus deep brain stimulation for generalized dystonia: Clinical and PET investigation. Neurology 1999;53(4):871–874.

25. Benabid AL, Pollak P, Gross C, Hoffman D, Benazzouz A, Gao DM, Laurent A, Gentil M, Perret J. Acute and long-term effects of subthalamic nucleus

stimulation in Parkinson's disease. Stereotact Funct Neurosurg 1994;62(1-4): 76–84.

26. Olanow CW, Freeman TB, Kordower JH. Neural transplantation as a therapy for Parkinson's disease. Adv Neurol 1997;74:249–269.

27. Hauser RA, Freeman TB, Snow BJ, Nawert M, Gauger L, Kordower JH, Olanow CW. Long-term evaluation of bilateral fetal nigral transplantation in Parkinson disease. Arch Neurol 1999;56(2):179–187.

28. Spangler WJ, Cosgrove GR, Ballantine HT Jr, Cassem EH, Rauch SL, Nierenberg A, Price BH. Magnetic resonance image-guided stereotactic cingulotomy for intractable psychiatric disease [see comments]. Neurosurgery 1996;38(6):1071–1076; discussion 1076–1078.

29. Mindus P. Present-day indications for capsulotomy. Acta Neurochir Suppl 1993;58:29–33.

30. Knight G. The orbital cortex as an objective in the surgical treatment of mental illness: The development of the stereotactic approach. Br J Surg 1964;51:114–124.

31. Barcia-Salorio JL, Barcia JA, Hernandez G, Lopez-Gomez L. Radiosurgery of epilepsy. Long-term results. Acta Neurochir Suppl (Wien) 1994;62:111–113.

32. Regis J, Bartolomei F, Rey M, Genton P, Dravet C, Semah F, Gastaut JL, Chauvel P, Peragut JC. Gamma knife surgery for mesial temporal lobe epilepsy. Epilepsia 1999;40(11):1551–1556.

33. Tasker RR, Vilela Filho O. Deep brain stimulation for neuropathic pain. Stereotact Funct Neurosurg 1995;65(1-4):122–124.

34. Tsubokawa T, Katayama Y, Yamamoto T, Hirayama T, Koyama S. Chronic motor cortex stimulation for the treatment of central pain. Acta Neurochir Suppl 1991;52:137–139.

35. Niizuma H, Yonemitsu T, Jokura H, Nakasato N, Suzuki J, Yoshimoto T. Stereotactic aspiration of thalamic hematoma. Overall results of 75 aspirated and 70 nonaspirated cases. Stereotact Funct Neurosurg 1990;55:438–444.

36. Niizuma H, Shimizu Y, Yonemitsu, T, Nakasato N, Suzuki J. Results of stereotactic aspiration in 175 cases of putaminal hemorrhage. Neurosurgery 1989; 24(6):814–819.

37. Lunsford LD. Stereotactic drainage of brain abscesses. Neurol Res 1987;9(4): 270–274.

38. Kondziolka D, Duma CM, Lunsford LD. Factors that enhance the likelihood of successful stereotactic treatment of brain abscesses. Acta Neurochir 1994; 127(1-2):85–90.

2

Stereotactic Frames: Technical Considerations

Ashwini D. Sharan and David W. Andrews

Thomas Jefferson University, Philadelphia, Pennsylvania, U.S.A.

1 INTRODUCTION

The term stereotaxis, derived from the Greek stereo- for "three-dimensional" and -taxic for "an arrangement," was coined by Horsley and Clarke in 1908 [1]. It was their use of a three-dimensional Cartesian coordinate system that provided the basis for all stereotactic systems used in modern day neurosurgery. Human stereotaxy was initially developed for the placement of deep lesions in patients with Parkinson's disease but lost favor with the development of dopamine agonist medications. The introduction of computed tomography (CT) renewed interest in stereotaxy and, together with the subsequent introduction of magnetic resonance imaging (MRI), broadened indications for stereotactic approaches dramatically as deeper areas of the brain could now be targeted with great accuracy. As radiosurgery developed, indications for the use of stereotactic frames broadened further. A thorough review of the history of stereotaxy and the development of frame-based systems can be found in Gildenberg and Tasker's definitive textbook [2]. This chapter will be devoted to three current frames systems, including technical aspects of frame application and target localization. Other frames will be described elsewhere in the book; our goal is to describe some of the theoretical underpinning for the use of stereotactic frames in the era of digital imaging.

2   GENERAL PRINCIPLES

The stereotactic approach to intracranial targets involves the rigid application of a stereotactic frame, a localizer, and an image data set derived from either CT, MRI, or angiography. With a fixed relationship between the patient's head and the fiducial localizers [3], any intracranial target can be reached with an optimal trajectory and great accuracy. The standard performance specifications for cerebral stereotactic systems, specified by the American Society for Testing and Materials, stipulate a mechanical accuracy below 1 mm [4]. Within a Cartesian coordinate system, the x- and y-axes refer to a medial–lateral and anterior–posterior location, respectively, whereas the z-axis refers to a base–vertex location. Many methods have been outlined to determine the z-axis, but the most popular method uses posts with an "N" shape configuration where the position of the oblique rod relative to the vertical rods defines the z plane of the slice [3]. Once the target is localized, the arc method is used to direct a probe to the selected target and carry out the remainder of the procedure. These features are discussed in more detail below.

2.1   Frame Application

With experience and assistance, a stereotactic frame application should take minimal time. Before applying the frame, the neurosurgeon must have a clear idea of the anatomical localization of the lesion and should bear in mind a suitable entrance point for the probe. When applying a Leksell frame for radiosurgery, the frame must be shifted as much as possible to center the lesion in Leksell space (Fig. 1A). Failure to do so may result in a collision with the collimation helmet. When using CT data, the surgeon must remember that the headpins may cause significant artifact, which may obscure the target if small, as might the beam-hardening artifacts of the temporal bone if the lesion is located in a low temporal or posterior fossa location. Frame application may be performed at the bedside or in the operating room and is most easily accomplished with the patient in the sitting position. Our preference is to sterilize the scalp with an alcohol or betadine prep without shaving hair. The assistant stands either behind or on the side of the patient and stabilizes the ring. The ring should be applied parallel to the cranial floor through the use of ear bars, but some frame parallax is acceptable. As one exception, Leksell frame application must be within 3°

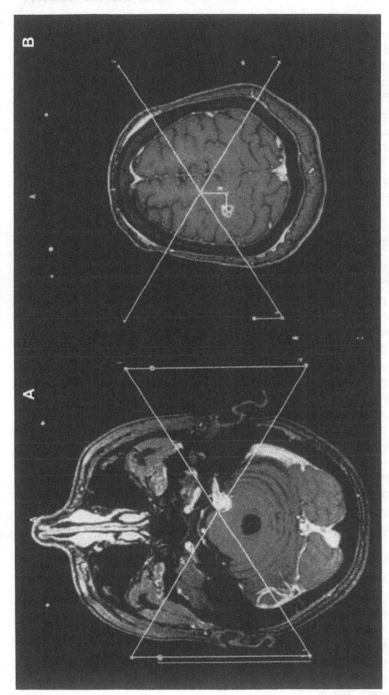

FIGURE 1 **A,** Axial gadolinium-enhanced T-1-weighted image with field-of-view including Leksell stereotactic coordinates. The frame was shifted to the patient's left to center an acoustic tumor in the stereotactic field for radiosurgery. Note the annotations that depict x, y, and z measurements. **B,** Axial gadolinium-enhanced T-1-weighted image with field-of-view including Leksell stereotactic coordinates for treatment of a right frontal brain metastasis.

of the coaxial imaging plane of Leksell Gamma Plan rejects further attempts at treatment planning for radiosurgery. We anesthetize the scalp and periosteum with a mixture of 9 parts 0.5% Marcaine (bupivicaine) and 1 part sodium bicarbonate, which reduces the burning sensation of the local anesthetic. With adequate local anesthesia, we have obviated the need for sedation. We prefer to place the two posterior pins first and then we place the anterior pins and hand tighten all four pins, before using the wrench, with a two-fingers method. During the frame application, the patient may be injected with intravenous contrast if the localization scan is to be performed immediately after the procedure. Otherwise, the patient can return to the bed with a pillow under the neck for comfort.

2.2   Target Localization for Stereotactic Biopsy

Imaging modality should depend on the modality that best demonstrates the lesion: either CT, MRI, or angiography. Basic principles that should be applied when planning a trajectory to target. The instrument's trajectory should avoid eloquent brain and breach only one pial surface to minimize the change of hemorrhage. This is particularly true for lesions near the sylvian fissure or pineal region. When possible, the instrument should penetrate the brain parallel to white matter tracts, especially when interested in brainstem lesions. Generally, the majority of the cerebrum, basal ganglia, thalamus, and brainstem can be approached with entry points anterior to the coronal suture. For lesions in the occipital, parietal, temporal lobe or the pineal region, a superior parieto-occipital approach is better. Temporal lesions may, additionally, be approached laterally and cerebellar lesions approached posteriorly.

  With the patient still in the scanner, it is important to ensure that all fiducial markers are visible on all images. With the advent of MRI-compatible localizers, MRI has provided superior target identification. Typically an axial T-1-weighted gadolinium-enhanced image will provide enough spatial information for target localization. For deep grey matter lesions, coronal and sagittal images provide ring and slide angles for isocentric frames (Fig. 2A and B). For brainstem lesions near midline, we recommend frontal lobe entry points with long-axis trajectories to avoid additional pial planes. For such cases, we obtain fiducial and target coordinates in all three orthogonal planes and average the three paired coordinates with the greatest spatial accuracy, eliminating the coordinate in each orthogonal plane which is, by definition, less accurate because of volume averaging. We always select a contrast-enhancing target if present, or abnormal signal visualized in a FLAIR sequence, if not.

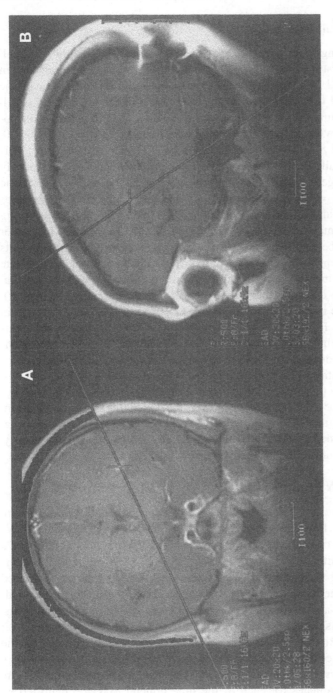

FIGURE 2 Patient with a small punctate contrast-enhancing lesion near speech that was discovered during evaluation for a new-onset seizure disorder. This lesion was biopsied and diagnosed as a pilocytic astrocytoma. **A,**
Coronal gadolinium-enhanced T-1-weighted image with annotation reflecting coronal angle of trajectory, which
will establish the slide angle on the CRW stereotactic frame. **B,** Sagittal gadolinium-enhanced T-1-weighted image
with annotation reflecting sagittal angle of trajectory, which will establish the ring or trunion angle on the CRW
stereotactic frame.

2.3 The Leksell Frame

After an inspiring visit with Spiegel and Wycis in Philadelphia, Leksell developed his first stereotactic frame [5]. His design included an arc system that was attached to a patient's head with pins such that the center of the arc corresponded to the selected target. The radius of the arc in the Leksell system is 190 mm, and stereotactic space is designated in a Cartesian coordinate system with center established, in millimeters, at x = 100, y = 100, and z = 100 and zero, by convention, is right, posterior, and superior. This elegant system allows the surgeon the opportunity to quickly and easily establish the target's coordinates on the MRI or CT monitor. The frame center at x and y = 100 is determined at the center of the intersecting lines drawn from the fiducial points at the corners of the localizing frame, as long as the frame is maintained in an orthogonal relationship with the scanner table. This may be confirmed with a carpenter's level; periodic adjustments of the frame attachment to the table may be needed. The Leksell z coordinate is established by measuring the distance from the ipsilateral superior fiducial coordinate to the diagonal coordinate and adding 40 mm (Fig. 1A and B). Alternatively, the images can be transferred by tape or ethernet to a surgical planning system. For Gamma Knife radiosurgery, we cross-check the treatment planning software determination (Leksell Gamma Plan) with the manually derived coordinates. If a lesion is left, posterior, and superior, for example, its location should be associated with x > 100, y < 100, and z < 100. For stereotactic surgery, the arc can be moved in the x, y, and z directions to allow for any entry point above the head ring, and the titanium frame is both CT and MRI compatible. Additionally, there is a localizer that can determine coordinates for angiographically obtained targets. Finally, there is no phantom frame with this system.

2.4 BRW/CRW Frames

In 1977, Theodore Roberts and a third-year medical student, Russel Brown, were responsible for developing the Brown-Roberts-Wells System (BRW) at the University of Utah [6]. This originally CT-based system consists of a skull base ring with carbon epoxy head posts that offers minimal CT interference. The ring is attached to the patient with screws that are tightened into the skull. The localizer unit is secured to the ring with three ball-and-socket interlocks and consists of six vertical posts and three diagonal posts, creating an "N" shaped appearance [7]. It is this latter "N" construct that establishes the axial CT plane relative to the skull base by calculating the relative distance of the oblique to the vertical rods. Target coordinates are established by first identifying the axial slice that best features the lesion. The x and y coordinates for each of the nine fiducial rods are identified on the CT or MRI monitor, as are the x and y coordinates for the target. All coordinates are entered into a laptop computer (the SCS1), which computes the target coordinates in BRW stereotactic space. The BRW system then further includes a movable arc and a probe holder. The arc guidance frame has four motions that create infinite different probe pathways, but for any trajectory, the computation must include entry coordinates [8]. Additionally, this system included a phantom base onto which the stereotactic frame including the arc could be placed to test the accuracy of the settings.

In the 1980s, Wells and Cosman simplified and improved the BRW by designing an arc guidance frame similar to the Leksell frame. The arc system directs a stereotactic probe isocentrically around the designated target, thus obviating a fixed entry point. The Cosman-Roberts-Wells (CRW) system included some of the same design elements as the BRW system, including a phantom frame, the same CT localizer, and the same probe depth fixed at 16 cm (Fig. 3A–C). New innovations included the introduction of MRI-compatible frames and localizers (Fig. 3A), and versatility in arc-to-frame applications that enabled inferior trajectories into the posterior fossa or lateral routes into the temporal lobe. For institutions with the Radionics OTS frameless image guidance system, target and trajectory calculations can now be performed with the OTS intraoperative workstation, which provides more flexibility than the SCS1 laptop.

2.5 COMPASS

The COMPASS system is specifically designed for volumetric tumor surgery and evolved from the Todd-Wells frame [9]. A removable head frame can be accurately replaced. This is particularly helpful if data acquisition and surgery are performed on separate days. There is, similarly, an arc frame with a 160-mm radius and 2° of freedom to allow a multitude of trajectories. There are localizer frames that are compatible with CT, MRI, and angiogram. Finally, the most unique aspect of the COMPASS system is that the head frame fits into a motor-controlled slide, which can move the head within a fixed arc-quadrant and allow computer control and volumetric surgery. This specialized frame-based system is discussed in much greater detail in Gildenberg and Tasker's Textbook of Functional and Stereotactic Neurosurgery [2].

3 WHICH FRAME IS "BEST?"

The quotes around the last word sum up the answer succinctly—there is no one "best" system or concept. Neurosurgeons or institutions seeking to purchase their first stereotactic frame may find various reasons for making a

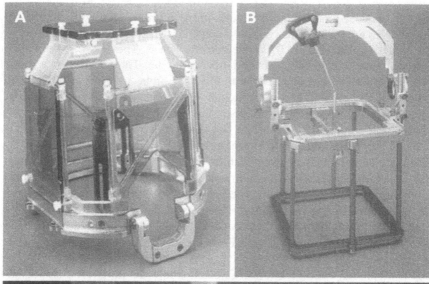

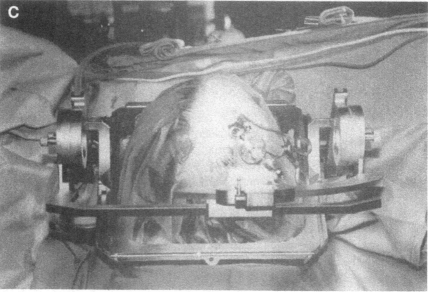

FIGURE 3 Cosman-Roberts-Wells (CRW) stereotactic system. **A,** MRI-compatible headring with attached Universal Compact Localizing Frame (UCLF). **B,** Rectilinear phantom pointer (RLPP) with CRW stereotactic frame calibrated to phantom target. The RLPP is also used for isocenter verification in the X-knife stereotactic radiosurgery system. **C,** Intraoperative view of CRW-based stereotactic biopsy for lesion in the right frontal lobe.

choice. These might include a factor as simple as familiarity with one device from one's training. Service from a vendor may be better in a particular region for a certain system. Also, as noted, this chapter does not provide a comprehensive list of all commercially available stereotactic frames. With the Leksell and Radionics CRW frames being the most commonly used devices, neurosurgeons may keep in mind the following:

1. The Leksell frame has a simpler system for instrument insertion to the desired target. No special measurements are necessary, as the zero point on the arc carrier is 19 cm from the target. It is lighter than the CRW frame. X, y, and z coordinates can be derived quickly from a two-dimensional image without a computer.
2. The CRW frame is accurate without the need for orthogonal positioning of the frame; patients may be scanned without rigid attachment of the frame to the table (although this may be desirable for other reasons, such as, eliminating head motion during a radiosurgical scan). It has a phantom base that can be sterilized and used in the operating room to confirm that accurate targeting has been planned. Although not the standard method, stereotactic coordinates can be derived directly from an image IF the scan was done with the frame in an orthogonal position.
3. These systems may be used as part of surgical navigation systems, wherein the stereotactic scans and frame coordinates are automatically read by the dedicated computer workstations, and target coordinates derived by clicking on the desired point on a particular image.

4 CONCLUSION

Modern CT and MR-guided stereotactic frames provide spatial accuracy for both stereotactic instrumentation and stereotactic radiosurgery. Despite the development and widespread use of frameless image-guidance systems, frame-based systems will remain an important tool in neurosurgical practice. For speed, ease, accuracy, and reliability, frames are the best method for performing point stereotaxis for biopsy and functional stereotactic neurosurgery.

REFERENCES

1. Horsely V, Clarke R. The structure and functions of the cerebellum examined by a new method. Brain 1908;31:45–124.
2. Tasker P, Gildenberg P, eds. Textbook of Functional and Stereotactic Neurosurgery. New York: McGraw-Hill, 1998.

3. Alker G, Kelly PJ. An overview of CT based stereotactic systems for the localization of intracranial lesions. Comput Radiol 1984;8:193–196.
4. American Society for Testing and Materials Committee F-4.05: Standard performance specifications for cerebral stereotactic instruments. Annual Book of ASTM Standards, F 1266-89. Philadelphia: 1990, pp 1–6.
5. Lunsford LD, Kondziolka D, Leksell D. The Leksell stereotactic system. In: Tasker PL, Gildenberg P, eds. Textbook of Stereotactic and Functional Neurosurgery. New York: McGraw-Hill, 1998, pp 51–64.
6. Roberts TS. The BRW/CRW stereotactic apparatus. In: Tasker PL, Gildenberg P, eds. Textbook of Functional and Stereotactic Neurosurgery. New York: McGraw-Hill, 1998, pp 65–71.
7. Cosman E. Development and technical features of the Cosman-Roberts-Wells (CRW) stereotactic system. In: Pell F, Thomas DGT, eds. Handbook of Stereotaxy Using the CRW Apparatus. Baltimore: Williams and Wilkins, 1994, pp 1–52.
8. Chin LS, Levy ML, Apuzzo MLK. Principles of stereotactic neurosurgery. In: Youmans JR, ed. Neurological Surgery. Philadelphia: WB Saunders, 1996, pp 767–785.
9. Kelly PJ. Stereotactic craniotomy. Neurosurg Clin N Am. 1990;1:781–799.

COMPANY INFORMATION

Radionics, Inc., USA Headquarters, 22 Terry Avenue, Burlington, MA 01803, (888) RSA-SERV, www.radionics.com

Elekta Instruments, Inc., 3155 Northwoods Parkway NW, Norcross, GA 30071, (800) 535-7355, www.elekta.com

COMPASS International, Inc., (formerly Stereotactic Medical Systems, Inc.), Cascade Business Park, 919 37th Avenue NW, Rochester, MN 55901, (507) 281-2143, www.compass.com

3

Stereotactic Surgery with the Radionics Frame

Michael Schulder
New Jersey Medical School, Newark, New Jersey, U.S.A.

1 INTRODUCTION

In the early 1980s Radionics, Inc. (Burlington, MA) was approached with a design for an innovative stereotactic frame that used computed tomography (CT) to directly target points within the brain. This device, the Brown-Roberts-Wells (BRW) frame, used a polar coordinate concept to define stereotactic space. A small computer with a simple menu was part of the system, thereby eliminating the need for strict orthogonality of the CT scan (a requirement of the Leksell arc-centered concept). The "picket-fence" configuration of the localizer was the key feature in this regard, as it allowed for calculation of the Z-coordinate (the height from the frame base, as opposed to the X and Y coordinates, which can be derived directly from a CT image).

The BRW frame was a great success, but further change was spurred by certain limitations. A direct approach to the posterior fossa was difficult because of the round base of the head ring. The polar coordinate system required the setting of four different angles on the arc itself, a process that could be cumbersome. A separate calculation was required for each new entry point. In 1988, introduction of the Cosman-Roberts-Wells (CRW) frame solved these problems, and the CRW design became the standard stereotactic frame made by Radionics [1].

At about the same time, a separate head ring for use with magnetic resonance imaging (MRI) scanners was introduced. Although functional, this tool was somewhat clumsy to use, and Radionics now makes one frame that is suitable for CT and MRI targeting. Application of the head ring, imaging, and use of the arc in the operating room are essentially the same as with the CRW frame, and these will be described in this chapter.

2 FRAME APPLICATION

In this era of frameless stereotaxy and emerging intraoperative imaging technologies, stereotactic frames still have their place. They are necessary for the performance of functional surgery, including placement of deep brain stimulators [2]. Brain biopsies arguably are done with the most accuracy and least time using a frame. Stereotactic radiosurgery is always done with a frame except in the unique case of the CyberKnife [3]. Craniotomies may be done in the frame, although frameless stereotaxy is much more suitable for this purpose [4].

The CRW frame is applied to awake adult patients (children younger than age 12 and the rare uncooperative adult are given general anesthesia). Oral sedation (2 tablets of Percocet and 5 mg of Valium) are administered 30 minutes before the procedure. The patient remains alert with this regimen, which usually eliminates much of the discomfort of frame application. The scalp is cleaned with alcohol swabs and the patient sits up. An assistant stands behind the patient, holds the stereotactic base ring, stabilizing his hands on the patient's shoulders. It is important to ensure that the patient's nose will clear the ring and the overlying localizer after application is completed. The surgeon must keep the target in mind and adjust the frame location accordingly. Local anesthesia (1% lidocaine without epinephrine) is injected through the posts, and the pins are inserted until finger tight. A gentle tug on the frame checks the placement.

3 IMAGING AND TARGETING

Scanning, most often with CT, is done. An adapter to the scan table, needed for radiosurgery image acquisition, is not necessary but may make scan interpretation and targeting easier. Axial scans with 3-mm slice thickness are obtained; if a lesion is known to enhance with contrast, this is given as well. Imaging for localization for functional surgery (e.g., targeting the Vim nucleus of the thalamus) should use the thinnest possible slices, usually 1 mm [5]. The scan field of view should be 34.5 to ensure inclusion of the localizer rods in the image. Gantry tilt should be avoided if a surgical navigation (SN) computer or the Radionics Stereo Calc program is to be used for image processing; if the dedicated Radionics "mini-computer" (MC) is used, then the gantry may be angled to optimize target visualization. This will be of use mainly for identifying the AC-PC line for functional targeting.

4 SURGERY

The images are transferred to the operating room computer and the rods identified. If the MC is used, then the surgeon must enter the coordinates for each rod and for the target on the slice of interest. If need be, registration with a nonstereotactic digital image [MRI, functional MRI, position emission tomography (PET), etc.) is done. Anteroposterior, lateral, and vertical settings for the stereotactic arc are derived. In the meantime, the patient is positioned, usually supine (or lateral for an occipital or posterior fossa approach) (Fig. 1). Local anesthesia with intravenous sedation is preferred for most patients, although children will require general anesthesia.

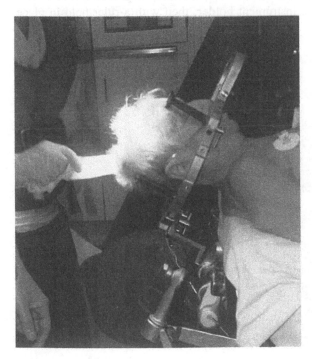

FIGURE 1 Patient positioned.

Use of the phantom base will add 5 or 10 minutes to the procedure but will give the surgeon assurance that the target will be reached using the spatial settings (Fig. 2). Sterilizing the base adds a measure of protection against infection. Coordinates are set on the phantom and arc, and a pointer is adjusted to the fixed depth from the probe holder to the target (17 cm). When the accuracy of the targeting is verified and the surgical field prepped and draped, the arc is transferred to the base ring. The arc-centered design of the CRW system allows for any entry point to be used, as long as it can be accessed through the arc and instrument holder. (Note that for temporal approaches, mounting the arc 90° to the usual orientation will give complete exposure of the area of interest).

A twist drill hole, burr hole, or craniotomy is then made, depending on the target and the surgeon's preference. The biopsy cannula or other instrument is fixed to the appropriate length, possibly shorter or longer than the arc radius, again depending on the clinical situation. The instrument is introduced to the desired depth and the patient is examined to rule out new neurological deficits (Fig. 3). Biopsies are then taken, or other manipulations (e.g., stimulation of a functional target) are done. To move the stereotactic instrument a set depth, measure to the protruding top of the tool from a fixed object, such as the instrument holder; then with a ruler held in place,

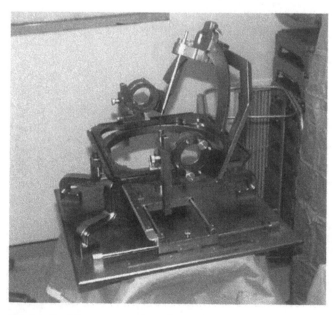

FIGURE 2   The arc on the phantom base in the operating room.

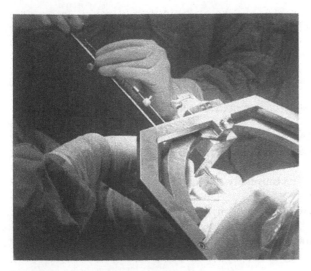

FIGURE 3 Insertion of a DBS electrode.

advance or withdraw the tool until the desired level is reached. Re-examine the patient after each change of instrument position. If a new deficit is noted, withdraw the instrument, close the incision, and obtain an emergency CT scan.

If a stereotactic biopsy is being done, frozen section confirmation that a lesional area has been targeted should be obtained; if not, specimens should be taken from different depths. If a different site needs to be targeted, this can be done quickly with an SN computer. Of course, the biopsy instrument must be withdrawn and the settings adjusted on the arc, although reconfirmation with the phantom base is not necessary. If the minicomputer was used, coordinates will need to be obtained during the surgery from the CT console—doable but cumbersome and time-consuming.

If bleeding is encountered during the procedure, irrigate patiently through the cannula. Periodically reinsert the stylet to dislodge any clot that may have formed at the cannula tip and that might falsely indicate that the hemorrhage has stopped. After the incision is closed, the patient is observed for several hours in the recovery room, a CT scan is obtained, and if no untoward findings are seen, he or she is observed in a regular hospital room overnight.

5 CONCLUSION

The CRW frame from Radionics remains a durable, versatile tool for stereotactic neurosurgery. Attention to detail, from frame application through imaging and the completion of surgery, will ensure a system that is safe and user friendly.

REFERENCES

1. P Gildenberg. The history of stereotactic neurosurgery. Neurosurg Clin N Am, 1:765–781, 1990.
2. PA Starr, JL Vitek, RA Bakay. Ablative surgery and deep brain stimulation for Parkinson's disease [see comments]. Neurosurgery 43(5):989–1013; discussion 1013–1015, 1998.
3. W Friedman, F Bova. The University of Florida radiosurgery system. Surg Neurol 32:334–342, 1989.
4. I Germano. The NeuroStation System for image-guided frameless stereotaxy. Neurosurgery 37:348–350, 1995.
5. R Maciunas, R Galloway, J Lattimer. The application accuracy of stereotactic frames. Neurosurgery 35:682–695, 1994.

4

Stereotactic Surgery with the Leksell Frame

Deon Louw

Foothills Medical Centre, Calgary, Alberta, Canada

1 LARS LEKSELL

It is well to reflect on the seminal contributions of Lars Leksell as we embrace new technology as a matter of course in the 21st century. A flurry of recent articles has appeared, for example, on the use of radiosurgery in trigeminal neuralgia. Few contemporary clinicians are aware that Leksell, in fact, pioneered this procedure in 1951, obtaining good results. He was also the first to perform intracavitary treatment of cystic craniopharyngiomas with phosphorus-32 [1]. Leksell is best known among stereotactic surgeons for developing the accurate and versatile frame that bears his name [2]. This was the result of ideas incubated under the influence of Spiegel and Wycis, with whom Leksell studied in 1947. He returned to Stockholm and furthered the already formidable reputation of the Karolinska Institute. During the next three decades, he continued to refine radiosurgery, developing the Gamma Knife with Borje Larson. His stereotactic frame was modified and updated until it became a standard neurosurgical tool. No less a luminary than Sugita felt that radiosurgery, stereotactic surgery and the operating microscope were the greatest neurosurgical technical advances of the 20th century. That Leksell pioneered two of these areas is a measure of his revolutionary influence

27

258

Louw

and serves as sobering inspiration to those who wish to follow in his footsteps.

2 FRAME AND COMPONENTS

Leksell's eloquent description of his system, as quoted by Lundsford et al. [3], is difficult to improve on. Essentially, it consists of a semicircular arc with a movable probe carrier. The arc is fixed to the patient's head in such a manner that its center corresponds with a selected cerebral target. The electrodes are always directed toward the center and, hence, to the target. Rotation of the arc around the axis rods in association with lateral adjustment of the electrode carrier enables any convenient point of entrance of the electrodes to be chosen, independent of the site of the target [4].

The model G base frame is rectangular and has dimensions of 190 mm × 210 mm (Fig. 1) [5]. A straight or curved front piece can be used; I prefer the latter, as it allows airway access in emergencies. Y coordinates are defined by supports attached to the y axes. Z coordinates are measured on vertical rings that are secured through the y supports. X coordinates are

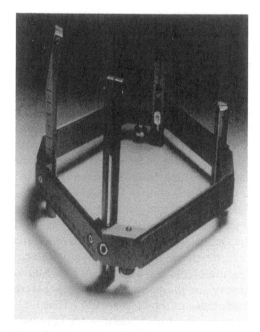

FIGURE 4.1   Leksell G base frame.

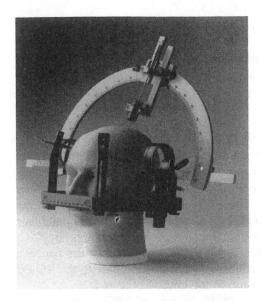

FIGURE 4.2   Z rings and arc attached to base frame.

entered on the arc, which in turn rotates around the z rings (Fig. 2). X, y, and z axes on the frame recapitulate the CT and MRI axes. The frame center coordinates are 100, 100, 100, whereas a hypothetical frame origin (x, y and z = 0) resides in the upper posterior right side of the frame. The semicircular arc attached to the base frame has a radius of 190 mm. Probes that are attached to the arc probe carrier, therefore, have a working distance of 190 mm, to ensure target access. Target coordinates can be confirmed by a lateral X-ray through the Z rings, the probe tip terminating at their center.

A variety of technical aids are available to attach to the arc. A twist-drill craniotomy set is widely used. Biopy systems, hematoma evacuation kits, and lesion-generating devices are available. There are also accessories for microsurgery, including laser beam localizers, endoscopic adapters, and brachytherapy catheter arrays. A software program called SurgiPlan has been allied to a computer workstation, allowing simulation of probe trajectories and verifying their safety [5]. The cost of the system we use in Calgary was US $82,000 in 1996, without any of the above accessories.

3   APPLICATION

General preoperative precautions are followed as in any stereotactic opera-tion [6]. In particular, normal coagulation profiles are clearly required. Anticoagulated patients receive intravenous heparin for 5 days before surgery. The frame is placed orthogonally to the midsagittal plane by advancing the ear bars symmetrically through the lowest side holes into the external auditory meati. Salcman suggests placing the frame off center, with the ear contralateral to the target abutting the side bar of the frame, if increased lateral travel is needed on the arc [7]. The meati are routinely inspected for the presence of microhearing aids before ear bar insertion. Ear bar insertion may cause the patient considerable discomfort. This can be reduced if assistants are available to stabilize the frame for the surgeon. This obviates the need to maximize ear bar penetration and allows the frame to freely rotate. Application of foam strips (Reston, 3M) to the ear bars before their insertion also reduces pain considerably [5]. The frame is tilted 15 degrees to the orbitomeatal plane and is inclined 6 degrees from the horizontal plane to parallel the plane of the anterior commissure-posterior commissure (AC-PC) line. Balancing the frame on a finger placed on the tip of the patient's nose is usually adequate approximation. Another useful guide to the AC-PC plane is a line drawn from the nasion to the inion.

The scalp is infiltrated with a 50:50 mixture of 1.0% lidocaine with 1:100 000 epinephrine and 0.5% plain bupivacaine. A 27-gauge needle is used to inject 3 to 5 ml of this solution through the pinholes. I have tried applying topical local anesthetic to the pin site areas 1 hour before scalp infiltration to minimize discomfort and have had an approximately 50% response rate so far. Mild sedation with midazolam or fentanyl may be needed, remembering that confusion should be avoided at all costs. Alternatively, propofol offers rapid emergence and is an excellent choice. It does require the availability of a dedicated anesthesiology team. After adopting the ear bar foam as championed by Lundsford et al., I apply the majority of frames without intravenous sedation. Of great practical importance is that the fiducial channels on the magnetic resonance (MR) localizer require fastiduous filling with a copper sulphate solution on a regular basis (Fig. 3). These channels are imperfectly sealed and lose enough fluid every few months to entrain air bubbles, which are capable of corrupting the fiducial markers on the MR images. It is imperative that the localizer be checked before application, as it is a costly and time-consuming exercise to discover degraded images after they have been generated. A table adaptor is also required for MR. This is secured to the base frame and fits into a slot in the MR table head. The objective is to stabilize the head and avoid excessive movement.

Unfortunately, this system does not work well for patients with thoracic kyphosis (not uncommon in elderly patients), as their limited neck extension precludes secure fixation in the table head slot. The best method to deal with this is to place one or more pillows under the patient's buttocks and

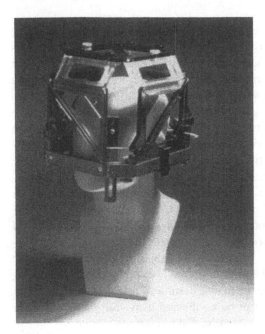

FIGURE 4.3 MR localizer.

hips, effectively flattening the kyphus. The head coil is then slid over the adaptor. It is vital that the MR alignment beam lights are then symmetrically superimposed on the lateral and anterior fiducial channels. Rotation of the adaptor screws is often required to accomplish this.

4 MR STRATEGIES

In general terms, attempts should be made to minimize distortion. Any hidden clips buried in long hair should be identified and removed. Impulse generators for deep brain stimulators should have their amplitude reduced to zero to prevent side effects. Higher field magnets are preferable, especially 1.5 Tesla and above. A protocol should be in place with the radiology department to ensure frequent calibration to minimize field heterogeneities. The Leksell frame is engineered to very high standards, and Burchiel et al. have indicated that its metallic purity is such that it induces little distortion relative to other commercially available frames [8].

Specific MR sequences are available in many articles and are beyond the purview of this chapter. T1-weighted sequences (thin cuts) reduce spatial distortion, and inversion recovery images sharply demarcate anatomical structures. Axial images are used to determine the x(lateral) and y(anteroposterior) target coordinates, whereas coronal scans define the x and z(vertical) coordinates. Cartesian principles are, therefore, used to create a three-dimensional address for a specific target. In functional cases in particular, it is helpful to generate axial images parallel to the AC-PC plane. Ideally, an image that contains both the AC and the PC in the same plane is available for study. The distance between the middle and basal fiducials is measured, and a discrepancy of 2 mm between the two sides of the frame is tolerated. Greater distances mandate frame realignment to the gantry. Diagonal lines between opposing anterior and posterior fiducials are drawn on the MR console, their crossing point indicating the frame center. A cursor is placed at this point and the coordinates recorded. A target is then selected (tumor or physiological) and its coordinates noted. The x and y frame coordinates for the target are then calculated by subtracting the frame center from the target coordinates. The z coordinate is determined by adding a constant of 40 to the distance between the basal and middle fiducials at the target plane. Frame coordinates can be confirmed using SurgiPlan software or a digitizer (Elekta Instruments, Atlanta, GA).

Acknowledgments

I would like to thank Kim Burchiel for teaching me all I know about the Leksell frame, and then some. Elekta also kindly provided us with images.

REFERENCES

1. L Leksell, K Liden. A therapeutic trial with radioactive isotopes in cystic brain tumors. In: Radioisotope Techniques, vol 1: Medical and Physiological Applications. London: HRI Stationery Office, 1951.
2. L Leksell. A stereotactic apparatus for intracerebral surgery. Acta Chir Scan 99: 229–233, 1949.
3. LD Lundsford, D Leksell. The Leksell system. In: Modern Stereotactic Neurosurgery. Boston: Martinus Nijhoff Publishing, 1988, pp 27–46.
4. L Leksell. Stereotaxis and Radiosurgery: An Operative System. Springfield, IL: Thomas, 1971.
5. LD Lundsford, D Konziolka, D Leksell. The Leksell Stereotactic System. In: R Tasker, P Gildenberg, eds. Stereotactic and Functional Neurosurgery, 1999, pp 51–63.
6. DF Louw, KJ Burchiel. Pallidotomy for Parkinson's disease. In M Appuzo, ed. Neurosurgical Care of the Elderly. Park Ridge, Il: American Association of Neurological Surgeons, 1999, pp 75–86

7. M Salcman, EH Bellis, W Sewchand, P Amin. Technical aids for the flexible use of the Leksell stereotactic system. Neurol Res 11:89–96, 1989.
8. Burchiel KJ, Nguyen T. MRI distortion and stereotactic neurosurgery using the Cosman-Roberts-Wells and Leksell frames. Stereotactic Funct Neurosurg 66(1–3):123–136, 1996.

5

Stereotactic Surgery with the Zamorano-Dujovny Frame

Lucía Zamorano, Ramiro Pérez de la Torre, and Fernando Díaz
Wayne State University, Detroit, Michigan, U.S.A.

1 INTRODUCTION

Modern stereotaxis implies that application of all space-defining devices to reach the selected target. The Zamorano-Dujovny (Z-D) stereotactic head frame (F. L. Fischer, Freiburg, Germany) was developed for several reasons: to provide a stable referencing system for several types of imaging studies, such as conventional X-rays, computed tomography (CT), magnetic resonance imaging (MRI), or digital subtraction angiography (DSA); freedom of choice for the surgeon on a patient's intraoperative position; fully sterile draping; and an unobstructed approach for using conventional neurosurgical and microsurgical intraoperative techniques [1,2].

Open stereotaxis provides a wide variety of applications with varying degrees of sophistication, ranging from a simple localization tool up to a highly complex system for surgical automation and robotic applications. Since its inception, continuous improvements and accessories have become necessary to accommodate evolving technology in the field of image-guided stereotaxis.

2 THE ZAMORANO-DUJOVNY STEREOTACTIC SYSTEM

The Z-D stereotactic system consists of an arc-centered frame, a carbon fiber base ring, and a localizer arc, also called an aiming bow. The system also accommodates multiple accessories and instruments, as well as optional software (Figs. 1 and 2).

2.1 Base Ring

The base ring acts as a reference system and intraoperative head holder. The base ring can be made of aluminum, which is CT and X-ray compatible, carbon fiber, which is compatible with all imaging modalities (CT, X-ray, MRI, positron emission tomography (PET), or titanium, which is CT, X-ray, MRI, and convergent beam irradiation (CBI) compatible. The Z-D unit includes an open base ring, three or four pin holders that can be positioned at any desired location, and a set of 18 pins in five different lengths. The ring opening and different pin lengths make it possible to place the ring in any chosen position (Fig 3). When the unit is in place on the patient's head the surgeon is provided with an unobstructed area within which to perform the craniotomy.

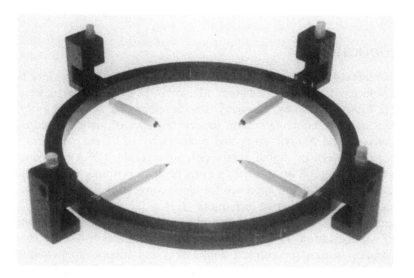

FIGURE 1 The carbon fiber ring, along with the posts and pins in pre-mounting position.

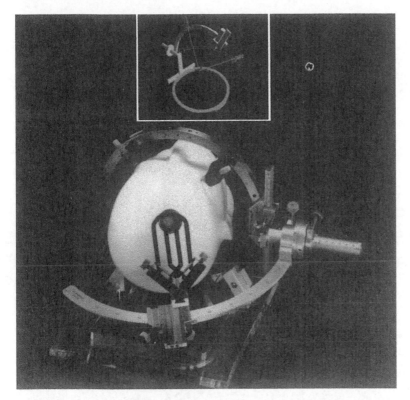

FIGURE 2 Phantom showing the superimposition of the retractors and the localizing unit for targeting.

2.2 The Localizer Arc

This unit consists of an arc quadrant that can be mounted in any of four positions on the base ring: at 0°, 90°, 180°, or 270°. The arc settings include three linear scales (a, b, c) and two angular scales (d, e). The first three correspond to the traditional x, y, and z spatial orientations. The last two are for modifying the entry point of the surgical trajectory according to the location of the lesion, vascular structures, and skull bone. The arc has two types of instruments holders, one for instruments 2 mm to 4 mm in diameter, and one for instruments 4 mm to 7 mm in diameter. The holders have a scale for depth adjustment. Several instruments can be adapted to the arc, including biopsy instruments (side-cutting and cup forceps), cannulae, hematoma evacuators, electrodes, endoscopes, brachytherapy plates, and especially important for open stereotaxis, stereotactic brain retractors (cylinder

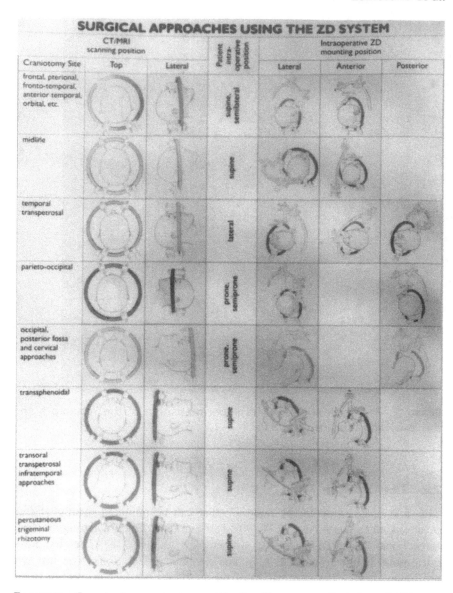

FIGURE 3 Surgical approaches with the Zamorano-Dujovny (Z-D) system. Notice the versatility of the system for standard neurosurgical approaches.

and speculum types). The biopsy instruments include forceps 1.4 mm in diameter, a probe with a lateral cutting edge, a Backlund spiral probe, and a biopsy and seed applicator set.

The stereotactic brain retractors consist of 2-cm and 3-cm diameter cylinders and 3-cm and 6-cm length specula that open from 0 to 5 cm in diameter; a reading displays the actual opening diameter. Both bivalve and quadravalve specula are available, as well as a bayonet-type design that allows free access to the surgical corridor (Fig. 2).

2.3 Attachments

The concept of the stereotactic head frame as a localization device has evolved into the head frame as a sophisticated carrier-equipment unit. The ease with which the frame, along with the arc quadrant, can be manipulated allows the integration of different devices according to surgical necessity. The most basic attachment, the biopsy needle, can share an instrument holder with biopsy forceps. The inner guide of the needle biopsy can be applied as a stylet through which to position ventricular catheters for hydrocephalus and, at same time, for brachytherapy. The rigid endoscope (Chavantes-Zamorano Neuroendoscope, Karl Storz, Tuttlingen, Germany) can be adapted to the stereotactic arc, along with rigid and flexible endoscopic instrumentation. Laser fibers can access the surgical corridor from the arc and be advanced to reach targets for specific applications.

3 IMAGING

During image acquisition, the base ring provides the attachment for the image localizers. Intraoperatively, the base ring acts as a head holder when used in conjunction with the Mayfield head holder and/or the Sugita adapter. For CT and MR imaging, adapters provide an isocentric relationship with the CT gantry and the MR imaging head coiler. Independent of the type of interfacing method selected between the imaging studies and the base ring (isocentric or localizing), the reference for target localization will be the center of the ring, which defines the point origin of the stereotactic space.

3.1 X-ray Localization

X-ray localization is performed using orthogonal X-ray tubes, which are securely mounted in a lateral and anteroposterior (AP) position and are aligned with the head ring of the stereotactic system. When the system is installed, the lateral AP tubes are positioned so that their central beam passes through the holes of the head ring at 0° and 180° (AP) and at 90° and 270°

(lateral). In order to limit magnification, the X-ray tubes should be mounted at a relatively large distance from the head ring. After the X-rays have been taken and developed, the coordinates for the x and z axes are obtained from the AP X-ray and the coordinates for the y and z axes for the target and trephination points are taken from lateral X-ray.

3.2 Angiographic Localization

Four quadrangular localizer plates are positioned and screwed to the head ring to allow X-ray views for localizing vascular structures. A fifth plate is used intraoperatively; when the Z-D localizer arc is mounted on the head ring, it takes the position where a localizing plate could be fastened. The Z-D setting module has two additional holes in which to insert localizer plate #5. After the X-ray films are taken, they are placed on a digitizing tablet; the desired target and trephination points are digitally determined and transferred automatically to a personal computer (PC) using the Angioloc 650 056 computer program. The program compensates for magnification error and determines the angle of incidence obtained from visible points on X-ray or angiographic films.

The Angioloc program includes an Angiorev program that accepts stereotactic coordinates already determined from CT or MRI scans and adds them to the X-ray/angiographic image. This proves important for stereotactic biopsy in a highly vascular area. The Angiorev program allows the surgeon to determine if the biopsy needle is likely to pierce a vessel on its way from the entry point to the target point.

3.3 CT, MRI, and PET Localization

For CT and PET localization, the head ring is attached to the CT adapter. Four specially designed plates are mounted and screwed to the ring (Fig. 1). The CT scan usually includes the alignment of the cursor of the gantry to the top of the arc in axial direction generating image acquisition in positive or negative direction according to the specific circumstances. Our setup parameters are to position the table at 175 mm, zeroing the gantry, and proceeding 200 mm forward.

For MRI localization, localizing plates are attached to the four quadrants that define the anatomical space, yielding a set of coordinates. Sequences and protocols can be flexible, according to the specific circumstances, but in general the authors use T_1-, T_2-, proton densities, and 2-mm slice thickness for tumor surgery with extra three-dimensional flash in functional cases.

4 SOFTWARE: THE PREOPERATIVE PLANNING PROCESS

The original concept of applying the frame to approach tumor resection has shifted to a more broad-based application in neurosurgery. Nevertheless, the majority of neurosurgical procedures begin with the preoperative planning process. We've developed PC-compatible software, the Neurosurgical Planning System (NSPS), that provides settings for mounting the Z-D localizer arc in any position. The extensive capabilities of the software allow the surgeon, during the preoperative planning process, to select imaging modalities interactively, define tumor volumes of interest, select entry and target points, and calculate the stereotactic coordinates that translate into a physical target.

The first set of coordinates are determined by the surgical approach, surface vessel pattern, and cortical brain anatomy. The second set of coordinates are chosen according to tumor pathology, biopsy specimen, and tissue sampling that includes pathological tissue and its interface with normal brain tissue.

5 ASSEMBLING THE Z-D FRAME-BASED SYSTEM FOR SURGERY

5.1 Mounting the Z-D Localizing Unit

The patient is prepared for mounting the Z-D unit: vital signs are monitored, an intravenous (IV) line is placed for sedation with Versed® 2 mg and Fentanyl® 100 mcg, and supplemental oxygen is provided. The ring is placed in the clamps of the head holder. The patient is put on the stretcher and carefully moved into the ring. The patient's head is positioned such that the ring is parallel to the obtitomeatal line.

The sites of pin placement are marked, and efforts are made to accommodate the frame at the same level. With the head frame in place, imaging studies are taken with the patient maximally positioned with regard to the lesion. The arc quadrant is mounted by fastening the basic carrier to the head ring. Then the ring slides into the axle mounting cross so the 1.1 numbers are exactly opposite. The right-angled drum axle is also inserted to the axle mounting cross. The aiming bow is positioned over the drum of the axle mounting cross. The aiming bow is turned by slightly pushing it until the guide pin locks in the guide groove. The instrument holder is positioned onto scale "E" on the arc of the aiming bow. The instrument carrier in inserted into the dovetail guide on the instrument holder and fastened to "0" on the depth control. An additional carrier is attached to the smaller dovetail guide and screwed down until it juts out at a 90° angle. A target point with a positive z coordinate (above the ring) is reached when the F. L. Fischer label on the fixation rail points in this direction.

By loosening one screw (D) on the stereotactic ring, the neurosurgeon can bring the localizer arc in and out of the surgical field to check the localization and the depth of the resection ("nonfixed" open stereotaxis). This feature is especially useful for craniotomies to treat superficial lesions located in eloquent areas of the brain. The nonfixed approach is also helpful for craniotomies of deep lesions using a microsurgical approach, allowing the neurosurgeon to operate using standard neurosurgical techniques while evaluating the intraoperative target localization. In addition, when a nonlinear pathway to a lesion is preferred, such as in transcallosal, lobe retraction, transoral, and skull base surgery, the surgeon performs the approach using microsurgical techniques and, when close to the target area, uses the d and e screw to guide the probe further along the defined surgical pathway.

For "fixed" open stereotaxis, useful for removing deep-seated lesions when a lineal transcortical or transcerebellar corridor is desired, the arc settings on the Z-D localizer unit (a,b,c,d,e) are kept fixed during the intracranial surgical procedure, and specially designed stereotactic brain retractors are mounted in the instrument holders. These consist of 2- and 3-cm diameter cylinders and a 6-cm long speculum; the last one opens from 0 to 5 cm in diameter. Both types of brain retractors are designed with a bayonet-type holder that allows an unobstructed surgeon's eye or microscope view line, as well as ample room for conventional surgical instruments like microinstruments, a laser, an ultrasonic aspirator, and others. The instrument holder scale allows continuous depth adjustment of surgical instruments (Fig. 4).

6 THE MULTIPLE APPLICATIONS OF THE Z-D FRAME

6.1 Z-D Frame in the Resection of Gliomas

Needle biopsy using the Z-D unit significantly enhances the information gathered by imaging studies regarding tumor dimensions, location, and depth. During biopsy, the forceps are inserted through a guide cannula, and the combined instrument is placed in the instrument carrier on the Z-D localizing arc.

We use the Z-D system with a real-time intraoperative digitization system to operate on gliomas [3]. Intraoperative digitizers are instruments through which a physical correlation between the image modality data (CT and MRI) and the patient's neuroanatomy is made so that intraoperatively, instruments can be tracked using an optoelectronic camera system. In the operating room, interactive image-guided surgery begins with instrument

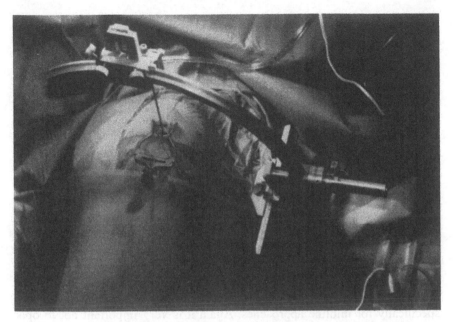

FIGURE 4 Intraoperatively, mounting the localizing unit and positioning the biopsy needle.

calibration using infrared cameras and a digitizing probe. When using the stereotactic frame as a reference point, the probe touches predefined points in circumferential fashion on the Z-D ring, establishing coordinates that match those derived from imaging studies and plotted using the NSPS software program during the preplanning process. Multiple trajectories can be chosen to approach the tumor sequentially in the resection, to aspirate cystic portions, for ventricular tapping, or to place a ventricular drain.

6.2 Brachytherapy

The planning process combines volume rendering and isodose planning to calculate number of catheters and seeds loading. Radioactive seeds can be placed subsequent to stereotactic biopsy. Inner coaxial catheters are preloaded with the seeds. The introduction of an external ventricular guide is accomplished following the guidelines. Subsequently, the catheter is glued to the bone continuing with the inner coaxial placement. Hemoclips are applied to secure it. Quality assessment protocols allows strict evaluation of postoperative placement [4].

6.3 The Z-D System in the Resection of Vascular Lesions

From all the group of arteriovenous malformations, cavernous angiomas are characterized by their clinical behavior, pseudocapsule formation, and from an origin intermingled at any level of the white matter where accurate localization is cumbersome. The biopsy needle can be advanced to locate the upper margin, depending on the size of the lesion, to continue with microsurgical dissection to resect in toto. Multiple lesions can be resected without increased morbidity and especially for seizure control [5].

6.4 Z-D Stereotactic Frame in Ventricular Approaches

This category of approaches deserves special mention, given the frequent distortion once the ventricle has been entered. The optimal approach is to select the target for sampling, ventricular catheter placement, or to bring the endoscope to the microsurgical field. We pay attention to the position of the patient, neutral in coronal approaches and completely lateral in temporal horn or occipital approaches. In the posterior fossa we use the prone position specifically for midline approaches. Again it is very important not to open the ventricle until we have available all equipment for the procedure. The stylet is used to guide the catheters marking 19 cm from the tip to the upper margin. We call attention to the fact that target zero is not in the tip of the needle but in the center of the slit aperture [6].

6.5 The Z-D Stereotactic Frame in Trigeminal Rhizotomy

Trigeminal neuralgia is another important application when targeting is essential, especially in transfacial pretrigeminal cistern approaches. Computed tomographic scan is the preferred imaging modality. The entry point can be selected in the 1 foramen to direct the needle. Electrodes can be inserted to confirm the position of the needle before lesioning with the radiofrequency generator (Neuro50, F. L. Fischer, Freiburg, Germany).

Acknowledgment

The authors wish to thank Julie Bedore for her editorial support and continuous assistance.

REFERENCES

1.   Zamorano L. The Zamorano-Dujovny Multipurpose Localizing Unit. Advanced Neurosurgical Navigation. New York: Thieme Medical Publishers, 1999, pp 255–266.

2. Zamorano L, Kadi M, Jiang Z, Díaz F. Zamorano-Dujovny multipurpose neurosurgical image-guided localizing unit: Experience in 866 consecutive cases of "open stereotaxis." Stereotac Funct Neurosurg 63:45–51, 1994.
3. Zamorano L, Pérez-de la Torre R. Stereotactic volumetric resection of malignant gliomas. In: Neurosurgical Operative Atlas, vol. 9. Park Ridge, Ill: American Association of Neurological Surgeons, 2000, pp 113–122.
4. Zamorano L, Bauer-Kirpes B, Dujovny M, Yakar D. Dose planning for interstitial irradiation. In: Computers in Stereotactic Neurosurgery. Boston: Blackwell Scientific Publications, 1992, pp 279–291.
5. Zamorano L, Matter A, Sáenz A, Buciuc R, Díaz F. Interactive image-guided resection of cerebral cavernous malformations. Comput Aided Surg 2:327–332, 1997.
6. Viñas F, Zamorano L, Lis-Planells M, Buciuc R, Díaz F. Interactive intraoperative localization during the resection of intraventricular lesions. Minim Invasive Neurosurg 39:65–70, 1996.

6

Stereotactic Surgery with the Patil Frame

Arun Angelo Patil
University of Nebraska Medical Center, Omaha, Nebraska, U.S.A.

1 INTRODUCTION

The Patil frame is designed to allow surgeons to measure coordinates directly on the scanner screen and obtain intraoperative images to confirm accuracy of the procedure. It is a center of the arc system and modification of the original Patil frame [1].

The frame (Fig. 1) consists of a fiducial plate, a head-ring, a base frame, two side stanchions, two pivot blocks, a yoke, an arc, several probe holders (for probes of different diameters) and several head pins (of different lengths). The fiducial plate is made of acetyl resin, the head holder of polycarbon, the head pins of titanium, and the remainder of the frame of anodized aluminum. The inferior surface of the fiducial plate has two grooves that serve as fiducial markers for computed tomography (CT) images: an outer groove that is parallel to and along the left margin of the plate, and an inner groove that is 45° to the outer groove and meets the outer groove at its caudal end. For magnetic resonance (MR) images, two tubes filled with paramagnetic solution (that serve as fiducial markers) are inserted in these grooves. The superior surface of the fiducial plate has attachments for the head ring and the base frame. The attachment for the head-ring is an elevated

47

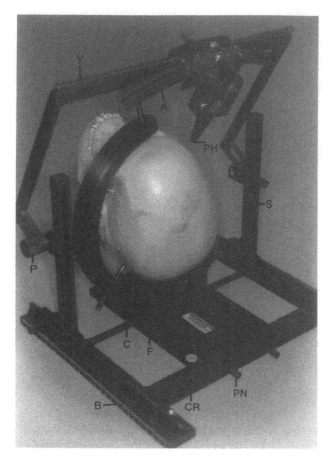

FIGURE 1 The Patil stereotactic system. A, arc; PH, probe holder; Y, yoke; S, side stanchion; P, pivot block; B, base frame; C, caudal cross bar; CR, cranial cross bar; PN, pin connecting the cranial cross bar to the fiducial plate; F, fiducial plate.

bracket. The head ring, which is C-shaped, is inserted into this bracket and secured by means of a screw. The base frame is attached to the fiducial plate by inserting its caudal crossbar into the transverse groove on the superior surface of the fiducial plate, and by means of two pins that connect the cranial crossbar of the base frame and the fiducial plate. The side stanchions are mounted on the sidebars of the base frame, the pivot blocks on the side stanchions, the yoke on the pivot blocks, and the arc on the yoke. The arc has a probe carrier into which the probe holder is inserted. The latter can slide along the length of the probe holder to change the depth of the probe. The system is arc centered and the radius of the arc is 21 cm. A 21-cm length probe is, therefore, used with this system. Zero for the Z coordinate (craniocaudal distance) is at a point where the two fiducial markers meet, zero for the Y coordinate (anterior-posterior distance) is the horizontal plane in which the two fiducial markers are located, and zero for the X coordinate (lateral distance) is in the vertical plane in which the left (outer) fiducial marker is located. Because the inner fiducial markers is at 45° to the outer fiducial marker, the distance between the two markers at any given point is equal to the perpendicular distance of that point from the meeting point of the markers.

2   METHOD

The procedure can be performed in the operating room or on the CT table. The head holder is attached to the fiducial plate, which in turn is attached perfectly horizontal and parallel to the CT table by means of a CT table interface. The head is fixed in the head holder by three head pins (Fig. 2). Special care is taken to avoid attaching the head pins in the plane in which the target is present. The CT table is set to a height at which the head and fiducial markers are both visible on a single CT image. The table height is noted and used for subsequent procedures. Serial CT images 3 mm in thickness at 1.5-mm intervals with a 25-cm field of view are then obtained through the area of interest. The gantry is not tilted. The image with the target is chosen (Fig. 3). Using the cursor of the scanner and measure distance mode, the angle of the coronal trajectory with the vertical is measured. Then the Y (perpendicular distance of the target from the horizontal plane of the fiducial markers), X (perpendicular distance of the target from the outer fiducial marker), and Z (distance between the two fiducial marker) coordinates are measured (Fig. 4). The base frame is then connected to the fiducial plate, the coordinates are adjusted, and the probe holder on the arc and the yoke on the pivot block are set at angles to allow safe passage of the probe. These angles can be chosen based on surface anatomy or on reconstructed images. A burr-hole is then made, a probe is placed at the target, and intraoperative scans are obtained to confirm accuracy of probe placement. When the procedure is performed in the operating room (e.g., during stereotactic craniotomy), after the coordinates are obtained, the fiducial plate is detached from the CT table and attached to the operating table interface.

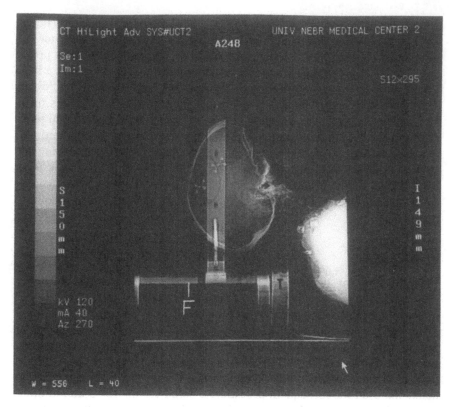

FIGURE 2 Scout image with the patient's head in the head holder (attached to the fiducial plate and computed tomographic table). **F,** fiducial plate; **T,** table interface.

During MR stereotaxis, MR fiducial markers are inserted into the fiducial grooves. Scans are obtained using the head coil of the MR scanner with the head holder and the fiducial plate attached to the patient's head. Coordinates are measured using the same technique used for CT images.

During linear accelerator radiosurgery, after coordinates are measured, the fiducial plate (with the head holder and the patient's head in it) is attached to the Linac table. The remainder of the frame is then attached to the fiducial plate, the coordinates are adjusted, the probe holder is set at zero position on the arc and the yoke is set perfectly vertical. The vertical positioning light is then aligned with the hole in the probe holder, and the side positioning lights are aligned with the center of the pivot blocks. This

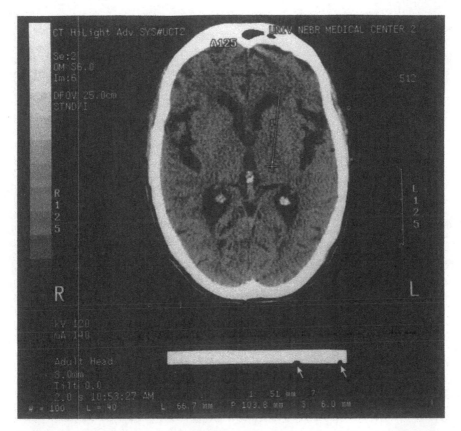

FIGURE 3 Computed tomographic image shows the thalamic target for deep brain stimulator (DBS) implant marked by a cursor. The coronal trajectory is marked by the line. The angle of this trajectory is displayed at the bottom of the image. The *arrows* mark the inner and outer **(left)** fiducial markers.

sets the target at the isocenter. The base frame (together with the components attached to it) are detached from the fiducial plate, and irradiation is started.

3 INDICATIONS FOR USING THE SYSTEM

The system can be used for functional neurosurgical procedures including implantation of deep brain stimulators, biopsy of intracranial lesions, brachytherapy, aspiration of cysts, aspiration of brain abscesses, stereotactic craniotomies, and radiosurgery.

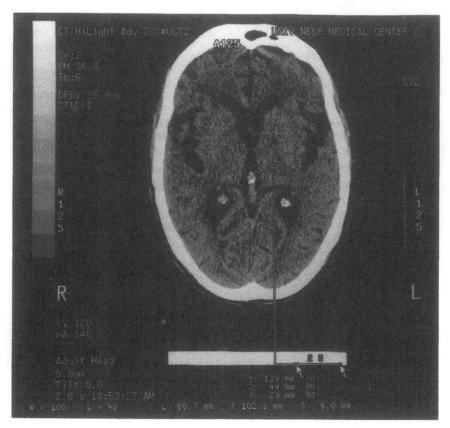

FIGURE 4 Computed tomographic image with coordinate measurements. The two *arrows* mark the fiducial markers. 1-Y coordinate (perpendicular distance from the target to the horizontal line joining the two fiducial markers), 2-X coordinate (perpendicular distance of the target from the outer fiducial marker), and 3-Z coordinate (distance between the two fiducial markers).

4 AREAS ACCESSIBLE BY THE SYSTEM

Intracranial areas including brainstem and other posterior fossa structures, pituitary fossa, all skull base structures, and C1 and C2 vertebra are accessible by this frame. The frame can be used in prone, lateral, or supine positions; transoral and transnasal procedures can be performed as well.

5 ACCURACY TESTING

Intraoperative scans can be obtained with this system because it is compact. Therefore, accuracy testing can be performed with each procedure. During coordinate measurements the scanner cursor is left on the screen to mark the target point. On the intraoperative image, the position of the probe tip in relationship to the cursor is viewed to determine the accuracy.

6 DISCUSSION

This is an arc-centered system in which the center of the arc is positioned on the target. It is, therefore, possible to approach the target using any desired trajectory, including transnasal and transoral trajectories, and to reach skull-base structures [2–4]. Because CT images used for the procedure are obtained with the gantry vertical, which is the vertical plane of the frame, coordinates can be directly measured on the scanner screen without need of a special computer or calculator, or the need to transfer data from the scanner to other computers. In addition, the scanner computer can be used for reconstructing images in different planes for complex trajectory planning. Because the system fits easily in the gantry of a CT scanner, it is feasible to obtain intraoperative scans to detect errors and correct them, thereby guaranteeing stereotactic accuracy [5,6]. Because of its compactness, it is possible to use CT images with a field of view of 25 cm. These images are larger than those obtained with the wider field of view required for other frames, and, therefore, have better accuracy and higher resolution. The system has a C-shaped open head holder, which makes it ideal for stereotactic craniotomy. Because of the simplicity of the system it is relatively inexpensive. In summary, this is a simple, accurate, versatile, and inexpensive system.

REFERENCES

1. Patil AA. Computed tomography (CT) plane of the target approach in CT stereotaxis. Neurosurgery 15:410–414, 1984.
2. Patil AA. Transoral stereotactic biopsy of the second cervical vertebral body: A case report with technical note. Neurosurgery 25:999–1002, 1989.
3. Patil AA, Kumar P, Leibrock L, Aarabi B. Stereotactic approach to skull base lesions. Skull Base Surgery 1(4):235–239, 1991.
4. Patil AA, Chand A. Modifications of transnasal and transoral stereotactic procedures. Acta Neurochir 34:46–50, 1995.

5. Patil AA. Intraoperative calibration of the Patil stereotactic system during computed tomography (CT) guided stereotactic procedures—a technical note. Stereotact Funct Neurosurg 56:179–183, 1991.
6. Patil AA, Kumar PP, Leibrock LG, Gelber B, Aarabi B. The value of intraoperative scans during computed tomography (CT) guided stereotactic procedures. Neuroradiology 34:451–456, 1992.

7

Frameless Stereotactic Systems: General Considerations

Marshall T. Watson, Jr.
University of Rochester, Rochester, New York, U.S.A.

Robert J. Maciunas
Case Western Reserve University, Cleveland, Ohio, U.S.A.

1 INTRODUCTION

Neurosurgeons continuously strive to improve the safety and effectiveness of their interventions. Stereotactic neurosurgery uses imaging modalities such as computed tomography (CT) and magnetic resonance imaging (MRI) to serve as spatial guides for the surgeon. These spatial guides provide patient-specific anatomical roadmaps which, although not a replacement for knowledge of neuroanatomy, aid the surgeon in successfully treating the patient.

The theory behind stereotactic neurosurgery is relatively simple. Three points define a volume in geometric space. If the same three points can be defined on a patient and on an image of that patient, then the three-dimensional space of that patient and image are known and can be defined relative to each other. Registration is the process whereby the location of any point on or within the patient is defined on the image, and vice versa. Stereotactic systems differ in the manner in which the spatial points are defined, the geometric coordinate spaces used, and the method to register the patient and image coordinate spaces.

Frame-based systems involve fixing a structure to the patient's head. The patient and frame are imaged together and the two spaces (patient and image) are registered. Points in the patient's space were defined based on how the frame hardware was designed, such as an x, y, z coordinate system, a radius and angle system, or some variation of the two. Today's frame-based systems are highly accurate and have become the gold standard for localization techniques. Frame-based systems are bulky and uncomfortable for the patient, however, and frames can obstruct the operative field. Most systems limit the surgeon to targets along a straight-line trajectory, and none offer real-time feedback.

Roberts et al. [1] and Friets et al. [2] introduced frameless stereotactic systems in the 1980s. Many different frameless stereotactic systems have been developed since that time. Some aspects are universal to all systems, frameless and frame-based alike. All systems must define points in the image and the patient and be able to map the two groups to each other.

2 POINT DEFINITION AND REGISTRATION

Two common methods for defining points are surface-based and point-based registration. Each offers a distinct set of advantages and disadvantages.

Surfaced-based registration fits a set of points from the contours of one image to a surface model from contours of the patient's head or from other images. An advantage of this system is that it allows retrospective registration from prior images. Its disadvantage, however, is that it is less accurate. Point-based registration involves selecting corresponding points in different images and on the patient. The coordinates of each set of points are defined, and then a geometric transformation is calculated between them; these points may be anatomical landmarks or may be applied artificial markers. Anatomical landmarks allow retrospective registration with existing images. Artificial extrinsic markers do not allow this, but have other advantages that have made them common in stereotactic guidance.

Extrinsic point registration allows greater accuracy than other registration methods. In addition, a calculation of the accuracy for each registration attempt is possible, giving the user a quantitated degree of accuracy. As long as a detectable marker can be manufactured, registration can theoretically be performed with any imaging modality.

Mobile markers and rigid markers are two types of extrinsic markers that are currently available. Mobile markers, which are taped, glued, or otherwise affixed to the patient's skin, have the advantage of ease and speed of application. They are, however, prone to error because the skin may move relative to the skull and intracranial contents during registration. Rigid markers eliminate this potential error, but are more difficult to apply and may be more uncomfortable for the patient because they are anchored to the patient's skull or other bony structure.

Three noncolinear points define a volume in space. Computer studies have analyzed the addition of more points to a registration system and its effect on registration error. It was found that four points increased registration accuracy over three, but that adding further points did not significantly improve accuracy [3]. However, if external mobile fiducials are to be placed, additional markers offer the benefit of redundancy should one or more markers become displaced. Fiducials should encompass the intracranial volume of interest and be noncolinear to ensure the most accurate registration possible. Small areas of hair shaving may be necessary.

3 IMAGING

Once the markers are positioned, the patient is imaged with one or more of several possible modalities. The imaging need not be either on the day of marker positioning or the day of surgery, although markers are more apt to be dislodged with time. Fiducial markers are commonly filled with a material that is visible on T1-weighted, T2-weighted, and proton-density MR images. MR angiography and venography, functional MR, and MR spectroscopy may be performed, as necessary. Fiducial markers for CT scans are easily available, and thin slice CT images (such as 3 mm) are usually obtained. Positron emission tomography (PET) and single photon emission computed tomography (SPECT) scans may be performed with fiducials that contain special materials.

4 INTRAOPERATIVE LOCALIZATION

It is necessary to determine the location of a point in space to register the patient and image spaces. A variety of devices have been developed that communicate the location of some device (wand, microscope, surgical instrument, etc.) relative to the patient to a computer, which then translates that position into image space. The Zeiss MKM microscope (Zeiss Corporation, Jena, Germany) combines a robotic arm mechanism and an optical microscope. The Neuronavigator (ISG Technologies, Toronto, Ontario, Canada, and FARO Medical Technologies, Miami, Florida) uses a passive localization arm, as does the OAS System (Radionics, Burlington, Massachusetts). The PUMA Industrial Robot (Westinghouse Electric, Pittsburgh, Pennsylvania) is an active robotic arm system. Stealth System (Bucholz;

Surgical Navigation Technologies, Boulder, Colorado) and the ACUSTAR I (Codman/JJPI, Raynham, Massachusetts) localize with infrared light-emitting diodes. The Utah Machine Vision System (Heilbrun) and the VISLAN System (Thomas; London, United Kingdom) use passive stereoscopic video [4–15].

All localizing systems have their disadvantages. Mechanical arms usually use either potentiometers, which are prone to drift, or digitizers, which are expensive, to determine the position of the tip relative to a fixed base. The arms, although simple, can be bulky. Sonic systems use the time delay between a pulse emission and its detection to calculate position. Although these systems are inexpensive and durable, they are prone to ultrasonic noise and require an unobstructed "line-of-site" between emitter(s) and detector. Magnetic systems detect position using magnetic waves and fields and, like mechanical arms, do not require an unobstructed line-of-site. A major disadvantage is the distortion that can be created by metal objects in or near the operative field. Optical systems, whether infrared emitters, fluorescent markers, or video cameras, all suffer from line-of-site difficulties [16].

The patient usually requires repositioning intraoperatively, and a system must be able to continuously monitor head positioning and adjust the registered coordinates rapidly, accurately, and in a minimally invasive manner. Detectors mounted to the table move with the head and fiducial markers and provide a simple and inexpensive solution. These detectors are often bulky and limit operative exposure and are not an ideal solution. Reference markers that communicate with a remote sensor, thus allowing tracking of the registered points, are another solution. If a marker is mounted on the head or head-holding assembly directly (such as the Mayfield head fixation device), head movement problems are minimized. A direct line-of-site must be maintained between the reference marker and remote sensor [16].

5 INTRAOPERATIVE VIDEO DISPLAY

Once the images have been registered with respect to the patient, they must be displayed in a meaningful manner. A high-resolution monitor with 512 × 512 pixel windows displays images in a variety of orientations and configurations. Color graphic overlays that represent the localizer position and trajectory are usually displayed relative to the on-screen images. The localizer position is usually updated on the screen at 20 frames per second. Real-time displays have become more common with increases in image processing speed and power and decreases in cost.

6 ACCURACY AND ERROR

Certain terms should be defined in discussions of any stereotactic system. Unbiasedness is a lack of skew. Precision is a tendency to approach a certain value. Observations may be precise (minimal spread from a mean value) but biased (that mean value is not the true value). Accuracy requires both unbiasedness and precision. In an article about three-dimensional digitizers, Wohlers describes the confusion about accuracy in his sidebar "How Accurate is Accurate?"

> Comparing the accuracy of 3-D digitizers can be confusing. The terms "accuracy," "precision," "resolution," and "repeatability" are often misused, misunderstood, misleading or just plain omitted. Buyer confusion also occurs when digitizer suppliers publish numbers related to the specific parts . . . that make up the system. This can be misleading. The precision of the system's mechanics does not reflect the accuracy of the process. In fact, the precision of the mechanics is . . . always better than the accuracy of the process [17].

The accuracy of any stereotactic system is influenced in an additive manner by the error introduced at each step. A system must correctly identify the location of each fiducial during the localization process and must then accurately map patient fiducials onto image fiducials (or image fiducials to image fiducials) during registration. The sum of the root mean square error of each fiducial location can be calculated and is related to the fiducial localization error. The surgeon needs to know that the structure he is pointing to in the patient is the same structure displayed on the image. Any error in this, the target registration error, cannot be calculated by the system and is not directly related to the registration error. The registration error number may be reduced by eliminating fiducial makers, but if the remaining markers are distant from the operative site, the accuracy of target localization may decrease. Anatomical landmarks, such as the lateral canthus, are useful guides for checking the system and avoiding errors.

The effect of tissue displacement between imaging and surgery and during surgery must also be considered. Movement of tissues is inevitable during surgery, and studies have shown as much as 1 cm of displacement of superficial brain tissues [18]. Deeper structures, such as those at the skull base or along the falx shift less than superficial structures, improving the accuracy of stereotactic systems at those regions. Steps can be taken to minimize the error caused by tissue displacement. Displacement is often greatest in the direction of gravity. Structures may shift downward along a given trajectory. Minimizing diuretic use does not seem to have an appreciable effect on displacement. Cerebrospinal fluid shunting can cause shifts of tissues in unpredictable directions, so its use should be avoided until after the primary approach has been made, if possible. Debulking of tumors in the "inside to outside" approach also yields significant tissue shifts; defining the outer margins of a tumor before proceeding with debulking may help to minimize this error [19–22].

Frameless stereotactic systems incorporate many of the advantages of frame-based systems without the discomfort and bulkiness of the frame. The systems differ in ease of use, cost, and availability, and at this time no one system is clearly superior to the others. The continued improvement in processor speed and cost and the advances in engineering promise exciting future developments in frameless systems.

The neurosurgeon considering the frameless stereotaxy for his practice has several options. Most commercially available systems (including those made by Medtronic/SNT, BrainLab, Radionics, and Leibinger) use optical infrared-based technology. By tracking a probe in a magnetic field, Cygnus offers a frameless stereotaxy device at a lower cost than the IR-based systems, but concerns regarding interference with ferromagnetic materials and resulting loss of accuracy have limited its appeal.

To make frameless stereotaxy a routine part of most neurosurgeons' operating room, certain criteria should be met:

1.   The system should accept standard CT and MRI scans from any standard imager. Scan data should be transferable to the operating room computer via portable media, such as optical disk, as well as over an ethernet connection (which would be the preferred method). Ability to run the system software on an office or home personal computer is useful to allow for convenient preoperative planning. Image fusion of CT, MRI, and any other appropriate digital studies (e.g., functional MRI or PET) should be possible.

Versatility is important as well. Most neurosurgical groups will want the ability to use frameless stereotaxy in the placement of spinal instrumentation; packages designed for ENT approaches may be useful for transsphenoidal approaches.

2.   The system should be as easy to use as possible. In practice, this means that the neurosurgeon should not have to supervise the imaging and data transfer himself; rather, a physician's assistant, nurse, or other "extender" should be able to manage the downloading of the scan and at least begin the registration process in the operating room. Ideally, the neurosurgeon will confirm the accuracy of the registration and use the information to plan the surgery itself.

During the operation, the system should be easily controllable from the sterile field or be easily manipulated by other operating room personnel, even those without significant experience in frameless stereotaxy.

3.   Cost must be kept in mind. A "fully-loaded" system typically will run between \$300,000 and \$400,000. Few, if any, physician groups will want to bear this cost themselves and will ask their affiliated hospital(s) to purchase a frameless stereotaxy device. Therefore, caveat emptor, as this purchase will have to service you for years to come. Note that the preoperative scans almost always will be done before admission to the hospital, allowing the facility to amortize the purchase costs of the unit by charging for these studies.

7   A NOTE ON INTRAOPERATIVE IMAGING

The desire to compensate for brain shift and to obtain tumor resection control has led to a strong interest in intraoperative imaging, especially with MRI (discussed elsewhere in this volume). Some of the intraoperative MRI (iMRI) units that are commercially available or under development incorporate frameless stereotaxic technology. In time, they may prove to be preferable to "standalone" units for certain operations, such as low-grade glioma resections or transsphenoidal removal of pituitary macroadenomas. However, it is far too early to suggest that, for the bulk of stereotactic approaches, the added cost and cumbersomeness of iMRI will make frameless stereotaxy obsolete. In fact, for navigation to fixed structures where updated imaging is relatively unimportant, such as parasaggital meningiomas and pituitary microadenomas, frameless stereotaxy will remain the ideal technology for the foreseeable future.

REFERENCES

1.   Roberts DW, Strohbehn JW, Hatch JF, Murray W, Kettenberger H. A frameless stereotaxic integration of computerized tomographic imaging and the operating microscope. J Neurosurg 65:545–549, 1986.
2.   Friets EM, Strohbehn JW, Hatch JF, Roberts DW. A frameless stereotaxic operating microscope for neurosurgery. IEEE Trans Biomed Eng 36:608–617, 1989.
3.   Maciunas RJ, Berger MS, Copeland B, Mayberg M, Selker R, Allen GS. A technique for interactive image-guided neurosurgical intervention in primary brain tumors. In: Maciunas RJ (ed). Neurosurgery Clinics of North America. Philadelphia: W.B. Saunders Company, 1996, pp 245–266.
4.   Drake JM, Joy M, Goldenberg A, Kreindler D. Computer- and robot-assisted resection of thalamic astrocytomas in children. Neurosurgery 29:27–33, 1991.
5.   Watanabe E, Watanabe T, Manaka S, Mayanagi Y, Takakura K. Three-dimensional digitizer (Neuronavigator): New equipment for computed tomography-guided stereotaxic surgery. Surg Neurol 27:543–547, 1987.

6. Watanabe E. The Neuronavigator: A potentiometer-based localization arm system. In: Maciunas RJ (ed). Interactive Image-Guided Neurosurgery. Park Ridge, IL: American Association of Neurological Surgeons, 1993, pp 135–148.

7. Oikarinen J, Alakuijala J, Louhisalmi Y, Sallinen S, Eng F, Helminen H, Koivukangas J. The Oulu neuronavigator system: Intraoperative ultrasonography in the verification of neurosurgical localization and visualization. In: Maciunas RJ (ed). Interactive Image-Guided Neurosurgery. Park Ridge, IL: American Association of Neurological Surgeons, 1993, pp 233–247.

8. Maciunas RJ, Galloway RL, Fitzpatrick JM, Mandara VR, Edwards CE, Allen GS. A universal system for interactive image-directed neurosurgery. Stereotact Funct Neurosurg 58:108–113, 1992.

9. Galloway RL Jr, Edwards CA II, Lewis JT, et al. Image display and surgical visualization in interactive image-guided neurosurgery. Optical Engineering 32: 1955–1962, 1993.

10. Barnett GH, Kormos DW, Steiner CP, Piraino D, Weisenberger J, Hajjar F, Wood C, McNally J. Frameless stereotaxy using a sonic digitizing wand: Development and adaptation to the Picker Vistar medical imaging system. In: Maciunas RJ (ed). Interactive Image-Guided Neurosurgery. Park Ridge, IL: American Association of Neurological Surgeons, 1993, pp 113–120.

11. Bucholz RD, Smith KR. A comparison of sonic digitizers versus light-emitting diode-based localization. In: Maciunas RJ (ed). Interactive Image-Guided Neurosurgery. Park Ridge, IL: American Association of Neurological Surgeons, 1993, pp 179–200.

12. Maciunas RJ, Fitzpatrick JM, Galloway RL, Allen GS. Beyond stereotaxy: Extreme levels of application accuracy are provided by implantable fiducial markers for interactive image-guided neurosurgery. In: Maciunas RJ (ed.). Interactive Image-Guided Neurosurgery. Park Ridge, IL: American Association of Neurological Surgeons, 1993, pp 259–270.

13. Maciunas RJ. Surgical aspects and general management of ganglion cell tumors. In: Apuzzo MLJ (ed). Benign Cerebral Gliomas. Park Ridge, IL: American Association of Neurological Surgeons, 1995, pp 427–444.

14. Heilbrun MP, McDonald P, Wiker C, Keohler S, Peters W. Stereotactic localization and guidance using a machine vision technique. Stereotact Funct Neurosurg 58:94–98, 1992.

15. Roberts DW, Friets EM, Strohbehn JW, Nakajima T. The sonic digitizing microscope. In: Maciunas RJ (ed.). Interactive Image-Guided Neurosurgery. Park Ridge, IL: American Association of Neurological Surgeons, 1993, pp 105–112.

16. Barnett GH, Steiner CP, and Roberts DW. Surgical navigation system technologies. In: Barnett GH, Roberts DW, and Maciunas RJ (eds). Image-Guided Neurosurgery Clinical Applications of Surgical Navigation. St Louis, MO: Quality Medical Publishing, Inc., 1998, pp 17–32.

17. Wohlers TT. 3 D digitizers. Comput Graphics World 15:73–77, 1992.

18. Hill DLG, Maurer CL Jr, Maciunas RJ, Barwise JA, Fitzpatrick JM, Wang MY. Measurement of intraoperative brain surface deformation under a craniotomy. Neurosurgery 43:514–528, 1998.

19. Gomez H, Barnett GH, Estes ML, Palmer J, Magdinee M. Stereotactic and computer-assisted neurosurgery at the Cleveland Clinic. Review of 501 consecutive cases. Cleve Clin Med 60:399–410, 1993.

20. Maciunas RJ, Berger MS, Copeland B, Mayberg MR, Selker R, Allen GS. A technique for interactive image-guided neurosurgical intervention in primary brain tumors. Neurosurg Clin N Am 7:245–266, 1997.

21. Berger MS, Deliganis AV, Dobbins J, Keles GE. The effect of extent of resection on recurrence in patients with low-grade cerebral hemisphere gliomas. Cancer 74:1784–1791, 1994.

22. Galloway RL, Maciunas RJ, Failinger AL. Factors affecting perceived tumor volumes in magnetic resonance imaging. Ann Biomed Eng 21:367–375, 1993.

8

Surgical Navigation with the BrainLAB System

Sagi Harnof and Roberto Spiegelmann

The Chaim Sheba Medical Center, Tel Hashomer, Israel and
The Sackler School of Medicine, Tel Aviv University, Tel Aviv, Israel

1 INTRODUCTION

The need to precisely localize targets within the brain and to refer them to important anatomical structures has occupied neurosurgeons since the early years of intracranial surgery. Craniometry, developed by neuroanatomists in the 19th century, was the first practical method of surgical navigation. It is still being used today as a crude but useful means to correlate the position of superficial brain anatomy with readily identifiable cranial hallmarks. Stereotaxis, first introduced by Horsley and Clarke in 1908 [1], represented the first big leap into deep brain localization. Advances in intracranial imaging and computer science enabled the evolution of stereotaxis, from a method that allowed the precise localization of a point in space in the human brain [2], to the capability of defining the whole contents of the head in a three-dimensional matrix [3–5]. This later development was crucial to intraoperative navigation. Computer reconstruction of images in different planes and three-dimensional rendering gave the neurosurgeon a display of anatomy that helps in the planning of surgical trajectories to deep-seated lesions and with the ability to "see" around the pathology to be treated. During the

65

1980s and early 1990s, several makers of stereotactic equipment developed computerized packages for volumetric stereotaxis in conjunction with stereotactic frames. Any frame reduces the working space available to the surgeon, particularly when the trajectory involves the lateral or posterior aspect of the skull. This limited the appeal of the newer computerized stereotactic systems, leading to the development of new approaches to neuronavigation.

There are two major paradigms for image-assisted neurosurgery: (1) real-time imaging, and (2) preoperative imaging. Real-time imaging is obviously the ideal approach to navigation, as it can correct for perioperative changes in the relative position and bulk of any pathology originated by the surgical procedure itself. Developments in this direction are mostly based on open MRI technology. Currently, these systems have disadvantages that compromise their widespread application: they are costly, require special sets of nonferromagnetic surgical instruments, and severely restrict the space available for optimal patient positioning and the neurosurgeon's freedom to maneuver. Issues of safety resulting from prolonged exposure of medical personnel to radiofrequency energy are still being debated. Preoperative image-based systems have the advantage of relative simplicity, reasonable cost, and the potential for hassle-free handling.

Methods for frameless stereotactic neuronavigation include encoder articulated arms, ultrasonic digitizers, robots, and infrared active or passive flash/camera systems. Their description is beyond the scope of this chapter. All these systems have minor problems in their integration to the regular operative suite environment.

Ideally, a neuronavigational system should allow the surgeon to work transparently, not being distracted by issues of instrument compatibility, detectors' line of vision, etc. An ideal system would recognize immediately any instrument handed to the surgeon, transforming it into a pointing device, so that during its use, the computer display would continue to update its anatomical rendering from the surgeon's point of view. This ideal is yet to be accomplished. The VectorVision system to be described here is a good step toward this goal.

2   THE SYSTEM

BrainLAB VectorVision is an intraoperative, frameless, image-guided navigation system. The system integrates preoperative computed tomographic/magnetic resonance imaging (CT/MRI) digital data, with real-time movement or position of surgical instruments. The navigation is based on reflective markers detected by infrared cameras [6].

The surgeon is able to point targets dynamically selected, in a frameless environment.

2.1   VectorVision Components

The whole system in use at our institution is contained within a trolley that can be easily rolled in and out of the operating room. The trolley contains the cameras, the cameras' controller, and the computer workstation. BrainLAB is now marketing a new version of the system (VectorVision 2). This new version, also based on the principle of easy transportation, has, aside from a sleek design, a touch-screen liquid crystal display that simplifies its use during surgery.

2.1.1   Cameras

Two infrared-emitting cameras are mounted on a holder at a fixed distance of 100 cm from each other (Fig. 1). Infrared detectors are arranged around each camera, so that they act both as source and detector of the infrared light. The angulation of each camera is adjustable, both in the horizontal and vertical planes, so that the position of the trolley can be modified within a certain range (90 to 200 mm).

2.1.2   Computer Workstation

The system is based on an alpha 433 MHz microprocessor (Digital Technologies), running on Windows NT® 4.0 operating system and containing the VectorVision® software. A cameras' controller represents the interface between the cameras and the computer (Fig. 1).

2.1.3   Reflective Markers

Reflective markers are plastic spheres with a glass-grain coating (Fig. 2). They reflect the infrared light emitted by the cameras. The detectors around the cameras read the reflection. These passive-reflective markers, first introduced by BrainLAB for navigation, are an important feature of the system. The lack of cables adds freedom for the surgeon during active navigation. These spheres can be mounted on any surgical instrument on a number of three-arm adapters (Fig. 2) with different geometries, which allow their separate recognition by the system. Thus, several instruments can work as pointers simultaneously. There is a basic pointer (Fig. 2), which is provided with two passive spheres and used for early registration. It may also be used for navigation throughout the procedure. All the reflective markers can be sterilized by gas or plasma. They have a limited lifetime of about ten procedures.

2.1.4   Mayfield Adapter

The Mayfield adapter has two components: a star-shaped tool to which three passive spheres are screwed and a fastener for the Mayfield headrest (Fig.

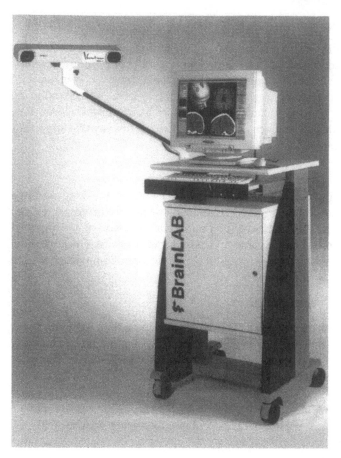

FIGURE 1   The working station.

3). The star-shaped tool locks into the fastener very precisely. This tool is essential for the navigation procedure. It acts as a reference for the system, provided that the patient's head does not move in relation to the Mayfield headrest during surgery. It has a calibration cone in its center, which allows for registration of normal instruments during surgery. The fastener may be applied to the Mayfield headrest under nonsterile conditions. The star-shaped tool may then be sterilely applied to the fastener for primary registration, and removed after registration is accomplished. The patient may be prepped and draped, and then the star-shaped tool reapplied to the fastener.

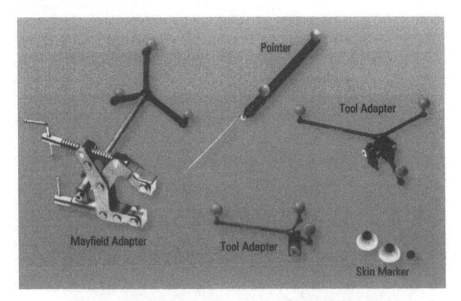

FIGURE 2   Reflective markers, skin markers, and Mayfield adapter.

2.1.5   Skin Markers

For preoperative imaging, skin fiducials are attached with double-sided tape to the patient's head. The fiducials have two components: a cone-shaped plastic, and three different metal markers: spherical for either MRI or CT scanning and hemispherical for registration in the OR (Fig. 2).

2.1.6   Microscope Interconnection

Only the Moller VM 900 microscope (J.D. Moller Optische Werke GmbH, Wedel, Germany) may be actively connected to the VectorVision system. The microscope is fitted with a special adapter containing reflective marker spheres. With this connection, the focus of the microscope is directed automatically to any place pointed to by one of the surgical instruments, freeing the neurosurgeon's hands from this task [7].

3   PREOPERATIVE PROCEDURES

For neuronavigation, the following steps are followed before actual surgery.

3.1   Preoperative Imaging

Preoperative imaging is obtained usually on the evening before surgery. The patient's head is shaved in all places where skin markers are applied. At

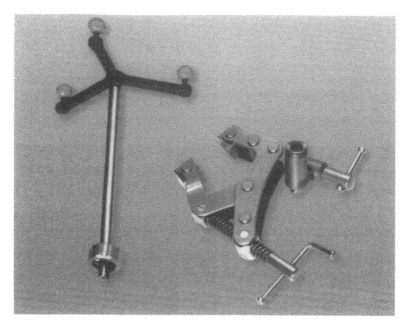

FIGURE 3 Mayfield adapter. The clamp is attached to the Mayfield holder under nonsterile conditions. The star-shaped tool may then be screwed to the clamp with sterile gloves and detached if needed. Accuracy of reattachment is within 0.1 mm.

least three markers should be used, but precision is enhanced with up to five markers. The position of the markers is dictated by several considerations: (1) Position of the lesion/target and the area of the planned skin incision; (2) The planned position of the head relative to the cameras; and (3) The prospective position of the Mayfield pins. Obviously, no skin fiducial should be applied in the area where the Mayfield pins will be applied, as Mayfield fastening (which is done before registration) will substantially displace the skin around the pins. In addition, the headrest itself may interfere with visualization or registration of the fiducials. All the fiducials should be easily seen by the cameras and, consequently, should be clustered on the side of the head that will be uppermost.

3.2 CT or MRI Scans

Scans are obtained, usually with contrast enhancement. A number of constrictions in imaging acquisition should be taken into consideration, as the BrainLAB software cannot recognize or process certain scanning formats.

The scan should be acquired without tilt. For better three-dimensional reconstruction, the slices should be as thin as possible and the scan should comprehend the entire head. The zoom factor should allow all skin markers to be visible. Scan parameters and the patient's head should remain constant during the scan. Slice overlap should be avoided (VectorVision software will not recognize overlapping slices as separate). The matrix should be set to either 256 × 256 or 512 × 512.

It is recommended to place the patient's head on a flat holder (such as the body holder), instead of the round-shaped head holder. This will enhance the usefulness of the three-dimensional view (the usual head holder will obscure the outline of the posterior-lateral aspects of the head in the three-dimensional reconstruction).

Imaging data are then transferred for processing to the VectorVision workstation using digital media or a communication network.

3.3 Preoperative Data Processing

The software provides a variety of options. Either CT, MRI, or both may be processed. An image-fusion module allows the surgeon to use both imaging modalities. In our experience, CT is sufficient for most navigations. The lesion and other areas of interest may be outlined so that they can be seen in 3D reconstruction. For the purpose of intraoperative navigation, the outlines may be switched off, so that true anatomical imaging can be used.

4 THE OPERATING ROOM

4.1 Positioning

There are several ways to organize the operating room. We use the cameras attached to the computer trolley, placing the trolley between the neurosurgeon and the anesthesiologist.

In any position, the trolley should be in the surgeon's visual field, and the cameras about 1 to 2 m from the patient's head. The two cameras can be moved freely as a unit during surgery. The cameras ought to have an unobstructed view of the star-shaped Mayfield adapter. When the operating microscope is to be used, the cameras are positioned as low as possible, so that the microscope will not interfere with their line of view.

4.2 Calibration

Calibration of the cameras can take place any time, although it is desirable to perform it in the final position for surgery. The procedure, which takes only a few seconds, is done with a special tool having two reflective markers.

As the tool is moved in front of the cameras, the software reads several markers' positions and displays the recommended working range.

4.3 Registration

The registration process includes digitizing the skin fiducials and the reference Mayfield headrest markers. This step is done after the Mayfield headrest is fixed to the head. The procedure can be done in a sterile or nonsterile manner (before or after the head is prepped and draped). We prefer the nonsterile method: the sterile star-shaped tool is handled with sterilized gloves, attached to the Mayfield headrest and angulated, so that the three reflective spheres are well within the field of view of both cameras. This is seen in an active window that opens in the computer display when the registration prompt is selected in the software. The skin fiducials are then digitized. The software gives a choice of automatic or manual registration. In the automatic mode, the software auto-detects the placement of each fiducial in the preoperative image and prompts the user to mark them on the patient's head. This is done with a nonsterile pointer. When the pointer touches the fiducial, the software digitizes the position of the spheres in the pointer. A color-coded window in the computer display changes color when the digitization is done. When all the fiducials have been digitized, the computer display becomes active, and an accuracy figure is given (if the accuracy is less than 5 mm, the software will reject the digitization). The whole procedure is completed in less than a minute. From this moment on, neuronavigation is active. Anytime the pointer is brought into the cameras' field of view, the computer display will show reconstructed axial, coronal, and sagittal images of the head centered at the pointer's tip.

The skin fiducials are no longer needed once registration has been completed. After their removal, the patient's head is prepped and draped as usual. The star-shaped tool is left above the drapes.

5 SURGERY

We use the split-screen mode during surgery, displaying coronal and sagittal views, as well as a choice between axial and three-dimensional view (Fig. 4). The three-dimensional view is useful to design the craniotomy flap. The other views are instrumental to navigation once the craniotomy is done. Obviously, changes in the geometry of the brain during surgery reduce the accuracy of the system. Common situations in which this may happen are brain shift after tumor debulking, brain shift after aspiration of cysts, aspiration or drainage of cerebrospinal fluid in hydrocephalic patients, and severe brain swelling/edema during surgery. All these situations may change brain

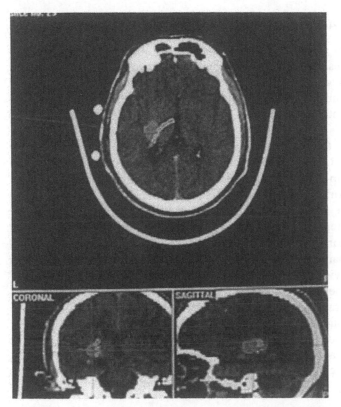

FIGURE 4   A typical display of the VectorVision system, with axial, coronal, and sagittal reconstructions during surgery, while the pointer is being introduced through a sylvian fissure approach to the target, a left basal ganglia cavernoma. The position of the internal capsule has been outlined. Surgery was done with the patient fully conscious.

configuration and make the system unreliable. We usually abort navigation under those circumstances. More unusual reasons for navigational failures are movement of the patient's head relative to the star-shaped tool and electric power shutdown during surgery. In the first situation, which takes place when the head falls from the Mayfield headrest, navigation needs to be aborted, unless another patient's head-contained reference system has been previously digitized [8]. In the event of an electric power shutdown, the system has an option named "recover" that can allow continuation of the procedure.

6 SURGICAL APPLICATIONS

The VectorVision system is accurate enough for almost all surgical localization procedures. We have not encountered a single case in which the
navigation failed to point to the target. The system advantages are the rapid
setup requiring only a few extra minutes in any procedure, the easy handling of the pointer tools devoid of cables, and well-designed software
tools.

   The pointer tool can be used to plan the skin incision and the bone
flap, and then to identify relevant anatomical structures. During tumor resection, it can help define tumor borders. Cavernous angiomas or small arteriovenous malformations deep in the brain are excellent cases for neuronavigation. With its three-dimensional and three-planar rendering, the
VectorVision system is of great help in designing and maintaining the best
approach to the target.

   Attached markers can be used to guide catheter into ventricles. In this
situation, it is advisable to use the transfrontal route. When using the trans-
occipital route, the markers attached to the far end of the catheter can fall
beyond the cameras' field of view.

   We have found neuronavigation ideally suited to assess the progress
of surgery when dealing with large skull-base meningiomas. Because the
remaining tumor attachment does not change its geometry during surgery,
the pointing tool can show the exact position of the surgeon's instruments
at any stage.

7 CONCLUSION

Neuronavigational systems such as VectorVision modestly increase the cost
and planning time of neurosurgical procedures by requiring additional imaging and hardware/software setups. They also require some time investment
in learning to deal with a computerized system. Nonetheless, the added
capabilities are worthwhile. The surgical procedure itself is better tailored
to the pathology: smaller skin incisions and craniotomy flaps result in less
postsurgical patient discomfort. This, in turn, may result in shorter hospi-
talization time. The surgeon enhances his/her confidence when dealing with
deep-seated intra-axial lesions, or large extra-axial tumors. There is no major
change in the immediate operative environment and no bulky added hardware compromising the surgeon's freedom.

   The VectorVision system also has a spinal module useful in the
planning and execution of fusion instrumentation, such as transpedicular
screw placing and plating. Its discussion is beyond the scope of this
article.

REFERENCES

1. Horsley V, Clarke RH. The structure and the function of the cerebellum examined by a new method. Brain 31:45–124, 1908
2. Spiegel EA, Wycis HT, Marks M, Lee AJ. Stereotaxic apparatus for operations on the human brain. Science 106:349–350, 1947.
3. Kelly PJ. Computer assisted stereotaxis: A new approach for the management of intracranial intra-axial tumors. Neurology 36:535–541, 1986.
4. Kelly PJ. Volumetric stereotactic surgical resection in intra-axial brain mass lesions. Mayo Clin Proc 63:1186–1198, 1988.
5. Kelly PJ, Alker GJ Jr, Goerss S. Computer-assisted stereotactic microsurgery for the treatment of intracranial neoplasms. Neurosurgery 10:324–331, 1982.
6. BrainLAB. User Manual. BrainLAB GmbH. Germany, 1996–1997.
7. Gumprecht HK, Lumenta CB. The operating microscope guided by a neuronavigation system: A technical note. Minim Invasive Neurosurg 41(3):141–143, 1998.
8. Gumprecht HK, Widenka DC, Lumenta CB. BrainLAB VectorVision Neuronavigation System: Technology and clinical experiences in 131 cases. Neurosurgery 44:97–105, 1999.

9

Surgical Navigation with the Voyager System

Gene H. Barnett

Brain Tumor Institute, The Cleveland Clinic, Cleveland, Ohio, U.S.A.

1 INTRODUCTION

Our early interest in development of a surgical navigation system arose from our background in computer-assisted frame stereotaxy [1,2] and the early development of "frameless stereotaxy" devices by Roberts et al. [3,4] and Watanabee et al. [5]. Roberts' group had devised a stereotactic surgical microscope using a sonic three-dimensional digitizer to locate the optical axis and focal point of the microscope in space. Because of the great uncertainty of each acquisition of the sonic digitizer, a stationary platform, such as the microscope, allowed for multiple acquisitions that would average out the "noise" and lead to acceptable accuracy. On the other hand, the Watanabees used a mechanical arm with analogue position sensors in the joints as the input device. This allowed for hand-held navigation, but constrained the user's freedom by the mechanical linkage.

   Don Kormos, Charles Steiner, and I set out to create a hand-held "wand" that did not require linkage but used sonic digitization as used by Roberts. Through painstaking experiments, we discerned that by placing the detectors (microphones) within a meter of the emitters (spark gaps) on the

77

wand and using an internal speed of sound reference (to compensate for temperature, humidity, etc.) we had a flexible, highly accurate digitizer suitable for use in the operating room [6–8]. Teaming up with Picker International (Highland Heights, Ohio), we developed the system into a Food and Drug Administration (FDA)-approved product (ViewPoint™) that was the first in North America to introduce wand-oriented views (i.e., orthogonal planes oriented to the axis of the pointing device), a visual method of target and trajectory guidance [9], and FDA approval for brain biopsy [10]. Ian Kalfas made important contributions that led to the system also being approved for spinal navigation [11], with *or without* spinal tracking. The system has proved versatile [12,13], cost effective [14], and useful for surgery of intra-axial tumors [15–20], meningiomas [19,21–23], sellar tumors [24], neuroendoscopy [25,26], brain biopsy [27], and related procedures [28].

Ultimately, the sonic digitizer was replaced by an active/passive infrared wand detected by a dual CCD camera; multiple and universal tools were developed; Picker International became Marconi Medical Systems, Inc. (Highland Heights, Ohio); and ViewPoint was renamed "Voyager." Today the Voyager system (Fig. 1) retains the ease of use that was the hallmark of the ViewPoint system but extends its versatility with multimodality navigation (i.e., image fusion), a more versatile display, and a more sophisticated platform.

2   SYSTEM SETUP

Voyager is composed of the dual CCD camera stand, the equipment rack with integrated flat panel light-emitting diode (LED) display and an (optional) outboard flat panel liquid crystal display (LCD) [7]. The camera stand houses a dual CCD infrared camera (Northern Digital Inc.) along with infrared emitters that allow for use of passive tools. The cameras may be oriented either horizontally or vertically, the latter allowing for a narrower line-of-sight corridor between the pointing devices and camera. Unlike some surgical navigation systems, Voyager allows for the camera to be plugged into the equipment rack after the computer has been "booted" up, without damaging the camera. The camera is currently filtered to allow it to operate in the presence of most commercial operating room and head lights.

The new equipment rack houses the system computer, uninterruptable power supply, camera adapter, keyboard, mouse, and the main flat panel display. System connections are also made here, including ethernet, camera, foot pedals, and cabling for active LEDs. Atop the rack is an extension arm that allows the display to be positioned close to the surgeon while keeping the rack out of the way. A working display on the rack allows the sophisticated software functions (beyond those performed with the foot pedals) to

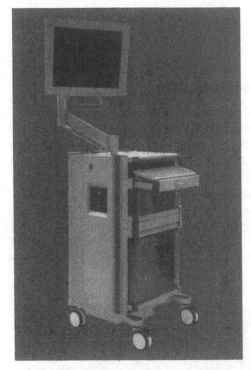

FIGURE 1 Voyager system composed of dual CCD camera, equipment rack with extendable flat panel liquid crystal display (LCD), and outboard flat panel LCD display.

be operated by someone else without moving the surgeon's display. As always, safety is paramount and the uninterruptable power supply serves to electrically isolate the system and maintain function, even in the event of external power loss. Even if the computer loses power, however, all registration information is retained and the surgery may proceed forward seamlessly.

3 SYSTEM USE

3.1 Image Loading

The initial step using the Voyager system is to load the patient's images. This is typically done over an ethernet system loading DICOM-compatible image files. The operator chooses whether one or more image sets is to be loaded and identifies them; the images are then imported (Fig. 2). If the images were previously loaded into Voyager, the patient file may be loaded instead of the raw image data.

3.2 Multimodality Correlation (Fusion)

When one or more image datasets are loaded, they must be correlated. Voyager allows for manual or automated fusion of data sets. The author prefers manual fusion, as it is fast, accurate, and totally under his control. Briefly, a 3 × 3 (or, optionally, a 2 × 2) workspace is presented in which one column represents image set 1; the second, image set 2; and the third is where the fusion is performed and displayed (Fig. 3). A useful technique is to assign the second dataset a color profile while the first set is left as a grayscale. Images may be magnified ("zoom") to facilitate the process. Images are then translated to roughly center the ventricular system, then rotated to align the ventricles and brainstem. This process is performed iteratively

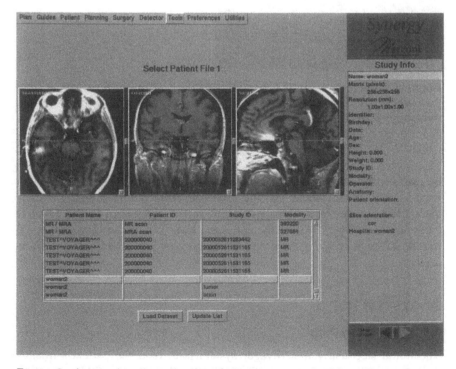

FIGURE 2 Image loading display of Voyager system. More than one type of image set may be imported for navigation.

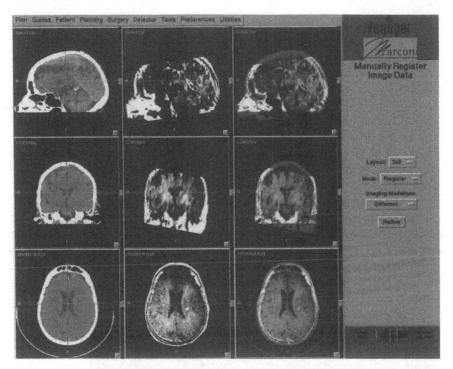

FIGURE 3 Multimodality correlation screen (fusion). Left column represents dataset 1, middle is dataset 2, and right is where fusion is performed and visualized.

until the desired result is obtained, usually in a few minutes or less. If the area of interest is remote from the ventricles, the surgeon may focus on that area, to locally refine the fusion, but this is rarely necessary.

3.3   Imaging and Registration

Voyager uses paired points to provide registration. For cranial use, these may be anatomical landmarks, applied scalp fiducials, or implanted "Accustar" skull fiducials. The latter routinely results in submillimetric registration accuracy. Fiducials and image acquisition may be performed from the day of surgery to weeks earlier. Fiducials are typically placed in a stereotypical array that are widely spaced about the patient's head, as this minimizes navigation error, not just registration error.

Thin slice (1–2 mm) computed tomogram (CT) or volume acquisition magnetic resonance imaging (MRI) (e.g., Siemens MPR) are preferred but may be augmented with other image data using the fusion process (above), such as nuclear medicine, other magnetic resonance imaging (MRI), MR angiography (MRA), magnetic resonance ventilation (MRV), fMRI, and medical radiation sciences (MRS). As such, if fiducials are used, only one of the image methods need visualize the fiducials. Imaging from spinal surgery typically is performed using thin slice CT.

Cranial surgery using Voyager should be performed using head tracking as provided by a dynamic reference frame (DRF). This allows the patient's head to be followed if it moves with respect to the camera, or vice versa. We routinely affix the DRF to a Mayfield head clamp that has been secured to the patient's head in such a way as to avoid displacing scalp fiducials. Ordinarily, the Mayfield is then secured to the operating room table to provide good surgical access while providing adequate cranial venous drainage and spinal alignment. The DRF may be secured to the body of the Mayfield or, uniquely, to a modified "C-arm" of the device, as the latter is least likely to move with respect to the patient's head during a case (Fig. 4). The DRF is positioned such that it is out of the surgeon's way, maintains

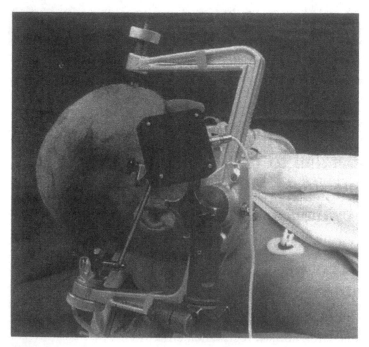

FIGURE 4   Optional fixation of dynamic reference display (DRF) to modified C-arm of Mayfield head fixation device minimizes fidelity of head tracking, as head may pivot with respect to main part of Mayfield device.

good line-of-sight with the camera, and will not be subject to undue traction by draping. Awake craniotomy is performed using the same setup, except that the Mayfield is applied using local anesthesia (Fig. 5), and the Mayfield clamp is NOT secured to the table, thereby allowing the limited freedom to move while maintaining accurate tracking using the DRF (Fig. 5). An unusual feature of Voyager is that it allows spinal surgery to be performed with *or without* use of a spinal DRF.

After creation of a registration set, the anatomical or scalp fiducials are defined. This is facilitated by visualizing the three-dimensional surface representation of the head and clicking on its surface near the point of interest. The actual location of the point is refined through use of the triplanar display and stored. The process is repeated for the remaining reference points. Each point is then touched with one of the wands [active infrared (IRED) or passive]. Fiducials that cannot be accessed or have been displaced can be inactivated. Spinal registration uses segmental (i.e., each vertebra) anatomical fiducials in a similar process, often using the tips of the spinal and transverse processes. Multiple registration sets may be created, including intraoperative sets that may be used for re-registration.

Registration error is typically less than 2 mm or 3 mm and submillimetric when using the Accustar fiducials. Larger errors may be reduced by

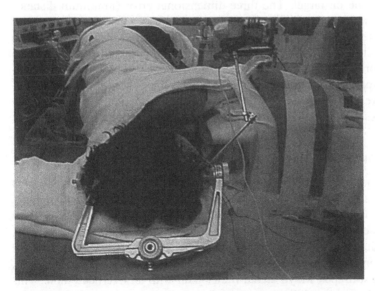

FIGURE 5 Setup for awake craniotomy. Mayfield clamp is not secured to the table allowing some head movement during surgery while tracking is maintained.

using the "Pin Point" function that tracks registration error as the user adjusts the position of the wand on the fiducial. Registration should always be checked by activating the system and ensuring that fiducials and anatomy are accurately localized.

3.4 Target and Trajectory Guidance

Voyager (then ViewPoint) was the first of the commercial surgical navigation systems to incorporate an intuitive, graphical means of target and trajectory guidance [9]. This was facilitated by its ability to display images oriented to the pointing device (e.g., wand). A target (with optional entry) point is defined by clicking on a point in the image and storing it as either a target or trajectory. If an entry point is also selected, the trajectory may then be previewed with two views, one showing the path of trajectory as it passes through the tissue and the other showing a plane perpendicular to the axis of the trajectory (Fig. 6). The depth of this plane is user selectable.

The method by which this technology is used to guide the surgeon has been previously described [9]. Briefly, when using target guidance alone, the one plane that is perpendicular to the pointing device (e.g., wand) *and* that also contains the target point (presented as a colored circle) is displayed. The projection of the wand is displayed as a different colored circle. One need only adjust the direction of the wand such that the two circles are concentric to be on target. The three-dimensional error (minimum distance between the trajectory and the target) is continuously presented. The course of the trajectory may be visualized on the two displayed planes that contain the wand. When a trajectory has been created, the perpendicular plane also shows the projection of the entry point, but more importantly, the wand-oriented displays and the three-dimensional display show the planned trajectory as well as actual axis of the wand. A few maneuvers are all that are usually necessary to make the wand align with the planned trajectory.

3.5 Intraoperative Use

The patient is draped in a conventional manner except that the DRF must have line of sight with the camera. We usually perforate the drape and apply a sterile, clear plastic bag over it. Care must be taken that the draping does not apply traction to the DRF during the case, even when the drapes become laden with fluid and blood, and that the DRF will not be struck by equipment or an assistant. The author prefers the scrub table to be placed to his right, mediated by a draped Mayo stand, rather than with an overhead table. This allows for placement of the camera at the patient's feet and out of the way of other equipment.

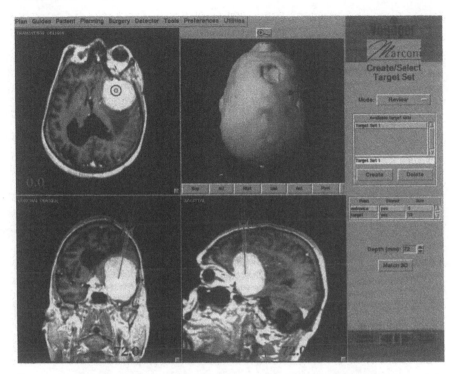

FIGURE 6 Display for target and trajectory guidance. **Top left** screen is plane containing target point and perpendicular to pointing device. **Bottom** row shows planes containing pointing device and projection of planned trajectory. **Top right** shows surface representation of the head with planned and actual trajectory. This system facilitates brain biopsy and related procedures.

If active wands are used, they are coupled to the navigation system. Passive wands are identified and then may be used. Universal adapters may be applied to instruments, (drills, probes, etc.), calibrated, then used. Many operating microscopes are used, but image injection is not supported.

Two general displays are used, irrespective of whether the case is cranial or spinal. The first is a presentation of axial, coronal, sagittal and three-dimensional surface images (Fig. 7). The cross-hairs show the position of the tip with respect to the anatomy. The system may be set to run continuously, or intermittently (such as when stepping on the foot pedal). The oblique display (Fig. 8) presents images that are steered by the pointing device—two contain the axis of the pointer, the other is the plane perpendicular to the tip of the wand. This depth may be adjusted up or down by

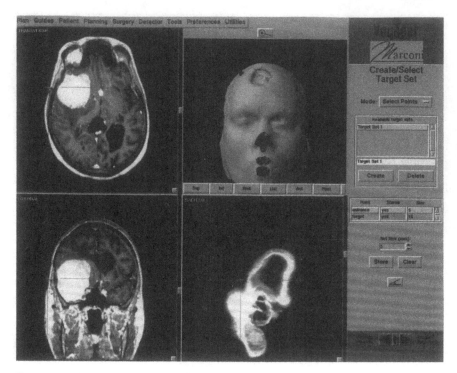

FIGURE 7   Typical triplanar display showing axial, coronal, and sagittal planes. This display provides localization function.

the foot pedal or be fixed at the depth of the target (if saved). The true and virtual positions of the tip are represented on the views that contain the wands. Navigation is then a straightforward process. Warnings are given if the wand, DRF, or both are out of view of the camera.

3.6   User Interface

The user interface may be customized so as to suit the different needs of multiple surgeons. The colors, dimensions, and transparency of various items may be individually selected and saved. For instance, a surgeon performing predominantly spine surgery using CT may elect to use red for the wand (i.e., virtual screw) for best visualization, whereas an intracranial surgeon using MRI may prefer yellow to represent the wand.

Each panel has independent adjustments for the display attributes of the various image datasets in use, or they may be applied to all displayed planes. The attributes are "remembered" when switching between different

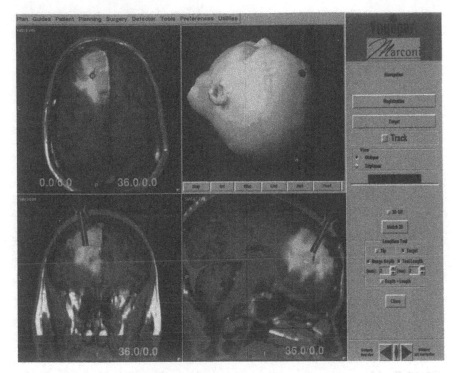

FIGURE 8 Typical oblique display where wand or pointing device "steers" the display. **Bottom** row shows two (orthogonal) planes including axis of wand. **Top left** shows a plane perpendicular to axis of pointer. **Top right** shows three-dimensional representation of head with projection of wand out of surface.

functions of the system. Each dataset may be individually windowed, leveled, and colorized within a panel (Fig. 9). The zoom function for that panel applies to all image sets displayed in that panel. Unlike some systems in which use of fused datasets may only be manipulated or used during planning, Voyager allows the relative contribution of the image data sets to be adjusted for better anatomical, physiological, or metabolic visualization during navigation.

4 SUMMARY

The Voyager navigation system is the product of evolutionary development that provides simple, yet flexible and powerful navigation in the head and

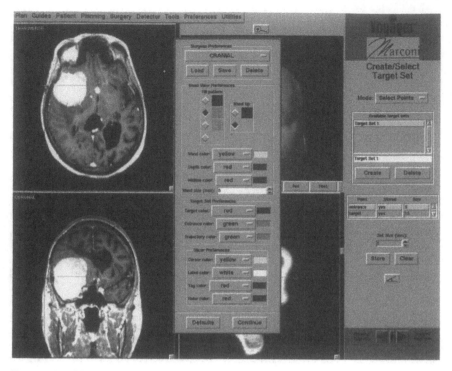

FIGURE 9   Many screen parameters may be adjusted for individual windows or the entire workspace. Colors and transparency of overlays may be stored as user preferences.

spine. The system and its creators have contributed several firsts to the field of surgical navigation and will continue to do so.

Acknowledgments

The authors acknowledge financial and research support from, as well as consulting agreements with, Marconi Medical Systems and DePuy Acromed.

REFERENCES

1. Barnett GH, McKenzie RL, Ramos L, Palmer J. Nonvolumetric stereotaxy-assisted craniotomy. Results in 50 consecutive cases. J Stereotact Funct Neurosurg 61:80–95, 1993.
2. Gomez H, Barnett GH, Estes ML, Palmer J, Magdinec M. Stereotactic and computer-assisted neurosurgery at the Cleveland Clinic. Review of 501 consecutive cases. Cleve Clin J Med 60:399–410, 1993.

3. Friets EM, Strohbehn JW, Hatch JF, Roberts DW. A frameless stereotaxic operating microscope for neurosurgery. IEEE Trans Biomed Eng 36:608–617, 1989.
4. Roberts DW, Strohbehn JW, Hatch JF, Murray W, Kettenberger H. A frameless stereotaxic integration of computerized tomographic imaging and the operating microscope. J Neurosurg 65:545–549, 1986.
5. Watanabe E, Watanabe T, Manaka S, Mayanagi Y, Takakura K. Three-dimensional digitizer (neuronavigator): New equipment for computed tomography-guided stereotaxic surgery. Surg Neurol 27:543–547, 1987.
6. Barnett GH, Kormos DW, Steiner CP, Weisenberger J. Intraoperative localization using an armless, frameless stereotactic wand. Technical Note. J Neurosurg 78:510–514, 1993.
7. Barnett GH, Steiner CP, Roberts DW. Surgical navigation system technologies. In: Barnett GH, Roberts DW, Maciunas RJ (eds.). Image-Guided Neurosurgery. Clinical Applications of Surgical Navigation. St. Louis, Missouri: Quality Medical Publishing, Inc., 1998.
8. Barnett GH, Steiner CP. Image-guided neurosurgery using sonic digitizers. In: Gildenberg PL, Tasker RR (eds.). Textbook of Stereotactic and Functional Neurosurgery. New York, New York: McGraw-Hill, 209–214, 1998.
9. Barnett GH, Steiner CP, Weisenberger J. Target and trajectory guidance for interactive surgical navigation systems. Stereotact Funct Neurosurg 66:91–95, 1996.
10. Barnett GH, Kormos DW, Steiner CP, Piraino D, Weisenberger J, Hajjar F, Wood C, McNally J. Frameless stereotaxy using a sonic digitizing wand: Development and adaptation to the Picker ViStar Medical Imaging System. In: Interactive Image Guided Neurosurgery. Neurosurgical Topics Series, AANS Publications, Park Ridge, Illinois, 17(10):113–119, 1993.
11. Kalfas IH, Kormos DW, Murphy MA, McKenzie RL, Barnett GH, Bell GR, Steiner CP, Trimble MB, Weisenberger JP. Application of frameless stereotaxy to pedicle screw fixation of the spine. J Neurosurg 83(4):641–647, 1995.
12. Barnett GH. Intracranial applications of surgical navigation systems. Perspect Neurol Surg 9(2):65–82, 1999.
13. Barnett GH. Stereotactic techniques in the management of brain tumors. Contemp Neurosurg 14(5):1–6, 1992.
14. Bingaman WE, Barnett GH. Social and economic impact of surgical navigation systems. In: Barnett GH, Roberts DW, Maciunas RJ (eds.). Clinical Applications of Surgical Navigation. Image Guided Neurosurgery. St. Louis, Missouri: Quality Medical Publishing, Inc., 1998.
15. Barnett GH, Kormos DW, Steiner CP, Weisenberger J. Use of a frameless, armless stereotactic wand for brain tumor localization with two-dimensional and three-dimensional neuroimaging. Neurosurgery 33:674–678, 1993.
16. Barnett GH, Walsh JG, Steiner CP, Weisenberger JP. One-year outcome data after resection of malignant glioma. In: Barnett GH, Roberts DW, Maciunas RJ (eds.). Image-Guided Neurosurgery. Clinical Applications of Surgical Navigation. St. Louis, Missouri: Quality Medical Publishing, Inc., 1998.

17. Barnett GH. Definition of functional anatomy. In: Barnett GH, Roberts DW, Maciunas RJ (eds.). Image-Guided Neurosurgery. Clinical Applications of Surgical Navigation. St. Louis, Missouri: Quality Medical Publishing, Inc., 1998.

18. Barnett GH. Minimal access craniotomy. In: Barnett GH, Roberts DW, Maciunas RJ (eds.). Image-Guided Neurosurgery. Clinical Applications of Surgical Navigation. St. Louis, Missouri: Quality Medical Publishing, Inc., 1998.

19. Barnett GH. Stereotactic craniotomy for excision of intracranial lesions. Atlas and Fascicles, Rengachary and Wilkins (eds.), 1997, in press.

20. Murphy MA, Barnett GH, Kormos DW, Weisenberger J. Astrocytoma resection using an interactive frameless stereotactic wand. An early experience. J Clin Neurosci 1:33–37, 1994.

21. Barnett GH, Kaakaji W. Intracranial meningiomas. In: Barnett GH, Roberts DW, Maciunas RJ (eds.). Image-Guided Neurosurgery. Clinical Applications of Surgical Navigation. St. Louis, Missouri: Quality Medical Publishing, Inc., 1998.

22. Barnett GH, Steiner CP, Kormos DW, Weisenberger J. Intracranial meningioma resection using interactive frameless stereotaxy-assistance. J Image Guid Surg 1:46–52, 1995.

23. Barnett GH. Surgical management of convexity and falcine meningiomas using interactive image-guided surgery systems. Neurosurg Clin N Am 7:279–284, 1996.

24. Barnett GH. Transsphenoidal hypophysectomy. In: Barnett GH, Roberts DW, Maciunas RJ, (eds.). Image-Guided Neurosurgery. Clinical Applications of Surgical Navigation. St. Louis, Missouri: Quality Medical Publishing, Inc., 1998.

25. Luciano MG, Rhoten RLP, Barnett GH. Hydrocephalus. In: Barnett GH, Roberts DW, Maciunas RJ (eds.). Image-Guided Neurosurgery. Clinical Applications of Surgical Navigation. St. Louis, Missouri: Quality Medical Publishing, Inc., 1998.

26. Rhoten RL, Luciano MG, Barnett GH. Computer-assisted endoscopy for neurosurgical procedures: Technical note. Neurosurgery 40(3):632–7, discussion, 638, 1997.

27. Barnett GH, Miller DW, Weisenberger J. Brain biopsy using frameless stereotaxy with scalp applied fiducials: Experience in 218 cases. J Neurosurg 91: 569–576, 1999.

28. Barnett GH, Miller DW. Brain biopsy and related procedures. In: Barnett GH, Roberts DW, Maciunas RJ (eds.). Image-Guided Neurosurgery. Clinical Applications of Surgical Navigation. St. Louis, Missouri: Quality Medical Publishing, Inc., 1998.

10

Surgical Navigation with the OMI System

William D. Tobler
University of Cincinnati and Mayfield Clinic and Spine Institute, Cincinnati, Ohio, U.S.A.

1 INTRODUCTION

Over the past decade, image-guided surgery has become one of the most exciting new technologies for the neurosurgeon. Advances in techniques and instrumentation have been rapid [1–9]. The Mayfield® ACCISS™ image-guided stereotactic workstation (OMI system) has been developed to meet the image-guided needs of the most demanding surgeons (Fig. 1). With the Mayfield ACCISS, the surgeon can perform stereotactic-guided craniotomies, transphenoidal and other ears, nose, throat (ENT)/skull-base procedures. The Mayfield ACCISS has the most rigid stereotactic platform in the image-guided field. The experienced stereotactic neurosurgeon can confidently use the Mayfield ACCISS for stereotactic procedures, eliminating the need for a traditional frame. Lastly, the requirements for spinal applications can be easily satisfied with this system.

This chapter describes the system and its components, fiducial placement, image acquisition, and surgical planning. It also defines its use in the operating room. The author also describes his surgical experience and recommendations for applications of the Mayfield ACCISS system and its unique components.

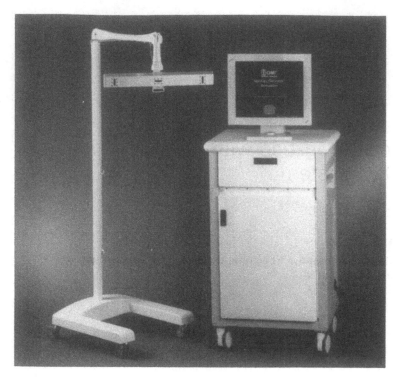

FIGURE 1   The Mayfield ACCISS system. Custom computer cart and infrared camera for optical tracking.

1.1   Description of the Mayfield ACCISS

The Mayfield ACCISS uses the Windows NT™ operating system, which provides the surgeon surprisingly fast and powerful computing capacity in a familiar and easy-to-use format. Placed in a customized cart, the system is positioned at the hand of the surgeon in the operating room. Its simple and user-friendly format eliminates the need and expense of a dedicated technician to run the system during surgery.

The Mayfield ACCISS is unique in the image-guided field because it uses both the commonly known optical tracking technology and the only small, light-weight (13.5 ounces) mechanical arm in the industry (Fig. 2). Unlike its cumbersome predecessors, the Mayfield ACCISS arm is easy to use. It has rigidity and stability, and eliminates the need for the infrared camera with floor stand and the dynamic reference frame (DRF) required with the more commonly used optical tracking systems.

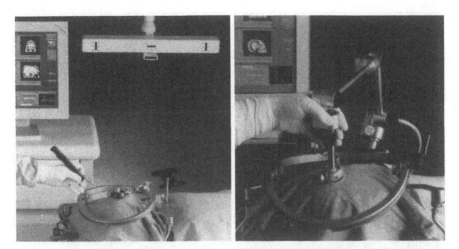

FIGURE 2 The Mayfield ACCISS dual digitizing system. **Left,** wireless active optical tracking systems with infrared camera. **Right,** mechanical arm system with the tip of the mechanical arm in the AccuPoint sphere for stereotactic targeting.

An active optical tracking system is a standard component of the Mayfield ACCISS. The power cable to the optical probes has been replaced by a disposable battery. The wireless custom probe comes with an adaptor that allows the interchange of multiple instruments, such as pointers and suction devices.

The AccuPoint™ sphere is a ball-and-socket device that can be used for generation and rigid fixation of a stereotactic trajectory (Fig. 3). It can be placed anywhere over the cranium for access to any stereotactic target. It is designed to be close to the entry point, which minimizes the length the probe must pass to reach its intended target.

The Mayfield ACCISS uses the Budde Halo™ retractor system for attachment of the mechanical arm, the optical tracking components, and the AccuPoint stereotactic device for cranial applications. These components can be placed anywhere around the 360° circumference of the halo to suit the needs and convenience of the surgeon (Figs. 2 and 3). Alternatively these components can be used without the halo retractor system.

2 FIDUCIAL PLACEMENT, IMAGE ACQUISITION, AND SURGICAL PLANNING

Adhesive fiducial markers are used almost exclusively, although implantable markers are commercially available. Anatomical landmarks can be used for

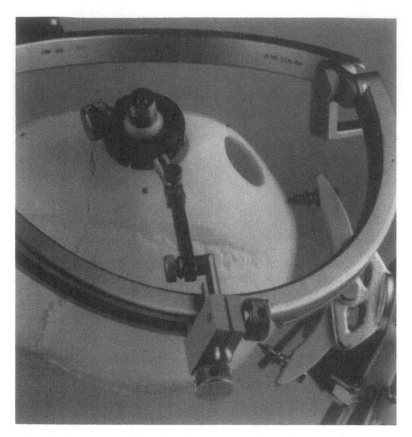

FIGURE 3 The stereotactic platform for the Mayfield ACCISS. It includes the rigid AccuPoint sphere which is attached to the Budde Halo retractor system.

ENT and spinal applications but are not recommended for cranial applications. Adhesive fiducials for cranial procedures can be applied by a technician, and the scan can be performed up to 7 days before the procedure, although no more than 2 to 3 days beforehand is recommended. The fiducial markers are placed around the area of interest and prepped into the surgical field so they can be easily accessed during the procedure to re-register or recheck the accuracy of registration. The software program finds the best fit between the location of the fiducials in patient space and the location of the fiducials on the image dataset and compensates to some degree for movement of an individual fiducial marker. Any fiducial marker identified with a large registration error can be easily eliminated from the registration process.

For this reason, five to seven fiducial markers are recommended for placement for every procedure. This technique has led to satisfactory or very good registration in nearly all cases including stereotactic procedures.

Computed tomography (CT) and magnetic resonance imaging (MRI) are the usual modalities for most surgical procedures. Standard formatting for CT requires image-acquisition with 3-mm contiguous slices and a 0° gantry tilt, although in certain cases 1.5-mm cuts may be desirable to improve accuracy. Volumetric MRI scans with contrast are usually performed for most tumors. Computed tomography is the usual modality used for spinal applications, because MRI poorly visualizes bone anatomy. Once acquired, these images can be downloaded to digital audio type (DAT) or directly transferred by ethernet to the workstation.

The Mayfield ACCISS uniquely coregisters images, which permits the surgeon to simultaneously navigate with a CT and MRI image (Fig. 4). This is especially advantageous in pituitary surgery, where identification of bone surfaces and tumor margins is important. Coregistration permits the measurement of postoperative stereotactic biopsy accuracy in a way never before possible (Fig. 5).

The virtual screw program is a useful adjunct for preplanning pedicle screw placement. One can measure and place the screws in a simulation of the surgical procedure. The workstation can store up to eight screws on a dataset.

2.1 Use of the Mayfield ACCISS in Surgery

With the Mayfield ACCISS system, the surgeon can choose to use either the mechanical arm or optical tracking system, depending on individual preferences. The mechanical arm system is ideal and the preferred digitizer for long procedures where the microscope is used. The presence of the microscope, assistant, scrub nurse, operating tables, and anesthesia setup creates a crowded space at the operating table and usually makes placement of the infrared camera and maintenance of unobstructed optical pathways throughout the duration of the procedure difficult. In this crowded environment, frequent disruption of optically tracked instruments occurs and occasionally the microscope has to be moved out of position in order to track the instrument. In this setting the mechanical arm functions in a superior fashion to the optical system completely eliminating this often frustrating problem.

The mechanical arm system is also preferred by the author for stereotactic procedures because of its greater stability and ability to provide along-the-probe views which display the trajectory to the lesion. By rotating the probe tip of the mechanical arm after it has been positioned into the rigidly

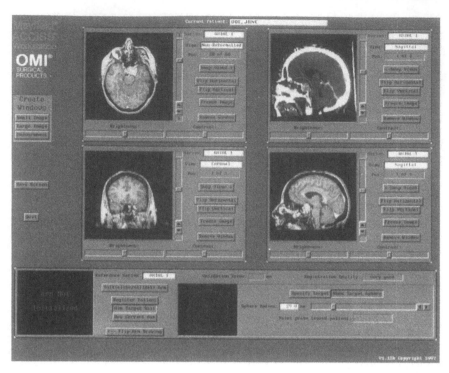

FIGURE 4 Coregistration of images for transphenoidal surgery allows one to navigate simultaneously on axial, coronal, and sagittal magnetic resonance imaging (MRI) and sagittal computed tomographic (CT) images. Any combination of images is possible. Note sagittal CT image **upper right** and its precise correlations with the sagittal image.

fixed AccuPoint sphere the along-the-probe view plane can be rotated and viewed at the workstation 360 degrees around the axis of the intended trajectory (Figs. 2 and 6). This provides the surgeon with the most complete anatomical understanding of the intended trajectory. This complete rotation through the 360° axis cannot be done with optical tracking technology. The AccuPoint sphere provides a rigid method for stereotactic targeting and is brought close to the target, which minimizes the potential for deflection of the probe and introduction of stereotactic error. Either the mechanical arm or the optical probe can be placed into the AccuPoint sphere for trajectory generation.

The Mayfield ACCISS can be adapted to the microscope. With the microscope as a pointer, it is used initially to locate the cranial flap and plan

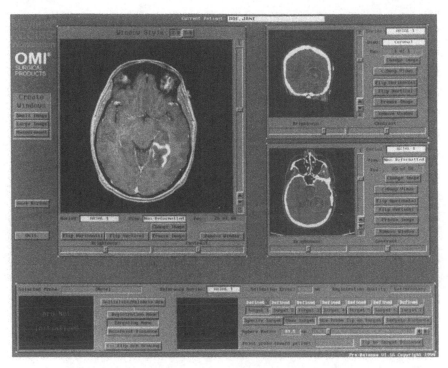

FIGURE 5 Sterostatic biopsy with postoperative coregistration. Small hemorrhage at biopsy site on postoperative computed tomographic (CT) coronal and axial view on right correlates with preoperative axial magnetic resonance imaging (MRI) image on **left**.

a trajectory to the lesion. As soon as the surgeon desires to use an instrument as pointer, the microscope ceases to function as a tracked instrument.

The optical tracking system is best used in cranial procedures in which the microscope is used in a limited capacity or not at all. It can also be used for stereotactic procedures. The optical tracking system is preferred for spinal procedures. The elimination of the wire to the optical probes has provided an additional degree of freedom while maintaining the high level of accuracy associated with active optical tracking systems.

The Mayfield ACCISS system has a distinct advantage imparted by its dual digitizing capabilities. If there is a failure at any time of the optical system because of malfunction of light-emitting diodes (LEDs), contamination of optical components that should not be autoclaved, or other technical problems, the mechanical arm can be activated in a short couple of

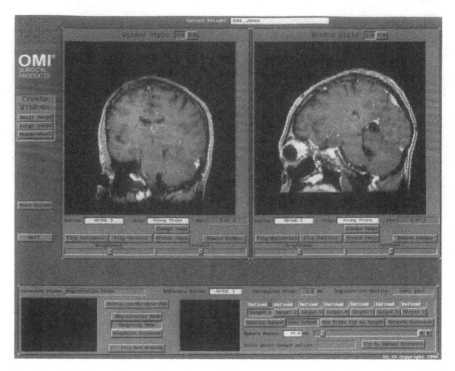

FIGURE 6 Along-the-probe views. One can rotate the view plane 360° around the axis of the probe (*solid yellow line*). Two such views are shown that provide the surgeon a clear picture of the trajectory to the lesion, which was a moderate grade thalamic glioma.

minutes. It requires a standard endoscope drape, and all its components, including pointer tips, can be autoclaved.

In addition, the availability of both tracking methods facilitates performing three or four image-guided procedures in the same day.

2.2 Surgical Experience with the Mayfield ACCISS System

Since its introduction in late 1994, the author has used the Mayfield ACCISS in approximately 300 image-guided assisted procedures (Table 1). A wide variety of applications has shown its versatility and dependability for the full gamut of image-guided neurosurgery with little if any time added to the procedure.

TABLE 1 Image-Guided Experience with the Mayfield ACCISS System

Craniotomy	
Metastases	57
Primary tumors	53
Extra-Axial tumors	34
Transphenoidal	8
Vascular lesions	8
Sterotaxis	
Tumor biopsy	67
Hematoma aspiration	16
Abscess aspiration	8
Catheter placement for shunt/cyst	10
Spine surgery	
Pedical screws	30
Miscellaneous	1
Total Cases	292

Resection of metastatic lesions can be accomplished efficiently and safely with image-guided surgery. A report of the first 41 patients operated on using the Mayfield ACCISS system showed an average time for the procedure of under 2 hours with minimal morbidity [10].

The Mayfield ACCISS for transphenoidal surgery eliminates the need for fluoroscopy. One can track the probe in the axial and coronal views as well as the sagittal view (Fig. 4). Even with the traditional use of fluoroscopy, one often struggles tracking the surgical instrument in a large tumor where the margins of the sella are poorly visualized. Both the CT (with its superb bone windows) and MRI can be simultaneously tracked in all three view planes. Removal of the fluoroscopy unit from the field is a welcome relief.

Stereotactic applications can be performed with accuracy and confidence. The rigidity of the AccuPoint sphere and the robust mechanical arm approximate the rigidity of stereotactic frames. More than 100 stereotactic procedures have been successfully performed with the Mayfield ACCISS and the AccuPoint sphere [11,12]. This includes stereotactic biopsy in 67 cases, aspiration of hematomas in 16 cases, and aspiration of intracerebral abscesses in eight cases. The diagnostic rates and complications for stereotactic biopsy with the Mayfield ACCISS are equivalent to the best results in the literature for stereotactic frames [11,13–16]. Coregistration of postbiopsy images confirms the efficacy of this methodology and provides doc-

umentation of stereotactic targeting in a way never demonstrated with stereotactic frame technology (Fig. 5).

The use of image-guided surgery in spinal applications has been more
limited than cranial applications in the author's experience of 31 cases. To
use the system for placement of pedicle screws, especially when a decompression has been performed and the pedicle can be palpated, is probably
not helpful but may be a good place for the beginner to gain experience. It
is certainly more beneficial in cases where pedicle screws are placed and no
laminectomy is performed. Patients with degenerative scoliosis, and those
who require pedicle screws in the thoracic and cervical region, present a
more compelling need for image-guided surgery.

The Mayfield ACCISS image-guided system has been integrated into
the Mayfield® Mobile SCAN™ portable CT, which provides the surgeon the
opportunity to obtain updated CT images during surgery. It also will allow
the surgeon to obtain spinal images in the prone position at the time of
surgery, eliminating concerns regarding spinal movement and the need for
segmental registration. The mechanical arm system has also been adapted
to and is compatible with intraoperative MRI systems. These adaptations
provide the surgeon solutions to many concerns about the limitations of
current image-guided surgery. These include the ability to obtain updated
images to correct for shift and to assess the amount of residual tumor in a
way that is superior to ultrasound.

3 CONCLUSION

Image-guided neurosurgery has many beneficial applications. The Mayfield
ACCISS has many unique features that distinguish it from others in addition
to its ease of use and economy for the neurosurgeon. First and foremost, it
is the only system with active, wireless optical tracking and mechanical arm
technology combined in one unit. This allows the surgeon to choose the
digitizer most suitable to the needs of an individual case. Second, the rigidity
of the AccuPoint sphere provides an unparalleled stereotactic capability for
an image-guided system. Third, the coregistration capability allows one to
use multimodality images during and after surgery. Fourth, the system is
reliable and so simple to use that additional personnel are not required to
operate the system for the surgeon. Lastly, the adaptation of the Mayfield
ACCISS to intraoperative CT or MRI ensures its utility as neurosurgeons
adopt these technologies.

REFERENCES

1. Barnett H, Kormos DW, Steiner CP, Weisenberger J. Intraoperative localization
    using an armless, framless stereotactic wand. J Neurosurg 78:510–514, 1993.

2. Gumprecht HK, Widenka DC, Lumenta CB. BrainLab VectorVision Neuronavigation System: Technology and clinical experience in 131 cases. Neurosurgery 44:97–105, 1999.

3. Guthrie BL, Adler JR Jr. Computer-assisted pre-operative planning, interactive surgery and frameless stereotaxy. Clin Neurosurg 38:112–131, 1992.

4. Guthrie BL. Graphic-interactive cranial surgery. Clin Neurosurg 41:489–516, 1994.

5. Roberts DW, Strohbehn JW, Hatch J, Murray W, Kettenberger H. A frameless stereotactic integration of computerized tomographic imaging and the operating microscope. J Neurosurg 65:545–549, 1986.

6. Rousu J, Kohls PE, Kall B, Kelly PJ. Computer-assisted image-guided surgery using the Regulus Navigator. Stud Health Technol Inform 50:103–109, 1998.

7. Sandeman DR, Patel N, Chandler C, Nelson RJ, Coakham HB, Griffith HB. Advances in image-directed neurosurgery: Preliminary experience with the ISG viewing wand compared with Leksell G Frame. Br J Neurosurg 8:529–544, 1994.

8. Smith KR, Frank DJ, Bucholz RD. The NeuroStation: A highly accurate minimally invasive solution to frameless stereotactic neurosurgery. Comput Med Imaging Graph 18:247–256, 1994.

9. Tobler WD. Image-guided Neurosurgery with the Mayfield ACCISS Workstation. Surgical Technology International VII. San Francisco: Universal Medical Press, Inc, 1998.

10. Tobler WD, Basham S. Efficacy of stereotactic craniotomy for metastatic disease. XIIth Meeting of the World Society for Stereotactic and Functional Neurosurgery. Lyon, France 1997.

11. Tobler WD. Frameless stereotactic biopsy, aspiration and catheter placement: Experience with 100 patients. In preparation.

12. Tobler WD, Basham S. Frameless stereotaxy for the aspiration of intracerebral hematomas. XIIth Meeting for the World Society of Stereotactic and Functional Neurosurgery. Lyon, France 1997:1.

13. Apuzzo MLJ, Chandrasoma PT, Cohen D, Zee CS, Zelman V. Computed imaging stereotaxy: experience and perspective related to 500 procedures applied to brain masses. Neurosurgery 20:930–937, 1987.

14. Mundinger F. CT sterotactic biopsy for optimizing the therapy of intracranial processes. Acta Neurochir Suppl 35:70–74, 1985.

15. Niizuma H, Otsuki T, Yonemitsu T, Kitahara M, Katakura R, Suzuki J. Experiences with CT-guided stereotactic biopsies in 121 cases. Acta Neurochir Suppl 42:157–160, 1988.

16. Ostertag CB, Mennel HD, Kiessling M. Stereotactic biopsy of brain tumors. Surg Neurol 14:275–283, 1980.

11

Surgical Navigation with the StealthStation

Michael Schulder
New Jersey Medical School, Newark, New Jersey, U.S.A.

1 INTRODUCTION

The availability of powerful computer workstations the size of a personal computer, along with new technology for tracking the position of a probe in 3-dimensional space, spurred certain far-seeing neurosurgical investigators to develop turnkey systems for navigation in neurosurgery. Dr. Richard Bucholz, a neurosurgeon at St. Louis University, saw the surgical potential in infrared digitizer tools. Together with a young engineer named Kurt Smith, he developed the system known as the StealthStation®. As with other frameless stereotactic (FS) devices, while the digitizing technology may be similar, the image rendering, user interface, means of maintaining stereotactic accuracy, essential hardware, and surgical tools are unique to this particular system.

2 SYSTEM DESCRIPTION AND USE

The StealthStation® system was designed by Surgical Navigation Technologies (Louisville, CO), now a division of Medtronic, Inc. (Minneapolis, MN). It has been described by Kurt Smith [1] and was independently evaluated by Germano [2]. System components include: a Unix-based Silicon

Graphics workstation, an infrared digitizer with active, infrared light emitting diodes (IRLED) or with passive reflector spheres, and infrared cameras (Polaris, Inc.); a dynamic reference frame that maintains registration accuracy even with movement of the patient or cameras; and a monitor with the StealthStation proprietary user interface. Software packages are available for cranial navigation, otolaryngological use (nasal sinus surgery, in essence), spinal surgery (for instrument insertion), functional stereotactic surgery, and certain orthopedic applications for limb surgery. These options make the StealthStation more attractive to hospitals as the system is more likely to be used and not gather dust—an important consideration for a device whose retail price is above $300,000.

Use of the StealthStation begins with preoperative imaging. The scan used for registration may be obtained with adhesive fiducial markers applied to the scalp in a manner that encompasses the volume of interest. It is possible to attempt registration with anatomical landmarks alone but at the New Jersey Medical School we have not found this to be sufficiently reliable. (SNT is developing a tool called the Fazer™ that will acquire a map of the patient's face using laser scanning, and provide registration; this may avoid the need for fiducials in the future.) The choice of MRI or CT will depend on the needs of the surgeon—when bony landmarks are the main concern then CT may be sufficient or ideal, but for most intracranial applications MRI will be the modality of choice. A scan may be obtained well in advance of surgery without fiducials and fused in the operating room (OR) to a different scan acquired with fiducials the day before operation. In any event, scans for the StealthStation must be obtained with zero gantry tilt, a slice thickness of 3 mm or less, no slice overlap or skip, and a field of view large enough to encompass the volume of interest.

Scan data is transferred to the OR workstation by an Ethernet connection or, if needed, by such removable media as optical disks ("sneakernet"). Image fusion of CT and MRI scans is easily done using the automated fusion program; functional data may be added in the same fashion [3]. Landmarks for registration (scalp markers or anatomical points) are numbered on a 3-dimensional image reconstruction. After the patient's head is secured in the head clamp, the dynamic reference frame (DRF) is attached to the clamp (see Fig. 1). Registration is then done using at least four fiducials. The program then provides an estimate of the accuracy of the mathematical match between the scan and physical space. This number is not a true estimate of registration accuracy, which must be verified using anatomical points before and during surgery. At this point, navigation may be used to plan an incision and approach for craniotomy or stereotactic biopsy.

The DRF is removed and the patient prepped and draped. A sterile DRF is placed (or the previous one sterilized and replaced), and maintenance

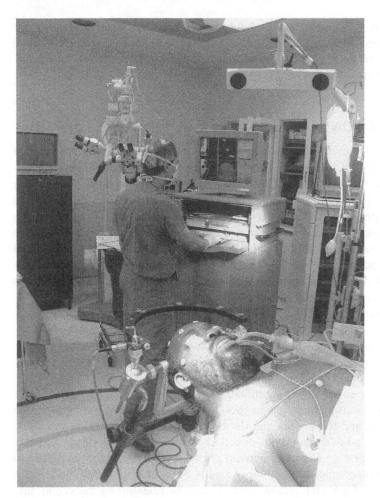

FIGURE 1 Patient positioned for transsphenoidal surgery with the StealthStation. Note placement of the dynamic reference frame, cameras, and monitor.

of registration accuracy is confirmed. During surgery, navigation is performed as desired. Draping the keyboard with a clear plastic sheet allows the surgeon to operate the computer if necessary. The operating microscope may be registered as a navigational tool, but often it is more convenient to use a wand with IRLEDs. Hardware and software tools for needle biopsy and functional targeting are available. Details are beyond the scope of this chapter but are based on the concepts and techniques of registration described above. Figures 2 and 3 show images from the StealthStation in use for transsphenoidal surgery. Images in Figure 2 were created with the Cranial program™, while Figure 3 shows the use of the Landmarx ENT™ package, which demonstrates the versatility of the StealthStation.

3 DISCUSSION

At the New Jersey Medical School we have used the StealthStation for over six years. At first, use of the StealthStation seemed like a cumbersome addition to the OR and added at least two hours to any procedure. With further experience the system became a completely routine part of surgery and its use is transparent to OR and radiology staff. All of the neurosurgeons in our group are comfortable with its use. Concerns have been raised that residents will come to rely on this technology to the abandonment of fundamental surgical principles; the obvious answer to this issue is that such fears have not prevented the incorporation of other advances such as CT and MRI scans into neurosurgical education.

The versatility of the StealthStation is one of its most appealing features. In this it is not unique but not all commercially available systems share this feature. The choice of using active IRLED probes or the passive probes with reflector spheres gives the surgeon yet another degree of freedom. Cost is comparable to other navigational devices.

Limitations of the StealthStation are to some extent generic for IRLED-based surgical navigation (SN) systems. A line of sight between the reference arc and the probes and the IR cameras is required. Downloading data may not go as smoothly as hoped in all cases. Shifting of the patient's scalp by positioning changes, or scalp pressure from the probe, may lead to registration inaccuracies. The biopsy arm is bulky and unwieldy, although a new device—the Vertek biopsy guide— will be released by the vendor and many of the ergonomic problems in the old arm should be solved. And of course, as with all SN systems that rely on preoperative datasets, brain shift will often render the intracranial registration inaccurate as surgery proceeds.

In May 2000 we began our experience with intraoperative imaging when we were the first North American site to install a PoleStar N-10 intraoperative MR (iMRI) MRI unit. This system, with its integrated navigational tool, provides the advantages of navigation updated by intraoperative images that eliminate concerns related to brain and lesion shift [4]. The promise of combining the best features of the StealthStation with the capabilities of the PoleStar N-10 is a new and exciting development, as surely SN in the near future will require the incorporation of new images. However, the utility of a stand-alone surgical navigation device without

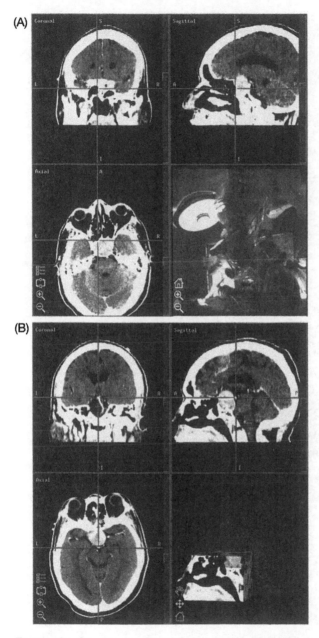

FIGURE 2　Screen images from transsphenoidal surgery for pituitary macroadenoma. (A) CT navigation shows probe at border of sella (OR view seen in lower right). (B) Probe points to basilar artery, just in back of eroded sella turcica.

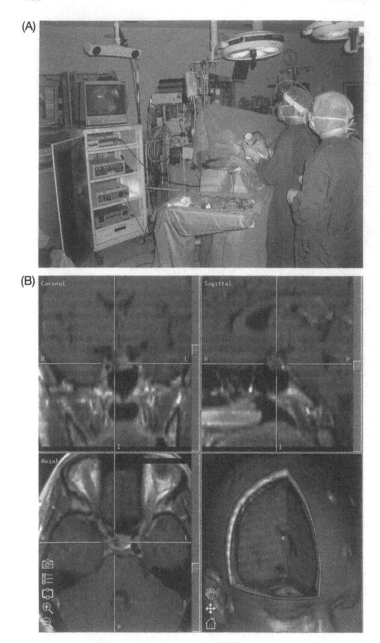

FIGURE 3 Endoscopic transsphenoidal navigation for microprolactinoma using the noninvasive Landmarx frame. (A) Setup and surgery. (B) Monitor view with probe in tumor bed on reformatted MRI.

iMRI or intraoperative CT will remain for patients undergoing a wide variety of surgery.

4 CONCLUSION

Surgical navigation with the StealthStation has become a routine part of many operating rooms. Little time is added to the procedure and, as with other advances in neurosurgical technology, a great deal of guesswork is eliminated in intracranial neurosurgery. The versatility of the StealthStation is a great advantage and in a relatively short time it can become a workhorse tool for any neurosurgeon. Even with the eventual incorporation of intra-operative imaging as an OR routine, the StealthStation will still have its place in the management of patients in whom intraoperative imaging is superfluous and as a system for updated navigation with newly acquired images.

REFERENCES

1. Smith KR, Frank KJ, Bucholz RD: The Neurostation—a highly accurate, min-imally invasive solution to frameless stereotactic neurosurgery. Computerized Medical Imaging and Graphics 18:247–256, 1994.
2. Germano I: The NeuroStation System for image-guided frameless stereotaxy. Neurosurgery 37:348–350, 1995.
3. Schulder M, Maldjian J, Liu W, et al.: Functional image-guided surgery of in-tracranial tumors in or near sensorimotor cortex. J Neurosurg 89:412–418, 1998.
4. Hadani M, Speigelman R, Feldman Z, Berkenstadt H, Ram Z: Novel, compact, intraoperative magnetic resonance imaging-guided system for conventional neu-rosurgical operating rooms. Neurosurgery 48:799–807, 2001.

12

Stereotactic Radiosurgery: Indications and General Technical Considerations

Michael Schulder
New Jersey Medical School, Newark, New Jersey, U.S.A.

1 INTRODUCTION

In 1951 Lars Leksell coined the term stereotactic radiosurgery (SRS) [1]. A ceaseless innovator, his goal was to develop a method for "the non-invasive destruction of intracranial . . . lesions that may be inaccessible or unsuitable for open surgery" [2]. The first procedures were done using an orthovoltage X-ray tube mounted on an early model of what is now known as the Leksell stereotactic frame, for the treatment of several patients with trigeminal neuralgia. After experimenting with particle beams and linear accelerators, Leksell and his colleagues ultimately designed the gamma knife, containing 179 cobalt sources in a hemispheric array (Figure 1). The first unit was operational in 1968 [3].

At the same time, work was continuing elsewhere with focussed heavy particle irradiation. Raymond Kjellberg spearheaded the use of proton beam treatments at the Harvard/Massachusetts General Hospital facility. A series of patients with arteriovenous malformations and pituitary tumors was amassed. Similar efforts were carried out in California (with helium ions) and Moscow [3]. Particle beams have the advantage of depositing their energy at a distinct point known as the Bragg peak, with minimal exit dose.

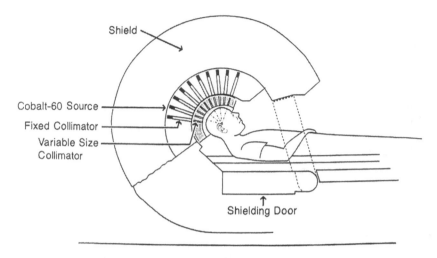

FIGURE 1 Schematic view of gamma knife.

In practice, the beams must be carefully shaped and spread in order to treat patients with intracranial lesions (Figure 2). The expense of building and maintaining a cyclotron has limited the use of heavy particle SRS to a few centers. (From Ref. 57 with permission of The McGraw-Hill Companies.)

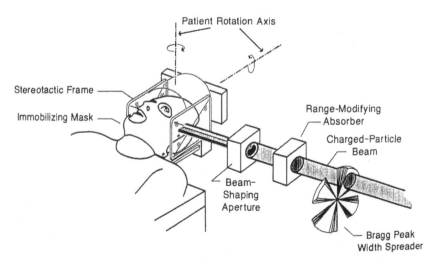

FIGURE 2 Spreading and shaping of particle beam for SRS with a particle beam accelerator. (From Ref. 57 with permission of The McGraw-Hill Companies.)

Through the 1970s SRS was used to treat intracranial targets that could be defined by plain X-rays or tomograms (e.g. acoustic neuromas arteriovenous malformations (AVMs), or the gasserian ganglion). The advent of computed tomography (CT) in the mid-70s opened up the possibility of direct targeting of tumors and other "soft tissue" targets inside the skull. As the potential horizons of SRS broadened other investigators were able to adapt linear accelerators (linacs) for SRS (Figure 3). These devices were more available (and less expensive) than gamma knives or heavy particle accelerators [4–7]. As clinical experience increased, publications appeared, indications broadened, and vendors became increasingly interested. A debate emerged regarding the merits of the gamma knife versus linac based SRS. Clinical and physics studies seemed to have settled the issue that SRS could be delivered effectively and accurately with either method [8–10].

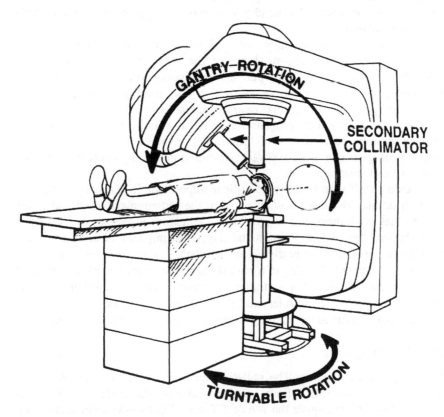

FIGURE 3 Diagram of linear accelerator, showing axes of rotation of couch and gantry. (From Ref. 57 with permission of The McGraw-Hill Companies.)

Currently, SRS is a routine part of neurosurgical practice, and should be part of resident education. Below is an overview of the current indications and technical considerations for SRS.

2 TECHNICAL CONSIDERATIONS

2.1 The Treatment Team

SRS, however it is delivered and planned, has a final common pathway—the delivery of ionizing radiation to a well-defined, relatively small volume. Many factors go into the safe and effective use of this technique, not the least of which is a multidisciplinary team. Besides the neurosurgeon, the active involvement of a medical physicist is required. This is the only person with the expertise to translate the virtual computer based SRS plan into the physical reality of irradiation. Quality assurance (QA) of the SRS device must also be maintained by the physicist; otherwise the plans will not match the actual treatment.

In the U.S. only radiation oncologists are permitted to sign off on a plan of therapeutic irradiation. However, the oncologist has much more to offer than a clerical role. Many patients undergoing SRS may have received fractionated radiation therapy in the past, or may need it in the future. They may have types of cancers that neurosurgeons have little experience with. Furthermore, radiation oncologists view SRS as a form of focussed radiation therapy as opposed to a form of "minimally invasive neurosurgery." Radiation oncologists can bring 100 years of radiation therapy experience to SRS planning and treatment.

Other staff members are of critical importance in the performance of SRS. A dedicated nurse, most often from the radiation oncology side, will ensure that equipment and any needed medication is prepared. He or she will sheperd the patient through the day, ensuring that discomfort is addressed as needed. Dosimetrists', an invaluable help, may be actively involved in treatment planning in a busy department where the physicists must attend to other duties. The radiation therapists must be familiar with the treatment equipment and understand the QA needs of the device. Their professionalism is crucial in ensuring a smooth experience for the patient.

2.2 Imaging

SRS is based on imaging. The radiation must be aimed at a specific target seen on CT and/or MRI. Some commercially available devices (e.g. Radionics X-Knife™) require the use of CT scanning even if other images are used. This is due to the presumed greater stereotactic accuracy of CT scanning [11]; however, other authors have demonstrated that MRI can be an accurate tool for radiosurgical targeting and use this method exclusively [12]. A stereotactic phantom should be scanned and the accuracy of the CT and MRI units verified. MRI is needed to adequately target lesions at the skull base and in the posterior fossa. Coronal MRI is of particular value to image the cerebral convexity and the optic chiasm.

Image fusion, available with most commercial systems, permits the registration of CT and MRI scans. Thus, patients can undergo MRI scanning in advance, limiting the length of time needed for scanning on the day of the procedure, and making it easier to schedule the SRS. If a question remains regarding the spatial accuracy of stereotactic MRI, image fusion can combine the reliability of CT with the improved anatomical resolution of MRI [13]. Any other digital image set can be incorporated, such as positron emission tomography (PET) or functional MRI [14]. AVMs are often best seen on contrast-enhanced CT [15]. For some patients catheter angiography is still necessary for AVM visualization. In these cases digital angiography can be used, but software to correct the spatial distortion inherent in digital X-rays must be installed and verified for accuracy.

2.3 Treatment

Patients arrive the morning of treatment, and in most institutions will be discharged at the end of the day. Oral sedation is administered (for instance Valium 5 mg) and an intravenous angiocath inserted for contrast injection. The stereotactic frame is then applied (unless treatment is planned with the CyberKnife™; see Chapter 21). This placement must ensure that 1) the treatment volume is above the base ring of the frame; 2) as much of the cranium as possible is included within the bounds of the localizer, so that dosimetry will be accurate; 3) there will be no obstruction to securing the frame to the scanning and treatment couches, especially in the back of the head; 4) the patient can eat and drink after the scan; 5) there is no scalp pressure from any part of the apparatus. Symmetrical placement is ideal, but not essential.

Scanning is performed with CT and/or MRI. Attaching the frame to the scan table prevents patient movement and ensures that the image will be in an orthogonal plane. Contrast should be injected if this will help visualize the target. Scan slice thickness should be 3 mm and the field of view adequate to encompass the localizer rods or panels. After the scan is done the patient waits, preferably in a comfortable private area until treatment.

2.4 Treatment Planning

The stereotactic scan is transferred electronically to the SRS planning computer. Image fusion is done if necessary, and the visual fit between scans is confirmed in 3 planes. Each slice is checked. If the software requires, or allows for 3-dimensional contouring of anatomical structures, these virtual models are used only to begin the planning—in the end the plan must be based on the 2-dimensional CT and/or MR images themselves.

The two main technical goals of SRS planning are to achieve *conformality* and a steep *dose gradient*. Conformality means that the prescription dose of radiation will match the borders of the target as closely as possible, so that the target/volume ratio (TVR) is as close to 1:1 as possible. This number should be less than 2 and certainly not more than 3. Of course, if it is less than 1 the target will be undertreated. A steep dose gradient means that the falloff of radiation outside the target will be rapid. Thus, the volume of brain receiving lower (but still significant) amounts of radiation will be as small as possible. A steep dose gradient will also protect critical structures, e.g. the optic chiasm, allowing for SRS use to treat lesions as close as 3 mm from the chiasm. Since more radiation falloff is inevitable, this can also be aimed as needed in a safer direction. For example, in patients with acoustic neuromas, it is preferable to place additional doses in the temporal bone rather than the brainstem by orienting beams in a craniocaudal fashion [16].

If SRS is administered using circular collimators (as with the Gamma Knife™ and "conventional" linac systems), a collimator large enough to encompass the treatment volume should be chosen. As the Gamma Knife™ has a maximum collimator size of 18 mm, often this will not be possible, in which case multiple treatment "shots" will be employed to fashion an ideal plan (Chapter 16). The maximum linac collimator size should be 40 mm, beyond which the volume treated will likely be too large for SRS. Rarely will a purely spherical treatment plan suffice, and even if a single linac collimator can be used for treatment, the beams must be angled, trimmed, or weighted in such a way as to conform to the target shape as much as possible [15]. Devices that use inverse planning such as the Peacock system (Chapter 20) or the CyberKnife™ are not limited by collimator size or shape; their quality assurance may be more complicated.

When the appearance of the treatment plan is satisfactory, as confirmed in 3 planes and multiple slices of the 2-dimensional images, the prescription dose is chosen. Here the goals are to deliver a dose that is safe and effective. In general, complications of SRS are directly related to increasing dose, volume, and target location, with volume the factor best understood [17,18]. Other factors, such as prior or anticipated fractionated radiation therapy, should be considered as well.

Practically speaking, balancing safety and efficacy means that treatment doses will lie somewhere between 10 Gy and 20 Gy for patients with tumors; occasionally a higher dose can be aimed at a small metastasis. Functional radiosurgical treatments will require a higher dose (such as maximum of 70 Gy for patients with trigeminal neuralgia); the very small target volume permits this to be done safely [19]. The difference between prescription and maximum doses must be kept in mind. The use of multiple collimators with overlapping treatment spheres may result in a maximum dose much higher than the prescription dose, depending on the SRS system being used. It must be ascertained that any major areas of overlap remain within the target volume. Coordination with the medical physicist is crucial to ensure that the translation from relative isodose shells, rendered in percentages of the maximum dose, and the actual, absolute dose in Gy is accurate. For patients with malignant disease in whom other radiation is needed, input from the radiation oncologist should be especially welcome.

2.5 Treatment

When it is time to turn the virtual treatment plan on the computer screen into a physical reality of delivered radiation, the strictest QA measures must be followed. The isocentric accuracy of any SRS system must be absolutely ensured—otherwise the high dose of radiation will go somewhere other than planned. Double and triple checking of stereotactic settings by multiple personnel is desirable. The physicist is responsible for verifying that the dose output of the treatment device is predicted.

The patient should lie as comfortably as possible for the treatment to avoid attempted head movement. Head fixation with the stereotactic frame (or with the mask in case of the CyberKnife™) is mandatory. After completion of the treatment and removal of the head ring, the patient may be discharged. Clinical and imaging followup will depend on the patient's status and the lesion treated. In general, patients with malignant disease will be seen sooner and imaged more often than those with benign tumors, AVMs, or with "functional" disorders.

3 INDICATIONS FOR SRS

SRS has evolved from an esoteric treatment to an option that should be offered to many patients with intracranial lesions. The older or more medically fragile the patient, the smaller the target. The more hazardous the surgical option, the more SRS should be offered as an alternative to surgery, or as the primary treatment. Radiobiology suggests that there is a particular advantage for single-session irradiation of benign tissues [20]. Thus, certain patients with AVMs, acoustic neuromas, and small cavernous sinus meningiomas are ideal candidates for primary SRS. Ample clinical evidence exists that SRS is an effective treatment for such lesions, with a morbidity rate less than surgery. The question is where to draw the line—e.g., should all patients with acoustic neuromas be offered SRS, or should this be reserved only for those considered elderly or medically infirm? Thus, the debate is not whether SRS is an effective treatment, but rather which patients are candidates for treatment.

At this time, patient choice is considered as valid an indication as any medical reason for SRS. However, it is up to the neurosurgeon to understand when SRS is a reasonable choice before presenting it to the patient as an option. For this reason some training in SRS and an understanding of the underlying physics and radiobiology are essential; guidelines for this have been published as a consensus statement by leading neurosurgeons, radiation oncologists, and physicists [21].

Increasing experience and documentation of its efficacy has fueled the expansion of indications for SRS. In truth the increase in SRS centers and practitioners may have played a role as well. There are more patients with malignant intracranial tumors than with benign lesions. There is evidence that SRS increases survival with maintained quality of life for patients with high grade gliomas, but this is an incremental improvement at best [22]. For a patient in good clinical shape with a "recurrent" glioma that is small enough to be targeted effectively and safely, SRS is a reasonable option. On the other hand, patients with metastatic tumors, especially single ones, may be better served by SRS compared to surgery. Tumors that are resistant to fractionated RT (e.g. melanoma) may be controlled with SRS [23].

The role of SRS in functional neurosurgery is being explored. For patients with trigeminal neuralgia, a condition where the target can be defined with great precision on MRI, SRS seems to be an effective option. For alleviation of pain or movement disorders, more uncertainty exists. Some encouraging reports have been published [24,25]. However, direct physiological target confirmation is lacking in SRS. For targets whose exact location may not be predictable with anatomic imaging alone (e.g. the Vim nucleus of the thalamus)—or more precisely, when effective lesion placement depends on physiological feedback—the best technique and indication for SRS remains to be determined.

The indications and technique of SRS with different tools and for different indications are discussed in detail in the chapters that follow.

4 CONCLUSION

SRS is an accepted and even ubiquitous part of contemporary neurosurgical practice. For the appropriate patients and in the proper hands, it provides minimally invasive, safe, and effective treatment. Neurosurgeons performing SRS should have the necessary skills and understanding of the basic principles underlying SRS, and be involved in every step of the procedure. With judicious use, SRS will remain an excellent primary and adjuvant treatment modality for many of our patients in neurosurgery.

REFERENCES

1. Leksell L. The stereotaxic method and radiosurgery of the brain. Acta Chir Scand 1951, 102:316–319.
2. Leksell L. Stereotactic radiosurgery. J Neurol Neurosurg Psyc 1983, 46:797–803.
3. Lunsford L, Alexander E, 3rd, Loeffler JS. General introduction: history of radiosurgery. In: Alexander E, 3rd, Loeffler JS, Lunsford LD, eds. Stereotactic Radiosurgery. New York: McGraw Hill, 1993, 1–4.
4. Betti O, Derechinsky V. Hyperselective encephalic irradiation with a linear accelerator. Acta Neurochir Suppl 1984, 33:385–390.
5. Columbo F, Benedetti A, Casentini L, et al. Linear accelerator radiosurgery of cerebral arteriovenous malformations. Neurosurgery 1989, 29:833–840.
6. Winston KR, Lutz W. Linear accelerator as a neurosurgical tool for stereotactic radiosurgery. Neurosurgery 1988, 22:454–464.
7. Friedman W, Bova F. The University of Florida radiosurgery system. Surg Neurol 1989, 32:334–342.
8. Phillips MH, Stelzer KJ, Griffin TW, et al. Stereotactic radiosurgery: a review and comparisons of methods. J Clin Oncol 1994, 12:1085–1099.
9. Schwartz M. Stereotactic radiosurgery: comparing different technologies. CMAJ 1998, 158:625–628.
10. Luxton G, Petrovich Z, Joszef G, Nedzi L, Apuzzo M. Stereotactic radiosurgery: principles and comparison of treatment methods. Neurosurgery 1993, 32: 241–259.
11. Walton L, Hampshire A, Forster D, Kemeny A. A phantom study to assess the accuracy of stereotactic localization using T1-weighted magnetic resonance imaging with the Leksell stereotactic system. Neurosurgery 1996, 38:170–178.
12. Kondziolka D, Dempsey P, Lunsford L, Kestle J, Dolan E, Tasker R. A comparison between magnetic resonance imaging and computed tomography for stereotactic coordinate determination. Neurosurgery 1992, 30:402–407.
13. Alexander EI, Kooy M, van Herk M, et al. Magnetic resonance image-directed stereotactic neurosurgery: use of image fusion with computerized tomography to enhance spatial accuracy. J Neurosurgery 1995, 83:271–276.
14. Schulder M, Vega J, Narra V, et al. Functional magnetic resonance imaging and radiosurgical dose planning. Stereotact Funct Neurosurg 1999, 73:38–44.
15. Friedman W, Bova F, Mendenhall W. Linear accelerator radiosurgery for arteriovenous malformations: relationship of size to outcome. Journal of Neurosurgery 1995, 82:180–189.
16. Mendenhall W, Friedman W, Bova F. Linear accelerator-based stereotactic radiosurgery for acoustic schwannomas. Int J Radiat Oncol Biol Phys 1994, 28: 803–810.

17. Flickinger JC. An integrated logistic formula for prediction of complications from radiosurgery. Int J Radiat Oncol Biol Phys 1989, 17:879–885.
18. Marks LB, Spencer DP. The influence of volume on the tolerance of the brain to radiosurgery. J Neurosurg 1991, 75:177–180.
19. Kondziolka D, Lusford L, Flickinger J, et al. Stereotactic radiosurgery for trigeminal neuralgia: a multiinstitutional study using the gamma unit. J Neurosurg 1996, 84:940–945.
20. Larson DA, Flickinger JC, Loeffler JS. The radiobiology of radiosurgery. Int J Radiat Oncol Biol Phys 1993, 25:557–561.
21. Consensus statement of stereotactic radiosurgery: quality improvement. Neurosurgery 1994, 34:193–195.
22. Sarkaria JN, Mehta MP, Loeffler JS, Buatti JM, Chapell RJ, Kinsella TJ. Stereotactic radiosurgery improves survival in malignant gliomas compared with the RTOG recursive partitioning analysis. Int J Radiat Oncol Biol Phys 1995, 30:164.
23. Somaza S, Kondziolka D, Lunsford LD, Kirkwood JM, Flickinger JC. Stereotactic radiosurgery for cerebral metastatic melanoma. J Neurosurg 1993, 79: 661–666.
24. Kondziolka D, Lunsford LD, Habeck M, Flickinger JC. Gamma knife radiosurgery for trigeminal neuralgia. Neurosurg Clin N Am 1997, 8:79–85.
25. Young R, Shumway-Cook A, Vermeulen S, et al. Gamma knife radiosurgery as a lesioning technique in movement disorder surgery. J Neurosurg 1998, 89: 183–193.

13

Stereotactic Radiosurgery for Benign Tumors

Gerhard Pendl and Oskar Schröttner
Karl-Franzens University Graz, Graz, Austria

1 INTRODUCTION

The use of stereotactic radiosurgery (SRS) to treat patients with benign tumors is still debatable. However, a consensus exists in favor of SRS for patients with high surgical and anesthesiological risk, patients of advanced age, and those who refuse open surgery for other reasons. Benign tumors in eloquent areas pose considerable surgical risks. Unrelated to a specific diagnosis, there are several important factors concerning patient assessment and SRS that should be taken into consideration before treatment. In all cases of radiosurgically treated tumors, the histological nature of the process should be evaluated. Variations of radiosensitivity of tumors and radiation tolerances of different structures within and outside the normal brain, mostly important for dose planning in different tumor locations, have to be taken into consideration. The volume of the tumor itself and the influence on the normal brain tissue around are important factors. The patient must be aware that the primary aim of treatment is to control the lesion and must be informed about possible risks of SRS. For example, SRS is strictly contraindicated in patients with compression of the optic apparatus (Fig. 1), or with signs of acute brainstem compression from cystic tumors.

All these factors should be borne in mind before using SRS to treat benign tumors, including meningiomas, acoustic or trigeminal schwannomas, benign tumors of the pituitary region, small, well-delineated, low-grade gliomas, hemangioblastomas, and glomus jugulare tumors.

1.1 Meningiomas

Patients with residual or recurrent meningiomas are often ideal candidates for radiosurgery especially those with skull base meningiomas in the parasellar region. For instance, many neurosurgeons still advocate extensive dissection for aggressive removal of cavernous sinus meningiomas (CSM), yielding "acceptable levels" of morbidity and mortality [1–5]. With open surgery, new neuropathies are reported in 18% to 43% of patients [4,6], and extensive resection of the cavernous sinus region carries a risk of permanent

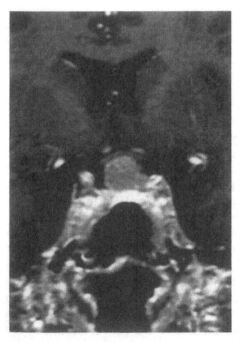

FIGURE 1   A 64-year-old female with recurrent sellar meningioma after open surgery 11 years before. Acute visual field defects within 6 weeks will not allow radiosurgery. Note the compression of the chiasm.

ocular palsy of about 20% [7]. The patient should be informed about these risks and the alternative of SRS.

Our own series of SRS for patients with CSM found no further cranial nerve deficit after treatment [8,9]; a report by Duma noted 6% transient deficits [10]. Although it is, of course, almost mandatory to have histological proof of the nature of a lesion to be treated by SRS, as computed tomography (CT) or magnetic resonance imaging (MR) may be misleading [11], such proof should not be obtained if this involves an unacceptable risk to the patient. This holds mainly for elderly or clinically disabled patients who are precluded from an open microsurgical approach. Figure 2A,B presents a case of a 69-year-old patient who refused open surgery despite VIth nerve palsy.

The radiosurgical prescription dose commonly used for meningiomas varies between 12 and 16 Gy. Decreasing the tumor dose to less than 12 Gy may defeat the therapeutical purpose of the radiosurgical procedure [12]. Therefore, patients in whom the optic nerves, chiasm, or tract are stretched, distorted, or displaced over the entire tumor surface should be excluded from SRS, as safe and effective doses cannot be delivered simultaneously by a single fraction dose plan under those circumstances [13]. Nevertheless, if surgery is required for visual pathway decompression or some other reason,

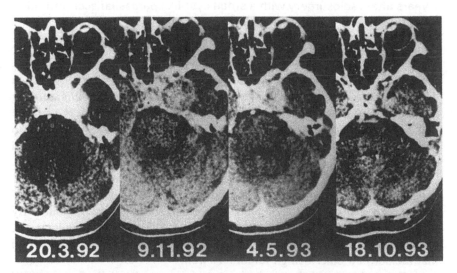

FIGURE 2   A, Gradual shrinkage of a parasellar meningioma of a 69-year-old female patient with VIth nerve palsy before treatment with 12 Gy at the 30% isodose volume. Shrinkage with radionecrosis occurred after slight enlargement 9 months after radiosurgery.

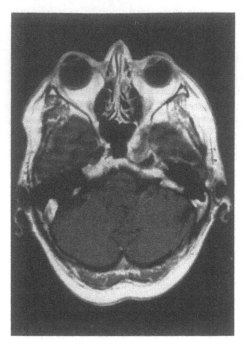

FIGURE 2   B, Magnetic resonance imaging control of patient in Figure 2A, 7 years after radiosurgery with a small cyst-like parasellar scar formation unchanged for 3 years.

the option of SRS means that the surgeon may be less aggressive when dissecting in the region of the optic apparatus or circle of Willis, leaving residual tumor for treatment with adjuvant SRS. Moreover there is evidence that SRS may control, even reduce, tumor size in meningiomas also with suboptimal doses less than 10 Gy, suggesting a further option in selected cases [14].

As some of the basal meningiomas are residual or recurrent tumors of considerable size and the growth rate is rather low, even these large volumes can be managed by SRS as a staged procedure separated by 6 months. By this method, the complications that are expected in treatment volumes of more than 3 cm in diameter will be minimized, if present at all—an option that includes all other benign tumors as well.

For patients with hemispheric meningiomas, the indication for SRS should be limited, as they have a greater risk of edema after treatment compared with those with basal meningiomas [15–17]. In these patients, the minimal risk of open surgery should be taken into consideration as well.

1.2 Acoustic Schwannomas

The typical imaging appearance of these tumors, along with the history of signs and symptoms, allows for their reliable diagnosis without biopsy. In dose planning for patients with these tumors, one must bear in mind the proximity of the facial and trigeminal nerves to the tumor surface, mandating a steep dose gradient of the marginal dose. Therefore, multiple small shots should be applied. The marginal dose itself should be 15 Gy in very small, 12 Gy in medium-sized, and 10 Gy in large tumors, especially if hearing can be preserved [18]. The growth of acoustic schwannomas can be controlled by SRS in 95% of patients with tumors with diameters up to 3 cm [18,19]. Figure 3 shows a 68-year-old woman with a medium-sized acoustic schwannoma in whom no visible tumor could be detected 2.5 years after SRS. Useful hearing was preserved.

The incidence of transitory facial and trigeminal nerve dysfunction after SRS is currently less than 2%, which is superior to the results of microsurgery [20]. After microsurgery, permanent trigeminal symptoms may occur in 11% of patients, and the incidence of persistent facial nerve paresis

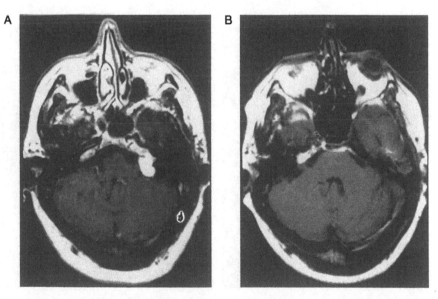

FIGURE 3 **A,** A 68-year-old woman with a 1.5 × 1.0-cm large acoustic schwannoma. Stereotactic radiosurgery with 12 Gy peripheral dose to the 50% isodose volume was applied. **B,** No visible tumor 2.5 years after radiosurgery. Useful hearing as before radiosurgery was preserved with no further neurological deficit.

varies between 0 and 35% correlating with tumor size [21,22]. Transitory hemifacial spasm, subsiding spontaneously, might occur as a side effect after SRS [18].

Rates of useful hearing preservation in the immediate postoperative period (defined as Gardner and Robertson classes I and II) are reported to be 100%, but decline to 62% to 70% after at least 2 years of follow-up. Similar rates of hearing preservation are reported only for selected small volume schwannomas after microsurgery [19,23,24].

Patients with neurofibromatosis type 2 (NF2) who still have useful hearing on both or either sides may be offered SRS as the optimal alternative to open surgery. Long-term follow-up of these patients has demonstrated that hearing loss may not be inevitable [24]. This is illustrated by our case of a 16-year-old female with large NF2 tumors. Because on the left side useful hearing was still preserved, SRS was applied on this side, followed by microsurgery with only partial resection to exclude any risk on the right side. Useful hearing could be preserved along with intact facial nerves on both sides (Fig. 4). In general, risk factors involving radiosurgical injury to cranial nerves increase with the irradiated length of the nerve, high total

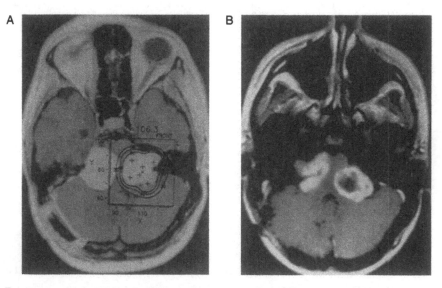

A   B

FIGURE 4   **A,** A 16-year-old female patient with NF2 tumors. Radiosurgical dose plan on the left neurofibroma: 10 Gy peripheral dose to 50% iso-dose volume. **B,** One year after stereotactic radiosurgery and microsurgical partial resection of the right neurofibroma showing central radionecrosis on the left side.

peripheral dose, and decreased conformality of the prescription isodose shell. This is especially the case in patients with intracanalicular tumors, in whom the use of multiple shots and relatively low marginal dose radiosurgical planning (on the order of 12 Gy) is mandatory [25,26].

Hydrocephalus induced by tumor compression may necessitate placement of a shunt before radiosurgery. Patients with large intracranial acoustic schwannomas who are not candidates for primary SRS because of brainstem compression should undergo tumor resection before SRS. In cases of cystic schwannomas, one should apply radiosurgery with caution, as the chance of increasing the cyst volume after radiosurgery is high. This can result in acute symptoms of brainstem compression, and open surgery for decompression might be needed as an emergency [27]. Cyst formation may also develop after SRS of larger acoustic schwannomas [28]. It may be appropriate to be cautious in advising radiosurgery for any intracranial tumor with a major cystic component [29].

Overall, however, the inevitable risks of open surgery—cerebrospinal fluid (CSF) leak, intracranial infection, and intraoperative and postoperative hemorrhage—can be avoided by SRS. Radiosurgery is also useful for treatment of recurrent tumors after microsurgery. The problems in performing microsurgery after SRS are sometimes discussed [22–30], although this has not been our observation.

1.3 Tumors of the Pituitary Region

Using SRS to treat patients with pituitary tumors is a challenging task. There is a risk of radiation damage to optic nerves, optic chiasm, or the hypothalamus, especially with larger tumors. The possibility of control of tumor growth and pituitary endocrinopathy without producing pituitary failure is a relatively new but promising aspect of radiosurgery [31].

Although SRS is not the preferred primary treatment for patients with hormonally active tumors, it has a role to play as an adjunct to treatment after failed microsurgery. Tumors may invade the cavernous sinus relatively far away from the optic apparatus. This makes a surgically awkward location a reasonable and safe indication for SRS. The carotid artery and nerves in the wall of the cavernous sinus tolerate those radiosurgical doses that are effective for controlling tumor growth. Residual tumors in this region can be controlled very reasonably by SRS [32–34]. Figure 5 presents a case of a 37-year-old man with a large recurrent prolactinoma after transsphenoidal surgery. After 3 years, no evidence of tumor was apparent, and his prolactin level was normal.

There is now evidence that a marginal dose of at least 25 Gy may normalize elevated hormone levels relatively soon after SRS [35–37]. Nev-

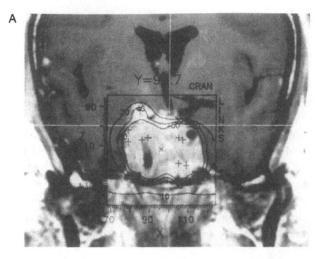

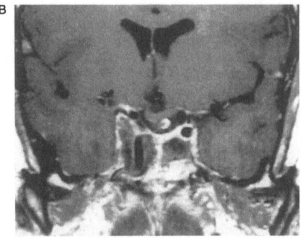

FIGURE 5   **A**, Large tumor mass of a prolactinoma with 45.2 cc volume. Dose plan with 10 Gy. **B**, Magnetic resonance imaging follow-up 3 years after stereotactic radiosurgery. No further evidence of vital tumor structures in the sellar region in accordance with the endocrinological situation.

ertheless, special heed must be taken of sparing critical structures from excessive radiation. Therefore, the radiosurgical dose plan has to be created with exact visualization of tumor, in relation to the normal pituitary gland, optic pathways, the cavernous sinus, and of the isodose lines and corresponding doses tangent to these critical structures. Doses up to 10 Gy to the optic apparatus are reported to be acceptable [32], but to avoid optic neuropathy, we recommend limiting this dose to no more than 8 Gy. If the chiasm is stretched over the tumor edge and subject to compression, primary microneurosurgery has to be performed for decompression; this can be followed by adjuvant radiosurgery. Patients should be followed up after SRS for at least 5 years to assess the effects on the endocrinopathy, to exclude pituitary failure, and to check visual function.

The tumor control rate for patients undergoing SRS for inactive and hormone-active pituitary adenomas (with peripheral doses ranging from 10 to 22 Gy) is as high as 98.3% [35,38–41]. The incidence of pituitary dysfunction ranges from 15% to 55% [36,42–44]. In 11% of 73 cases, improvement of pituitary function is reported [38]. Moreover, with sophisticated doses that deliver less than 9 Gy to the optic apparatus, patients will avoid radiation-induced visual damage [38]. The endocrinological cure rate in patients with hormonally active adenomas may be up to 57% [36,38].

1.4 Craniopharyngiomas

For selected patients, in whom microsurgery may not be appropriate, SRS may be a viable option [45,46]. In those with cystic craniopharyngiomas, intracystic bleomycin, initially described by Takahashi in 1985 [47], has proved effective in preparing these tumors for radiosurgery after shrinkage. With SRS, the radiation field can be closely tailored to the tumor volume, keeping the radiation dose to the surrounding hypothalamic region and optical structures to a minimum. After bleomycin instillation, radiosurgery may achieve volume reductions of the residual tumors in 74% of patients [48,49]. The prescription dose should be kept within 12 to 18 Gy. In these reports, SRS resulted in no mortality and no significant morbidity. Figure 6 shows a cystic craniopharyngeoma, which had been stereotactically punctured and treated by instillation of bleomycin into the evacuated cyst. Shrinkage of the craniopharyngioma could be observed 3 months later and SRS was then applied. Four years later, only a small area of tumor tissue in front of the chiasm could be noted, which is stable in size up to now. Vision has remained normal since before evacuation.

1.5 Glomus Jugulare Tumors

With rare exceptions, glomus jugulare tumors are histologically benign, non-secreting paragangliomas. They have a well-known predilection for local invasion of the surrounding structures, such as the middle ear, jugular vein, clivus, internal carotid artery, cavernous sinus and cranial nerves [50]. De-

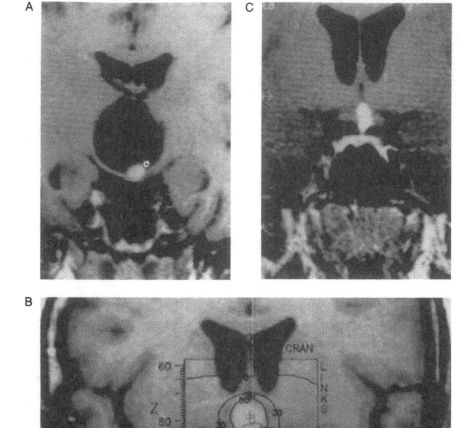

FIGURE 6 **A,** Craniopharyngioma cyst of 3.5-cm diameter, bulging into the third ventricle. Calcified nodule at the base of the tumor cyst. **B,** Dose planning for stereotactic radiosurgery of the remaining small volume of the craniopharyngioma after bleomycin treatment to the evacuated cyst with 9 Gy to the 50% isodose volume. **C,** Control magnetic resonance imaging 4 years after stereotactic radiosurgery with residual calcified small tumor nodule near the chiasm.

spite advances in neuroimaging and microsurgical techniques, some of these lesions defy radical resection because of their critical location. If complete excision is inadvisable owing to concerns of postoperative morbidity, the residual glomus tumor should be treated by SRS. The optimal dose for these tumors has not yet been established. Nevertheless, we recommend using a prescription dose above 18 Gy to achieve tumor control. This dose should be delivered while minimizing the amount of radiation received by the brainstem [51,52]. With this strategy in mind, no complications are reported to occur after SRS of glomus juglare tumors [52].

1.6 Miscellaneous Lesions

Stereotactic radiosurgery has become a well-accepted adjuvant or even primary treatment option to reduce risk and to improve outcome for patients with midline lesions located within the thalamus, hypothalamus, pineal region, and even brainstem. In midline tumors, especially in the brainstem, the marginal dose should not exceed 14 Gy [53]. Low-dose radiosurgery to critically located hamartomas of the hypothalamus may be effective for tumor arrest and suppression of epileptic activity [54]. In general, SRS may be used in lesional epilepsy by incorporating epileptogenic areas outside the tumor into the dose plan [55,56].

REFERENCES

1. F Lesoin, M Jomin. Direct microsurgical approach to intracavernous tumors. Surg Neurol 28:17–22, 1987.
2. LN Sekhar, EM Altschuler. Meningiomas of the cavernous sinus. In: O Al-Mefty, ed. Meningiomas. New York: Raven Press, 1991, pp 445–460.
3. A Sephernia, M Samii, M Tatagiba. Management of intracavernous tumors. An 11-year experience. Acta Neurochir (Wien) 53(suppl):122–126, 1991.
4. F DeMonte, HK Smith, O Al-Mefty. Outcome of aggressive removal of cavernous sinus meningiomas. J Neurosurg 81:245–251, 1994.
5. O DeJesus, LN Sekhar, HK Parikh, DC Wright, DP Wagner. Long-term follow-up of patients with meningiomas involving the cavernous sinus: Recurrence, progression, and quality of life. Neurosurgery 39:915–920, 1996.
6. DK Kim, J Grieve, DJ Archer, D Uttley. Meningiomas in the region of the cavernous sinus: A review of 21 patients. Br J Neurosurg 10:439–444, 1996.
7. DM Long. Comment to Suzuki M, Mizoi K, Yoshimoto T: Should meningiomas involving the cavernous sinus be totally resected? Surg Neurol 44:12–13, 1995.
8. G Pendl, O Schröttner, S Eustacchio, K Feichtinger, J Ganz. Stereotactic radiosurgery of skull base meningiomas. Min Invas Neurosurg 40:87–90, 1997.
9. G Pendl, O Schröttner, S Eustacchio, JC Ganz, K Feichtinger. Cavernous sinus meningiomas—what is the strategy: Upfront or adjuvant Gamma Knife surgery? Stereotact Funct Neurosurg 70(suppl 1):33–40, 1998.

10. CM Duma, LD Lunsford, D Kondziolka IV, GR Harsh, JC Flickinger. Stereotactic radiosurgery of cavernous sinus meningiomas as an addition or alternative to microsurgery. Neurosurgery 32:699–705, 1993.
11. H Nakatomi, T Sasaki, S Kawamoto, T Fujimaki, K Furuya, T Kirino. Primary cavernous sinus malignant lymphoma treated by gamma knife radiosurgery: Case report and review of the literature. Surg Neurol 46:272–279, 1996.
12. JC Ganz, EO Backlund, FA Thorsen. The results of Gamma Knife surgery of meningiomas, related to size of tumor and dose. Stereotact Funct Neurosurg 61(suppl 1):23–29, 1993.
13. A Morita, RJ Coffey, RL Foote, D Schiff, D Gorman. Risk of injury to cranial nerves after gamma knife radiosurgery for skull base meningiomas: Experience in 88 patients. J Neurosurg 90:42–49, 1999.
14. K Nakaya, M Hayashi, S Nakamura, S Atsuchi, H Sato, T Ochial, M Yamamoto, M Izawa, T Hori, K Takaura. Low-dose radiosurgery for meningiomas. Stereotact Funct Neurosurg 72(suppl 1):67–72, 1999.
15. S Nakamura, H Hiyama, K Arai, K Nakaya, H Sato, M Hayashi, T Kawamata, M Izawa, K Takakura. Gamma knife radiosurgery for meningiomas: Four cases of radiation-induced edema. Stereotact Funct Neurosurg 66(suppl 1):142–145, 1996.
16. JC Ganz, O Schröttner, G Pendl. Radiation-induced edema after Gamma Knife treatment for meningiomas. Stereotact Funct Neurosurg 66(suppl 1):129–133, 1996.
17. S Vermeulen, R Young, F Li, R Meier, J Raisis, S Klein, E Kohier. A comparison of single fraction radiosurgery tumor control and toxicity in the treatment of basal and nonbasal meningiomas. Stereotact Funct Neurosurg 72(suppl 1):60–66, 1999.
18. G Noren. Gamma Knife radiosurgery for acoustic neurinomas. In: PL Gildenberg, RR Tasker, eds. Textbook of Stereotactic and Functional Radiosurgery. New York: McGraw-Hill, 1998, pp 835–844.
19. F Unger, C Walch, K Haselsberger, G Papaefthymiou, M Trummer, S Eustacchio, G Pendl. Radiosurgery of vestibular schwannomas: A minimally invasive alternative to microsurgery. Acta Neurochir (Wien) 141:1281–1286, 1999.
20. G Noren, D Greitz, A Hirsch, I Lax. Gamma Knife surgery in acoustic tumors. Acta Neurochir (Wien) 58(suppl):104–107, 1993.
21. BE Pollock, LD Lunsford, D Kondziolka, JC Flickinger, DJ Bissonette, SF Kelsey, PJ Jannetta. Outcome analysis of acoustic neuroma management: A comparison of microsurgery and stereotactic radiosurgery. Neurosurgery 36:215–229, 1995.
22. M Samii, C Matthies. Management of 1000 vestibular schwannomas (acoustic neuromas): The facial nerve preservation and restitution of function. Neurosurgery 40:684–695, 1997.
23. OK Ogunrinde, DL Lunsford, DS Kondziolka, DJ Bissonette, JC Flickinger. Cranial nerve preservation after stereotactic radiosurgery of intracanalicular acoustic tumors. Stereotact Funct Neurosurg 64(suppl 1):87–97, 1995.
24. G Noren. Long-term complications following gamma knife radiosurgery of vestibular schwannomas. Stereotact Funct Neurosurg 70(suppl 1):65–73, 1998.

25. ME Linskey, JC Flickinger, LD Lunsford. Cranial nerve length predicts the risk of delayed facial and trigeminal neuropathies after acoustic tumor stereotactic radiosurgery. Int J Radiat Oncol Biol Phys 25:227–233, 1993.
26. S Vermeulen, R Young, A Posewitz, P Grimm, J Blasko, E Kohler, J Raisis. Stereotactic radiosurgery toxicity in the treatment of intracanalicular acoustic neuromas: The Seattle Northwest gamma knife experience. Stereotact Funct Neurosurg 70(suppl 1):80–87, 1998.
27. G Pendl, JC Ganz, K Kitz, S Eustacchio. Acoustic neurinomas with macrocysts treated with Gamma Knife radiosurgery. Stereotact Funct Neurosurg 66(suppl 1):103–111, 1996.
28. Y Kwon, SK Khang, CJ Kim, DJ Lee, BD Kwun. Radiologic and histopathologic changes after gamma knife radiosurgery for acoustic schwannomas. Stereotact Funct Neurosurg 72(suppl 1):2–10, 1999.
29. MS Kim, SI Lee, JH Sim. Brain tumors with cysts treated with Gamma Knife radiosurgery: Is microsurgery indicated? Stereotact Funct Neurosurg 72(suppl 1):38–44, 1999.
30. WH Slattery III, DE Brackmann. Results of surgery following stereotactic irradiation for acoustic neuromas. Am J Otol 16:315–319, 1995.
31. JC Ganz. Gamma Knife applications in and around the pituitary fossa. In: Gamma Knife Surgery. A Guide for Referring Physicians. Wien: Springer-Verlag, 1993, pp 122–142.
32. KA Leber, J Berglöff, G Langmann, M Mokry, O Schröttner, G Pendl. Radiation sensitivity of visual and oculomotor pathways. Stereotact Funct Neurosurg 64(suppl 1):233–238, 1995.
33. RB Tishler, JS Loeffler, LD Lunsford, C Duma, E Alexander, HM Kooy, JC Flickinger. Tolerance of cranial nerves of the cavernous sinus to radiosurgery. Int J Radiat Oncol Biol Phys 27:212–215, 1993.
34. RB Tishler, JS Loeffler, LD Lunsford, C Duma, E Alexander III, H Kooy, JC Flickinger. Cranial neuropathies following radiosurgery for cavernous sinus lesions. Int J Radiat Oncol Biol Phys 27:215–221, 1993.
35. JC Ganz. Gamma knife treatment of pituitary adenomas. In: AM Landolt, ML Vance, PL Reilly, eds. Pituitary Adenomas. New York: Churchill Livingstone, 1996, pp 461–474.
36. YJ Lim, W Leem, TS Kim, BA Rhee, GK Kim. Four years' experiences in the treatment of pituitary adenomas with gamma knife radiosurgery. Stereotact Funct Neurosurg 70(suppl 1):95–109, 1998.
37. AM Landolt, D Haller, N Lomax, S Scheib, O Schubiger, J Siegfried, G Wellis. Stereotactic radiosurgery for recurrent surgically treated acromegaly. Comparison with fractionated radiotherapy. J Neurosurg 88:1002–1008, 1998.
38. M Mokry, S Ramschak-Schwarzer, J Simbrunner, JC Ganz, G Pendl. A six year experience with the postoperative radiosurgical management of pituitary adenomas. Stereotact Funct Neurosurg 72(suppl 1):88–100, 1999.
39. JC Ganz, E-O Backlund, FA Thorson. The effects of gamma knife surgery of pituitary adenomas on tumor growth and endocrinopathies. Stereotact Funct Neurosurg 61(suppl 1):30–37, 1993.

40. JC Ganz. Gamma knife treatment of pituitary adenomas. Stereotact Funct Neurosurg 64(suppl 1):3–10, 1995.
41. BE Pollock, D Kondziolka, LD Lunsford, JC Flickinger. Stereotactic radiosurgery for pituitary adenomas: Imaging, visual and endocrine results. Acta Neurochir (Wien) 62(suppl):33–38, 1994.
42. M Degerblad, T Rähn, G Bergstrand, M Thoren. Long term results of stereotactic radiosurgery to the pituitary gland in Cushing's disease. Acta Endocrinol Copenhagen 112:310–314, 1986.
43. I Morange-Ramos, J Regis, H Dufour, JM Andrieu, F Grisoli, P Jaquet, JC Peragut. Short term endocrinological results after gamma knife radiosurgery of pituitary adenomas. Stereotact Funct Neurosurg 70(suppl 1):127–138, 1998.
44. M Thoren, T Rähn, B Hallengren, PH Kaad, KO Nilsson, H Ravn, M Ritzen, KE Petersen, D Aarskog. Treatment of Cushing's disease in childhood and adolescence by stereotactic pituitary irradiation. Acta Paediatr Scand 75:388–395, 1986.
45. T Kobayashi, T Tanaka, Y Kida. Stereotactic gamma radiosurgery of craniopharyngioma. Pediatr Neurosurg 21(suppl 1):69–74, 1994.
46. L Steiner, C Linquist, M Steiner. Radiosurgery. In: L Symon, L Calliann, F Cohadon, J Lobo Autunes, F Loew, H Nornes, E Pastar, JD Pickard, AJ Strong, MG Yasarpil, eds. Advances and Technical Standards in Neurosurgery. Vol 19. Wien, New York: Springer, 1993, pp 19–102.
47. H Takahashi, S Nakazawa, T Shimura. Evaluation of postoperative injection of bleomycin for craniopharyngioma in children. J Neurosurg 62:120–127, 1985.
48. M Mokry. Craniopharyngiomas—a six year experience with Gamma Knife radiosurgery. Stereotact Funct Neurosurg 72(suppl 1):140–149, 1999.
49. E-O Backlund. Treatment of craniopharyngiomas. The multimodality approach. Pediatr Neurosurg 21(suppl):82–89, 1994.
50. JD Green, DE Brackmann, CD Nguyen, MA Arriaga, FF Telischi, A De la Cruz. Surgical management of previously untreated glomus jugulare tumors. Laryngoscope 104:917–921, 1994
51. R Liscak, V Vladyka, B Wowra, A Kemeny, D Forster, JA Burzaco, R Martinez, S Eustacchio, G Pendl, J Regis, W Pellet. Gamma Knife radiosurgery of glomus jugulare tumor—early multicentre experience. Acta Neurochir (Wien) 141:1141–1146, 1999.
52. S Eustacchio, K Leber, M Trummer, F Unger, G Pendl. Gamma Knife radiosurgery for glomus jugulare tumors. Acta Neurochir (Wien) 141:811–818, 1999.
53. J Legat, M Morkry, K Leber, O Schröttner, G Pendl. Gamma knife radiosurgery for midline lesions. Kitakanto Med J 1:41–50, 1998.
54. F Unger, O Schröttner, K Haselsberger, E Körner, R Ploier, G Pendl. Gamma Knife radiosurgery in hypothalamic hamartomas with medically intractable epilepsy and precocious puberty: Report of two cases. J Neurosurg 92:726–731, 2000.

55. CJ Whang, Y Kwon. Long-term follow up of stereotactic Gamma Knife radiosurgery in epilepsy. Stereotact Funct Neurosurg 66(suppl 1):349–356, 1996.

56. O Schröttner, HG Eder, F Unger, K Feichtinger, G Pendl. Radiosurgery in lesional epilepsy: Brain tumors. Stereotact Funct Neurosurg 70(suppl 1):50–56, 1998.

57. E Alexander, JS Loeffler, DL Lunsford, eds. Stereotactic Radiosurgery. New York: McGraw-Hill, 1993.

14

Stereotactic Radiosurgery: Gliomas

Jay S. Loeffler

Massachusetts General Hospital and Harvard Medical School, Boston, Massachusetts, U.S.A.

Alan C. Hartford

Northeast Proton Therapy Center, Boston, Massachusetts, U.S.A.

1 INTRODUCTION

Stereotactic radiosurgery for the treatment of primary malignant gliomas is counterintuitive. Radiosurgery provides a high dose of ionizing radiation to a small, well-defined volume of tissue, whereas gliomas tend to be large, diffuse, and infiltrating. Nevertheless, standard therapeutic approaches in the management of gliomas yield discouraging results, with the majority of patients diagnosed with glioblastoma multiforme (GBM) suffering local recurrence and dying within a year of diagnosis, and with survival beyond 2 years being rare. Nearly 80% of GBM recurrences occur within 2 cm of the primary site after conventional therapies [1]. In this context, either by retarding or preventing recurrence, dose escalation in areas with greatest tumor cell density may offer significant benefit for the individual patient while sparing normal functioning brain tissue lying on the periphery.

2 MANAGEMENT OF PRIMARY GLIOMAS USING STEREOTACTIC RADIATION

Clinical experiences with focal boost techniques include trials of brachytherapy, stereotactic radiosurgery, and fractionated proton radiotherapy, each

137

designed to escalate dose to well-defined volumes within the target tumor tissue. Major series are summarized in Table 1.

2.1 Stereotactic Brachytherapy

During the 1980s, stereotactic brachytherapy yielded encouraging results as a treatment for selected patients with recurrent disease. These results led to the use of iodine-125 (I-125) brachytherapy as boost technique for primary glioblastoma, with early results suggesting a substantial increase in survival when compared with historical controls [2]. Larger series also demonstrated encouraging results, with patients receiving additional median boost doses between 50 and 60 Gy after surgical biopsy or resection and external beam irradiation of 60 Gy in 30 to 33 fractions (Table 1).

A large series from the University of California at San Francisco (UCSF) demonstrated a 3-year survival rate of 22% within median survival of 20 months for 106 patients with primary glioblastoma [3]. A subgroup of these patients was enrolled in the Northern California Oncology Group (NCOG) Study 6G-82-2. These patients received hydroxyurea during the external beam irradiation, and thereafter, adjuvant procarbazine, lomustine (CCNU), and vincristine chemotherapy (PCV) for 1 year [4]. Although 30 of the 64 GBM patients on this trial were excluded from receiving brachytherapy, mostly because of intercurrent death or tumor progression, for all enrolled patients the median survival was 67 weeks, with nine patients alive after 2 years' follow-up, and three alive after 3 years. Among the 34 GBM patients who did receive brachytherapy, the median survival was 88 weeks.

Similarly, at the Joint Center for Radiation Therapy, 56 patients were treated with surgery, limited field external beam radiotherapy to 60 Gy, and brachytherapy for an additional 50 Gy. These were compared to a set of 40 historical controls with similar clinical and radiologic characteristics [5]. Median survival for the brachytherapy group was 18 months, compared with 11 months for the historical control group.

One randomized trial addressed the value of I-125 brachytherapy as a boost for treatment for high-grade glioma. The Brain Tumor Cooperative Group Trial 87-01, published in abstract form, demonstrated an improvement in median survival for eligible patients who underwent stereotactic implant boost [6]. More than 250 patients (87% with the diagnosis of GBM) were randomized to receive 60 Gy brachytherapy or to be observed, after external beam irradiation and carmustine chemotherapy (BCNU). The median survival for those randomized to receive I-125 brachytherapy was 16 months versus 13 months for the control group, with the reoperation rates similar for the two groups (50% and 42%, respectively).

TABLE 1 Stereotactic Radiation Boost for Primary Glioblastoma Multiforme

Institution	Median minimum boost	Diameter size limit (cm)	Median boost volume (cm^3)	Patient number	Median survival (months)	Survival at 2 years (%)	Reoperation rate (%)
Brachytherapy							
UCSF (3)	52.9 Gy	< 6 cm	N/S	106	20	39%	38%
JCRT (5)	50.0 Gy	≤ 5 cm	22 cm^3	56	18	34%	64%
BTCG (6)	60.0 Gy	N/S	N/S	125	16	N/S	50%
Sterotactic radiosurgery							
JCRT, Wisconsin, and Florida (14)	12.0 Gy	≤ 4 cm	10.0 cm^3	96	21	38%	29%
Pittsburgh (15)	15.5 Gy	< 3.5 cm	6.5 cm^3	45	20	41%	19%
Harvard (16)	12 Gy	≤ 4 cm	9.4 cm^3	78	20	36%	50%
Fractionated proton radiotherapy (10 fractions/ week for 5 weeks)							
MGH-HCL (19)	33.5 CGE (total dose 93.5 CGE)	≤ 5 cm	36 cm^3	23	20	34%	57%

N/S, not stated.

2.2   Stereotactic Radiosurgery

The encouraging results of stereotactic brachytherapy, which enabled the escalation of radiation dose within a well-defined volume beyond the capabilities of conventional external-beam techniques, led to several centers applying techniques of stereotactic radiosurgery (SRS) to the management of patients presenting with GBM tumors. Stereotactic radiosurgery provided another radiation therapy technique for marked dose escalation while avoiding some of the potential risks of the brachytherapy implant procedure in patients with serious coexisting morbidities or tumors located in relatively inaccessible or eloquent regions of the brain. This early experience with SRS for GBM tumors suggested benefits comparable to those seen with stereotactic brachytherapy, with several GBM patients surviving beyond 2 years at rates higher than what would be expected for conventional therapies [7–9]. However, other data suggested the observed survival benefit accruing from SRS for glioma patients might be ascribable to selection factors, particularly a smaller total target volume for the SRS boost, rather than to improved outcomes after radiosurgery [10–12].

In the early 1990s, recursive partitioning analysis of several Radiation Therapy Oncology Group (RTOG) studies yielded detailed information about selection factors that influenced the prognosis for glioma patients (Table 2) [13]. Given the importance of these selection factors in the survival of conventionally treated patients—including age, performance status, and extent of resection—subsequent studies of the efficacy of SRS boost treatments controlled for these prognostic factors (Table 3) [14–16].

Using the RTOG analysis, one series from the Joint Center for Radiation Therapy (JCRT), the University of Wisconsin, and the University of Florida examined a combined group of 96 patients with GBM, along with an additional 19 patients with anaplastic astrocytoma, partitioned into prognostic classes III through VI [14]. As shown in Table 3, the relative risk of death for SRS-treated patients was about half that of the RTOG patients, for prognostic groups III through V.

Similarly, 65 patients at the University of Pittsburgh underwent SRS as part of their initial management plans for histologically proven anaplastic astrocytoma or glioblastoma [15]. The patients who were included had a contrast-enhancing tumor diameter size (the disease targeted for SRS boost) that was limited to less than 3.5 cm, although the study did include tumors in sensitive locations such as the diencephalon and brainstem. Like the JCRT/Wisconsin/Florida study, for patients with RTOG groups III, IV, and V, SRS yielded about a doubling of the survival rate at 2 years (Table 3). Although neither RTOG class nor extent of resection appeared predictive in this study, multivariate analysis did show age, Karnofsky score of 70 or higher, and histology to be important predictors of survival.

TABLE 2 RTOG Definitions of Prognostic Classes for Malignant Glioma Patients with Estimated Survival Rates Using Standard Therapies (13)

Prognostic class	GBM patients	Anaplastic astrocytoma patients	Survival at two years
I	N/A	Age < 50; normal mental status	76%
II	N/A	Age ≥ 50; KPS ≥ 70; more than 3 months of symptoms	68%
III	Age < 50; KPS ≥ 90	Age < 50; abnormal mental status	35%
IV	Age < 50; KPS < 90 —or— Age ≥ 50; KPS ≥ 70; at least partial surgical resection; able to work	Age ≥ 50; KPS ≥ 70; no more than 3 months of symptoms	15%
V	Age ≥ 50; along with: KPS < 70; normal mental status —or— KPS ≥ 70; at least partial surgical resection; not able to work —or— KPS ≥ 70; biopsy only and dose > 54.4 Gy	Age ≥ 50; KPS < 70; normal mental status	6%
VI	Age ≥ 50; along with: KPS < 70; abnormal mental status —or— KPS ≥ 70; biopsy only and dose ≤ 54.4 Gy	Age ≥ 50; KPS < 70; abnormal mental status	4%

RTOG, Radiation Therapy Oncology Group; KPS, Karnovsky Performance Status; GBM, glioblastoma multiforme.

TABLE 3 Comparison of 2-Year Survival Rates (%), Stratified by RTOG-Defined Risk Groups: III, IV, V, and VI

Series stratified by risk group	III	IV	V	VI
Historical controls—RTOG standard risk groups (13)	35% (175)	15% (457)	6% (395)	4% (263)
SRS—combined experience of Wisconsin, JCRT, and Gainesville (14)	75% (24)	34% (35)	21% (43)	(3 pts included in class V)
SRS—Univ. of Pittsburgh (15)	73% (13)	24% (11)	26% (24)	0% (2)
SRS—JCRT (16)	58% (27)	23% (29)	23% (22)	N/A
Fractionated treatment—MGH-HCL (19)	57% (7)	43% (7)	22% (9)	N/A

Numbers of patients in each group at time of diagnosis are shown in parentheses. **RTOG**, Radiation Therapy Oncology Group; **SRS**, Stereostatic Radiotherapy; **JCRT**, Joint Center for Radiation Therapy; **MGH-HCL**, Massachusetts General Hospital–Harvard Cyclotron Laboratory.

Shrieve and coworkers found similar results for 78 patients with GBM tumors treated with SRS boost after attempted surgical resection and standard postoperative radiation therapy [16]. Patients were eligible for SRS treatment if tumors measured no more than 4 cm in diameter with contrast enhancement, excluding edema. Seven patients showed no enhancing tumor on the postoperative imaging studies, in which cases the surgical cavity was treated with a 5-mm margin. Again, similar to the results from Pittsburgh, SRS showed a substantial improvement in 2-year survival rates, when compared with the RTOG historical control groups (Table 3).

2.3 Fractionated Stereotactic Radiotherapy

Although several studies have investigated alternative fractionation schemes as attempts to achieve radiobiological advantages with high doses in the treatment of glial neoplasms [17,18], only one study has investigated the use of fractionated radiotherapy to boost gliomas beyond more conventional dose levels to the higher levels that may be biologically comparable to stereotactic radiosurgery or brachytherapy. A phase I/II protocol at the Massachusetts General Hospital (MGH) studied 23 GBM patients treated with a mixture of photons and protons to doses above 90 cobalt gray equivalents (CGE), treating two fractions a day with a minimum 6-hour interfraction interval, for a total of 5 weeks [19]. Conventional volumes received a median dose of 64.8 CGE, and volumes considered at highest risk for harboring residual disease were boosted to a median total dose of 93.5 CGE. Although 10 patients showed no residual gadolinium enhancement after resection and another eight had residual enhancing volumes ranging from 0.1 to 1.0 cm^3, across all patients the median volume receiving the high-dose boost was 36 cm^3. This high-dose boost volume encompassed the remaining surgical cavity on the earliest postoperative imaging study, as well as any remaining gadolinium-enhancing tissue.

Stratifying by RTOG prognostic group, the results of this study were roughly comparable to the various SRS series (Table 3). The reoperation rate, however, was relatively high (13/23 = 57%). Of these 13 patients five underwent biopsies subsequent to radiation therapy, five underwent one resection, whereas three underwent multiple resections. Among the 15 patients with pathological material available for analysis subsequent to radiation therapy, all showed evidence of extensive tumor necrosis, but 60% also showed evidence of tumor persistence or recurrence. The median survival for patients showing only tumor necrosis was 29 months, as compared with 16 months for those also with pathological evidence of tumor recurrence ($P = 0.01$). In only one of the nine pathologically documented recurrences was tumor found within the 90-CGE volume, although among all 23 patients, 18

(78%) developed new enhancement on MR imaging within the high-dose target volume, suggesting that most of these imaging changes represented tissue necrosis rather than tumor recurrence.

2.4 Indications for SRS in the Treatment of Primary High-Grand Gliomas

In summary, in comparison with conventional radiation therapy, following maximal surgical debulking with SRS provides a survival benefit for appropriately selected patients. Major series demonstrate survival rates that appear almost double those achieved with conventional radiation therapy. This likely benefit of SRS has persuaded the neuro-oncology community to pursue a phase-III trial, RTOG 93-05, randomizing GBM patients with less than 4-cm tumors (all of whom receive BCNU chemotherapy) between (1) standard radiation therapy versus (2) radiosurgery followed by standard radiation therapy. To date, more than 250 patients have been randomized, and the results are pending.

Some commentators suggest that within each RTOG risk group, there may be further patient selection effects that account for the observed differences in survival rates, particularly for patients with residual contrast-enhancing tumor volumes that are small or non-existent. However, the results of the proton-dose escalation study argue against this objection. Among these 23 patients 10 (43%) had no postoperative gadolinium enhancement. Therefore, in terms of residual enhancing tumor, this study represents a subgroup more favorable than those patients in the study by Shrieve et al., in which only 7 of 78 patients had no postoperative gadolinium tumor enhancement [16], and more favorable than those in the study of Kondziolka et al., in which (the authors imply that) all GBM patients evinced some enhancement [15]. There was only one documented recurrence in the high-dose volumes treated with protons. These treatment volumes were substantially larger than the SRS median boost volumes in the two other studies, yet the survival benefits by RTOG risk classification were comparable to those achieved with SRS (Table 3). Thus, the clinical benefits that could be achieved with 90 CGE using fractionated therapy to larger volumes with smaller tumors— benefits that were confirmed on pathological review—were comparable to the clinical benefits achieved with SRS boosts to smaller volumes with *larger* tumors. Together, these points argue against the suggestion that the benefits to SRS boost treatment seen in Table 3 are ascribable only to selection effects attributable to target tumor volume.

For very large targets with postoperative enhancement beyond 3.5 to 4.0 cm in diameter, the likelihood of radiosurgical complications increases. For these cases, however, the MGH proton study demonstrates that fractionated conformal irradiation can be clinically delivered to larger volumes while maintaining high pathologic complete response rates in the high-dose volume. Further investigations are indicated in this regard, such as RTOG 98-03, a phase I/II radiation study investigating fractionated dose escalation from 66 Gy up to 82 Gy, applying conformal radiation technologies to the treatment of large supratentorial GBM tumors.

3 THE MANAGEMENT OF RECURRENT GLIOMAS

There are several treatment options for patients with recurrent malignant gliomas, including reoperation, radiosurgery, interstitial implantation, and chemotherapy [20]. Historically, chemotherapy has been the standard therapy for recurrent gliomas, yet results are discouraging. For example, Levin et al. reported a 55% response rate to combination chemotherapy for recurrent GBM disease with a median time to progression of 23 weeks [21]. Overall, tumor location, size, the patient's overall condition, and the prior therapeutic history each plays a role in the choice of appropriate modality.

3.1 Surgery for Recurrent Gliomas

One series from UCSF showed that in younger patients with higher Karnofsky scores and with large, surgically accessible, recurrent tumors that caused deficits from compression rather than infiltration, reoperation contributed to high quality postoperative survival [Karnovsky Performance Status (KPS ≥ 70) as well as to overall survival, with a median overall survival of 36 weeks after reoperation [22]. A more recent series confirmed a median survival of 36 weeks for patients selected for reoperation, along with a median high-quality survival period of 18 weeks, compared with total median survival of 23 weeks after first tumor progression for patients not undergoing reoperations [23]. Postoperative improvements in KPS scores (28% of patients) were slightly more likely than declines in KPS scores (23% of patients), with these improvements most likely in those patients who had symptomatic recurrences.

3.2 Stereotactic Radiosurgery for Recurrent Disease

Stereotactic radiosurgery also has a role in the management of recurrent glial tumors after standard therapeutic approaches. First presented in 1995, the results of RTOG 90-05 demonstrated that the incidence of severe central nervous system (CNS) toxicity in previously irradiated brain tissues subsequently treated with SRS for recurrence was a function of both the target volume and the prescribed dose. Nevertheless, the incidence of complications could be maintained at an acceptable, low level while providing clinically meaningful doses to malignant tissues. There were chronic, severe CNS toxicities in 14% of patients who had 3.1 to 4.0-cm tumors treated to 15.0 Gy, in 20% of patients who had 2.1 to 3.0-cm tumors treated to 18.0 Gy, and in 10% of patients who had up to 2.0-cm tumors treated to 24.0 Gy [24].

Similar to results from the reoperation series, studies of SRS for recurrent gliomas have shown median survivals after SRS treatment across all treated patients that range from 7 to 10 months [25–29]. In a series from Boston, comparison of patients undergoing SRS and those receiving stereotactic brachytherapy suggested the two modalities had similar survival benefits [27]. For SRS, the median actuarial survival from time of treatment for recurrence was 10.2 months, whereas for brachytherapy the median actuarial survival after treatment was 11.5 months. Patients receiving SRS had somewhat smaller tumor volumes compared with brachytherapy (median 10.1 cm^3 vs 29 cm^3). Among the SRS patients, younger age and a tumor volume less than 10.1 cm^3 were predictive of better outcome; however, for brachytherapy patients, patient age was predictive of outcome, whereas tumor volume, interval from initial diagnosis, and tumor dose were not. Of 86 patients treated with SRS, 19 (22%) required subsequent reoperation, whereas 14 of 32 patients (44%) required reoperation after brachytherapy; furthermore, the outcomes after SRS were independent of a need for reoperation. This comparison suggests that, for patients qualifying for SRS at time of recurrence, and particularly for younger patients with limited-volume tumor recurrences, SRS is the preferred therapeutic option. For larger tumors or irregularly shaped volumes, other modalities may be more appropriate.

3.3 Fractionated Stereotactic Radiation Therapy for Recurrent Gliomas

Some recent data suggest that fractionated stereotactic radiation therapy (SRT) may be of benefit for patients otherwise unsuitable for SRS. Cho and colleagues evaluated 71 patients with recurrent high-grade gliomas: 46 patients received single-fraction SRS (median 17 Gy to the 50% isodose surface), and 25 received fractionated SRT (37.5 Gy in 15 fractions to the 85% isodose surface) [30]. Patients in the SRS group had more favorable prognostic factors than those in the SRT group, including median age (48 vs 53 years), median KPS (70 vs 60), and median tumor volume (10 vs 25 cm^3), but median survival times were comparable for the two groups: 11 months for the SRS group and 12 months for the SRT group. Late complications developed in 14 (30%) of the 46 SRS patients but in only 2 (8%) of the 25 SRT patients, suggesting the SRT dose-fractionation schemes were less toxic than the SRS plans.

There may be a role for chemotherapy, in combination with fractionated stereotactic radiation therapy (SRT), in the treatment of recurrent glial tumors. One pilot study treated 14 patients with recurrent glioblastoma that had median tumor volumes of 15.7 cm^3, using fractionated stereotactic radiation therapy along with Taxol as a radiation sensitizer [31]. Taxol was given once per week for 4 weeks, with an SRT treatment delivered immediately after each Taxol infusion. The median radiation dose per week was 6.0 Gy at the 90% isodose line, for a median total dose of 24 Gy in four fractions. The median survival from time of treatment for recurrence was 14.2 months, but with a short minimum follow-up of 10 months. The fractionated radiation dose appeared well-tolerated, with only four patients undergoing reoperation. These data suggest that, for large volume recurrences not surgically accessible or amenable to SRS, there may be a role for fractionated SRT, perhaps in conjunction with systemic chemotherapy. Further studies are required.

4 CONCLUSION

Stereotactic radiosurgery is effective in the treatment of selected primary and recurrent glial neoplasms. After maximal tumor resection, in conjunction with a standard course of radiation therapy, SRS boost likely improves survival for patients in RTOG risk classes III, IV, and V. We anticipate RTOG 93-05 will confirm this survival benefit. For primary tumors with anatomically amenable, well-defined postoperative residual volumes less than 4 cm in diameter, SRS is the preferred radiation boost technique, whether using Linac radiosurgery, the Leksell Gamma Knife, or proton radiosurgery. For larger lesions, irregular volumes, or difficult anatomical constraints, other boost techniques may be considered, including brachytherapy, fractionated stereotactic irradiation, or proton radiotherapy. For focally recurrent GBM disease, patients with small (less than 3 cm in diameter), radiographically distinct lesions may benefit from SRS. Larger lesions, especially those adjacent to eloquent cortex or critical white matter pathways, must be evaluated with caution. Although SRS offers another tool in the treatment of high-grade gliomas, these tumors continue to present a serious therapeutic challenge, and overall results are still dismal. Further innovations in dose-delivery, targeting, and adjuvant treatments are required.

REFERENCES

1. KE Wallner, JH Galicich, G Krol, E Arbit, MG Malkin. Patterns of failure following treatment for glioblastoma multiforme and anaplastic astrocytoma. Int J Radiat Oncol Biol Phys 16:1405–1409, 1988.

2. JS Loeffler, E Alexander, III, PY Wen, WM Shea, CN Coleman, HM Kooy, HA Fine, LA Nedzi, B Silver, NE Riese, PM Black. Results of stereotactic brachytherapy used in the initial management of patients with glioblastoma. J Natl Cancer Inst 82:1918–1921, 1990.
3. CO Scharfen, PK Sneed, WM Wara, DA Larson, TL Phillips, MD Prados, KA Weaver, M Malec, P Acord, KR Lamborn, SA Lamb, B Ham, PH Gutin. High activity iodine-125 interstitial implant for gliomas. Int J Radiat Oncol Biol Phys 24:583–591, 1992.
4. PH Gutin, MD Prados, TL Phillips, WM Wara, DA Larson, SA Leibel, PK Sneed, VA Levin, KA Weaver, P Silver, K Lamborn, S Lamb, B Ham. External irradiation followed by an interstitial high activity iodine-125 implant "boost" in the initial treatment of malignant gliomas: NCOG study 6G-82-2. Int J Radiat Oncol Biol Phys 21:601–606, 1991.
5. PY Wen, E Alexander III, PM Black, HA Fine, N Riese, JM Levin, CN Coleman, JS Loeffler. Long term results of stereotactic brachytherapy used in the initial treatment of patients with glioblastomas. Cancer 73:3029–3036, 1994.
6. SB Green, WR Shapiro, PC Burger, et al. A randomized trial of interstitial radiotherapy (RT) boost for newly diagnosed malignant glioma: Brain Tumor Cooperative Group (BTCG) trial 8701 [abstract]. Proc Annu Meet Am Soc Clin Oncol 13:A486, 1994.
7. JS Loeffler, E Alexander III, WM Shea, PY Wen, HA Fine, HM Kooy, PM Black. Radiosurgery as part of the initial management of patients with malignant gliomas. J Clin Oncol 10:1379–1385, 1992.
8. MP Mehta, J Masciopinto, J Rozental, A Levin, R Chappell, K Bastin, J Miles, P Turski, S Kubsad, T Mackie, T Kinsella. Stereotactic radiosurgery for glioblastoma multiforme: Report of a prospective study evaluating prognostic factors and analyzing long-term survival advantage. Int J Radiat Oncol Biol Phys 30:541–549, 1994.
9. D Gannett, B Stea, B Lulu, T Adair, C Verdi, A Hamilton. Stereotactic radiosurgery as an adjunct to surgery and external beam radiotherapy in the treatment of patients with malignant gliomas. Int J Radiat Oncol Biol Phys 33:461–468, 1995.
10. WJ Curran Jr, AS Weinstein, LA Martin, JS Nelson, TL Phillips, K Murray, AJ Fischbach, D Yakar, JG Schwade. Survival comparison of radiosurgery-eligible and -ineligible malignant glioma patients treated with hyperfractionated radiation therapy and carmustine: A report of Radiation Therapy Oncology Group 83-02. J Clin Oncol 11:857–862, 1993.
11. JM Buatti, WA Friedman, FJ Bova, WM Mendenhall. Linac radiosurgery for high-grade gliomas: The University of Florida experience. Int J Radiat Oncol Biol Phys 32:205–210, 1995.
12. JE Masciopinto, AB Levin, MP Mehta, BS Rhode. Stereotactic radiosurgery for glioblastoma: A final report of 31 patients. J Neurosurg 82:530–535, 1995.
13. WJ Curran Jr, CB Scott, J Horton, JS Nelson, AS Weinstein, AJ Fischbach, CH Chang, M Rotman, SO Asbell, RE Krisch, DF Nelson. Recursive parti-

tioning analysis of prognostic factors in three radiation therapy oncology group malignant glioma trials. J Natl Cancer Inst 85:704–710, 1993.

14. JN Sarkaria, MP Mehta, JS Loeffler, JM Buatti, RJ Chappell, AB Levin, E Alexander III, WA Frieman, TJ Kinsella. Radiosurgery in the initial management of malignant gliomas: Survival comparison with the RTOG recursive partitioning analysis. Int J Radiat Oncol Biol Phys 32:931–941, 1995.

15. D Kondziolka, JC Flickinger, DJ Bissonette, M Bozik, LD Lunsford. Survival benefit of stereotactic radiosurgery for patients with malignant glial neoplasms. Neurosurgery 41:776–785, 1997.

16. DC Shrieve, E Alexander III, PM Black, PY Wen, HA Fine, HM Kooy, JS Loeffler. Treatment of patients with primary glioblastoma multiforme with standard postoperative radiotherapy and radiosurgical boost: Prognostic factors and long-term outcome. J Neurosurg 90:72–77, 1999.

17. M Werner-Wasik, CB Scott, DF Nelson, LE Gaspar, KJ Murray, JA Fischbach, JS Nelson, AS Weinstein, WJ Curran Jr. Final report of a phase I/II trial of hyperfractionated and accelerated hyperfractionated radiation therapy with carmustine for adults with supratentiorial malignant gliomas. Radiation Therapy Oncology Group Study 83-02. Cancer 77:1535–1543, 1996.

18. C Fallai, P Olmi. Hyperfractionated and accelerated radiation therapy in central nervous system tumors (malignant gliomas, pediatric tumors, and brain metastases). Radiother Oncol 43:235–246, 1997.

19. MM Fitzek, AF Thornton, JD Rabinov, MH Lev, FS Pardo, JE Munzenrider, P Okunieff, M Bussiere, I Braun, FH Hochberg, ET Hedley-Whyte, NJ Liebsch, GR Harsh IV. Accelerated fractionated proton/photon irradiation to 90 cobalt gray equivalent for glioblastoma multiforme: Results of a phase II prospective trial. J Neurosurg 91:251–260, 1999.

20. DA Larson, WM Wara. Radiotherapy of primary malignant brain tumors. Sem Surg Oncol 14:34–42, 1998.

21. V Levin, S Phuphanich, H Liu, V DaSilva, J Murovic, A Choucair, M Chamberlain, M Berger, M Seager, RL Davis, P Silver, PH Gutin, CB Wilson. Phase II study of combined BCNU and 5-fluorouracil, hydroxyurea, and 6-mercaptopurine (BHFM) for the treatment of malignant gliomas. Cancer Treat Rep 70:1271–1274, 1986.

22. GR Harsh IV, VA Levin, PH Gutin, M Seager, P Silver, CB Wilson. Reoperation for recurrent glioblastoma and anaplastic astrocytoma. Neurosurgery 21: 615–621, 1987.

23. FG Barker II, SM Chang, PH Gutin, MK Malec, MW McDermott, MD Prados, CB Wilson. Survival and functional status after resection of recurrent glioblastoma multiforme. Neurosurgery 42:709–723, 1998.

24. E Shaw, C Scott, L Souhami, R Dinapoli, JP Bahary, R Kline, M Wharam, C Schultz, P Davey, J Loeffler, JD Rowe, L Marks, B Fisher, K Shin. Radiosurgery for the treatment of previously irradiated recurrent primary brain tumors and brain metastases: Initial report of radiation therapy oncology group protocol (90-05). Int J Radiat Oncol Biol Phys 34:647–654, 1996.

25. MC Chamberlain, D Barba, P Kormanik, WMC Shea. Stereotactic radiosurgery for recurrent gliomas. Cancer 74:1342–1347, 1994.
26. WA Hall, HR Djalilian, PW Sperduto, KH Cho, BJ Gerbi, JP Gibbons, M Rohr, HB Clark. Stereotactic radiosurgery for recurrent malignant gliomas. J Clin Oncol 13:1642–1648, 1995.
27. DC Shrieve, E Alexander III, PY Wen, HA Fine, HM Kooy, PM Black, JS Loeffler. Comparison of stereotactic radiosurgery and brachytherapy in the treatment of recurrent glioblastoma multiforme. Neurosurgery 36:275–284, 1995.
28. MW McDermott, PK Sneed, SM Chang, PH Gutin, WM Wara, LJ Verhey. Results of radiosurgery for recurrent gliomas. In: D Kondziolka, ed. Radiosurgery. Basel: Karger, 1996, pp 102–112.
29. M van Kampen, R Engenhart-Cabillic, J Debus, M Fuss, B Rhen, M Wannenmacher. The radiosurgery of glioblastoma multiforme in cases of recurrence. The Heidelberg experiences compared to the literature. Strahlenther Onkol 174: 19–24, 1998.
30. KH Cho, WA Hall, BJ Gerbi, PD Higgins, WA McGuire, HB Clark. Single dose versus fractionated stereotactic radiotherapy for recurrent high-grade gliomas. Int J Radiat Oncol Biol Phys 45:1133–1141, 1999.
31. G Lederman, E Arbit, M Odaimi, E Lombardi, M Wrzolek, M Wronski. Fractionated stereotactic radiosurgery and concurrent taxol in recurrent glioblastoma multiforme: A preliminary report. Int J Radiat Oncol Biol Phys 40:661–666, 1998.

15

Stereotactic Radiosurgery: Arteriovenous Malformations

Kelly D. Foote and William A. Friedman
University of Florida, Gainesville, Florida, U.S.A.

1 INTRODUCTION

The most devastating presentation associated with arteriovenous malformations (AVMs) of the brain is intracerebral hemorrhage. Numerous natural history studies have demonstrated a substantial (3% to 4% per year) risk of hemorrhage in patients harboring AVMs [1–5]. Several treatment modalities (microsurgery, radiosurgery, or endovascular therapy) are available that may eliminate the lesion before a hemorrhage can occur—or recur, in the case of a hemorrhagic presentation. When an AVM is amenable to safe microsurgical resection, this therapy is preferred because it offers immediate cure and elimination of hemorrhage risk. When the surgical morbidity is judged to be excessive, radiosurgery offers a reasonable expectation of delayed cure.

When an AVM is treated with radiosurgery a pathologic process appears to be induced that is similar to the response-to-injury model of atherosclerosis. Radiation injury to the vascular endothelium is believed to induce the proliferation of smooth-muscle cells and the elaboration of extracellular collagen. This leads to progressive stenosis and obliteration of the AVM nidus (Fig. 1) [6–10], thereby eliminating the risk of hemorrhage.

The advantages of radiosurgery—compared to microsurgical and endovascular treatments—are that it is noninvasive, has minimal risk of acute

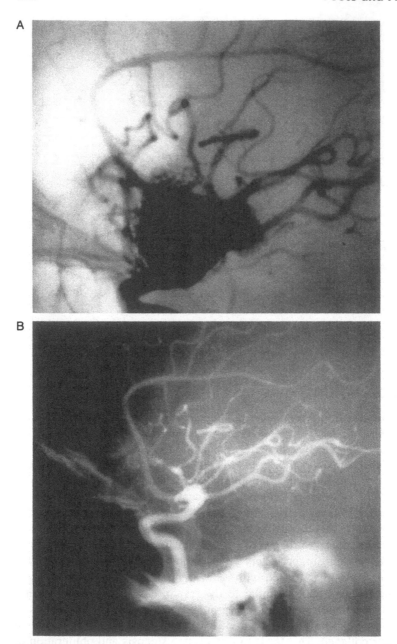

FIGURE 1   Before and after radiosurgery for arteriovenous malformation
(AVM). **A,** This patient received 17.5 Gy to the margin of the nidus of
this left frontotemporal AVM. **B,** On follow-up angiography 3 years later,
the lesion has been completely obliterated.

complications, and is performed as an outpatient procedure requiring no recovery time for the patient. The primary disadvantage of radiosurgery is that cure is not immediate. Thrombosis of the lesion is achieved in the majority of cases, but it commonly does not occur until 2 or 3 years after treatment. During the interval between radiosurgical treatment and AVM thrombosis, the risk of hemorrhage remains. Another potential disadvantage of radiosurgery is possible long-term adverse effects of radiation. Finally, radiosurgery has been shown to be much less effective for lesions over 10 cc in volume. For these reasons, selection of an appropriate treatment modality depends on multiple variables, including perceived risks of surgery and predicted lielihood of hemorrhage for a given patient.

2 AVM RADIOSURGERY TECHNIQUE

The technical methods of radiosurgery have been described at length in other publications [11], but a brief description of radiosurgical techniques that apply specifically to AVM treatment is in order. The fundamental elements of any successful radiosurgical treatment include the following: patient selection, head ring application, stereotactic image acquisition, treatment planning, dose selection, radiation delivery and follow-up. All of these elements are critical, and poor performance of any step will result in suboptimal results.

2.1 Patient Selection

Open surgery is generally favored if an AVM is amenable to low-risk resection (e.g., low Spetzler-Martin grade, young healthy patient) or is felt to be at high risk for hemorrhage during the latency period between radiosurgical treatment and AVM obliteration (e.g., associated aneurysm, prior hemorrhage, large AVM with diffuse morphology, venous outflow obstruction).

Radiosurgery is favored when the AVM nidus is small (<3 cm) and compact, when surgery is judged to carry a high risk or is refused by the patient, or when the risk of hemorrhage is not felt to be extraordinarily high.

Endovascular treatment, although rarely curative alone, may be useful as a preoperative adjunct to either microsurgery or radiosurgery.

The history, physical examination, and diagnostic imaging of each patient are evaluated, and the various factors outlined above are weighed in combination to determine the best treatment approach for a given case.

2 Head Ring Application

The techniques for optimal head ring application for AVM radiosurgery are no different from those for other target lesions, and are described in detail elsewhere [11].

2.3 Stereotactic Image Acquisition

The most problematic aspect of AVM radiosurgery is target identification. In some series (see below), targeting error is listed as the most frequent cause of radiosurgical failure. The problem lies with imaging. Angiography very effectively defines blood flow (feeding arteries, nidus, and draining veins), however, it does so in only two dimensions. Using the two-dimensional data from stereotactic angiography to represent the three-dimensional target results in significant errors of both overestimation and underestimation of AVM nidus dimensions [12,13]. Underestimation of the nidus size may result in treatment failure, whereas overestimation results in the inclusion of normal brain within the treatment volume. This can cause radiation damage to normal brain, which, when affecting an eloquent area, may result in a neurological deficit. To avoid such targeting errors, a true three-dimensional image database is required. Both contrast-enhanced computed tomography (CT) and magnetic resonance imaging (MRI) are commonly used for this purpose.

Diagnostic (nonstereotactic) angiography is used to characterize the AVM, but because of its inherent inadequacies as a treatment planning database, stereotactic angiography has been largely abandoned at our institution. We use contrast-enhanced stereotactic CT as a targeting image database for the vast majority of AVMs. Our CT technique uses rapid infusion (1 cc/sec) of contrast while scanning through the AVM nidus with 1-mm slices. The head ring is bolted to a bracket at the head of the CT table, assuring that the head/ring/localizer complex remains immobile during the scan. This technique yields a very clear three-dimensional picture of the nidus. Alternative approaches use MRI/MRA, as opposed to CT. Attention to optimal image sequences in both CT and MRI is essential for effective AVM radiosurgical targeting.

2.4 Treatment Planning

The primary goal of AVM radiosurgery treatment planning is to develop a plan with a target volume that conforms closely to the surface of the AVM nidus while maintaining a steep *dose gradient* (the rate of change in dose relative to position) away from the nidal surface to minimize the radiation dose to surrounding brain. A number of treatment planning tools can be used to tailor the shape of the target volume to fit even highly irregular nidus shapes. Regardless of its shape, the entire nidus, not including the feeding arteries and draining veins, must lie within the target volume (the "prescription isodose shell"), with as little normal brain included as possible (Fig. 2).

Another goal of dose planning is to manipulate the dose gradient so that critical brain structures receive the lowest possible dose of radiation, to

avoid disabling complications. In addition, many radiosurgeons strive to produce a treatment dose distribution that maximizes uniformity (homogeneity)
of dose throughout the entire target volume. A detailed discussion of the
methodology of dose planning is beyond the scope of this chapter, but can
be found elsewhere [11].

2.5 Dose Selection

Various analyses of AVM radiosurgery outcomes (described below) have
elucidated an appropriate range of doses for the treatment of AVMs. Minimum nidal doses lower than 15 Gy have been associated with a significantly
lower rate of AVM obliteration, whereas doses above 20 Gy have been
associated with a higher rate of permanent neurological complications. We
prescribe doses ranging from 15 Gy to as high as 22.5 Gy to the margin of
the AVM nidus, nearly always at the 70% or 80% isodose line. The selection
of a dose within this range is made based on the volume of the nidus, as
well as the eloquence and radiosensitivity of surrounding brain structures.
Lower doses are prescribed for larger lesions and lesions in eloquent areas.

2.6 Radiation Delivery

The process of radiation delivery is the same for any radiosurgical target,
but careful attention to detail and the execution of various safety checks and
redundancies are necessary to ensure that the prescribed treatment plan is
accurately and safely delivered [11]. When radiation delivery has been completed, the head ring is removed, the patient is observed for approximately
30 minutes, and then discharged to resume her/his normal activities.

2.7 Follow-up

Standard follow-up after AVM radiosurgery typically consists of annual
clinic visits with MRI/MRA to evaluate the effect of the procedure and
monitor for neurological complications. If the patient's clinical status
changes, she/he is followed more closely at clinically appropriate intervals.

Each patient is scheduled to undergo cerebral angiography at three
years postradiosurgery, and a definitive assessment of the success or failure
of treatment is made based on the results of angiography (see below). If no
flow is observed through the AVM nidus, the patient is pronounced cured
and is discharged from follow-up. If the AVM nidus is incompletely obliterated, appropriate further therapy (most commonly repeat radiosurgon on
the day of angiography) is prescribed, and the treatment/follow-up cycle is
repeated.

3   REPORTED EFFICACY OF AVM RADIOSURGERY

Many series have evaluated rates of AVM thrombosis after radiosurgery
[10,14–29]. Overall reported rates of successful angiographic AVM obliteration range from 56% to 92% (Table 1). The rate of obliteration is strongly
correlated with AVM size. For example, among the 153 AVM radiosurgery
patients who have undergone 3-year follow-up angiography at the University

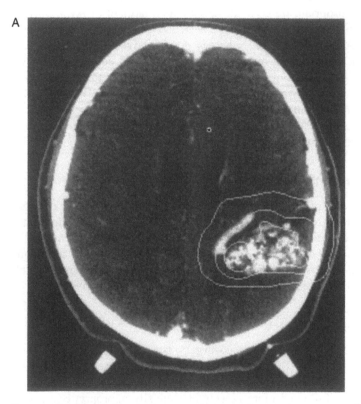

A

FIGURE 2   Treatment plan, contrast-enhanced computed tomography
(CT). This 43-year-old male presented with seizures and refused surgical
intervention in favor of radiosurgery. His treatment plan, based on a
contrast-enhanced CT database, is shown here (**A**, Axial; **B**, Sagittal; **C**,
Coronal). Note the conformality of the innermost (70%) isodose line to
the arteriovenous malformation (AVM) nidus in all planes. The 35% and
14% isodose lines are also shown. This 7-isocenter plan delivered 15.0
Gy to the 70% isodose shell. The total AVM nidus volume treated was
12 cc.

of Florida, rates of angiographic cure according to AVM volume were as follows: < 1 cc—82%; 1–4 cc—81%; 4–10 cc—73%; > 10 cc—42%. Similar trends have been reported by most groups [14,15,20,24].

4 WHY DOES RADIOSURGERY FAIL?

Synthesis of the published studies addressing etiologies of AVM radiosurgical failure [17,21,30–33] leads to several useful conclusions. The dose delivered to the periphery of the AVM (D_{min}) is the most significant predictor

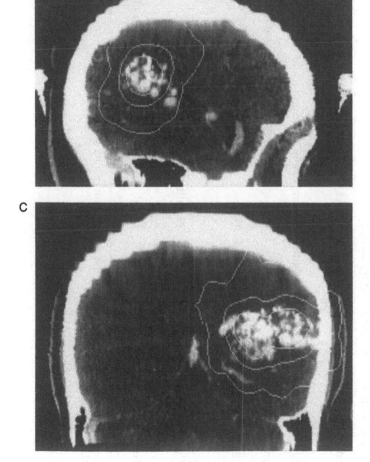

FIGURE 2 Continued

TABLE 1 Major AVM Radiosurgery Series

First author	Yamamoto (28)	Pollock (21)	Karlsson (17)	Steinberg (24)	Colombo (16)	Friedman
Radiosurgical device	Gamma Knife	Gamma Knife	Gamma Knife	Proton beam	LINAC	LINAC
Number of patients	40	313	945	86	180	407
Angiographic cure rate	65%	61%	56%	92%	80%	65%
Complications						
Permanent radiation induced	3 patients (7.5%)	30 patients (9%)	5%	11%	4 patients (2%)	7 patients (2%)
Hemorrhage	None	8 fatal	55 patients	10 patients	15 patients, 5 fatal	26 patients, 5 fatal

When a group had multiple reports, the most recent results are listed.
AVM, Arteriovenous malformation.

of successful obliteration, provided that the nidus is completely encompassed by the prescription isodose shell (targeting error is an important cause of failure and is commonly caused by inadequate imaging/angiography). Large lesion volume and high Spetzler-Martin grade are also predictors of failure, although less significant than D_{min}. The importance of AVM location and patient age are unclear. Based on our experience [30], lower rates of AVM obliteration can be expected at peripheral doses below 15 Gy and for lesion volumes greater than 10 cc.

5 COMPLICATIONS

5.1 Hemorrhage after Radiosurgery

The issue of AVM hemorrhage after radiosurgical treatment has been examined by several groups [14,16,20,22,24,34–38]. It has been reported that radiosurgery decreases the risk of hemorrhage even with incomplete AVM obliteration [34]; however, most reports have shown no postradiosurgical alteration in bleeding risk [39,40] from the 3% to 4% per year expected based on natural history [1–5]. This suggests that radiosurgery offers no protective effect unless complete obliteration is achieved.

Several groups have reported an increased risk of AVM hemorrhage with increasing AVM size or subtotal irradiation [16,34,39]. In our series [39], a strong correlation between AVM volume and the risk of hemorrhage was also found. Ten of the 12 AVMs that bled were more than 10 cc in volume. It is also noteworthy that in this study, neither age nor history of prior hemorrhage correlated with the incidence of hemorrhage.

Ten of the 12 AVMs that bled also had associated "angiographic risk factors" for bleeding, including arterial aneurysms, venous aneurysms, venous outlet obstruction, and periventricular location. Pollock et al. [40] found a significant correlation between the incidence of postradiosurgical hemorrhage and presence of an unsecured proximal aneurysm and recommended that such aneurysms be obliterated before radiosurgery.

The Pittsburgh group [41] also recently studied factors associated with bleeding risk of AVMs and found three AVM characteristics to be predictive of greater hemorrhage risk: (1) history of prior bleed, (2) presence of a single draining vein, and (3) diffuse AVM morphology. Based on the presence or absence of these risk factors, they stratified AVM patients into hemorrhage risk groups and recommended that predicted hemorrhage risk be used to help determine appropriate management of patients with AVMs. For example, patients with a high predicted hemorrhage risk would be considered less attractive candidates for radiosurgery because of their greater risk during the latency period between treatment and cure.

5.2 Radiation-Induced Complications

Acute complications are rare after AVM radiosurgery. Several authors have previously reported that radiosurgery can acutely exacerbate seizure activity. Others have reported nausea, vomiting, and headache occasionally occurring after radiosurgical treatment [42].

Delayed radiation-induced complications have been reported by all groups performing radiosurgery. Observed rates of permanent postradiosurgical neurological deficit range from 2% to 4%, and transient deficits have been observed in 3% to 9% of patients [20,25,43,44]. Symptoms are location dependent and generally develop between 3 and 18 months after treatment. Symptomatic patients are commonly treated with a several-week course of oral steroids, and nearly all improve. The use of peripheral doses greater than 20 Gy have been associated with a higher frequency of permanent neurological deficits [43].

In addition to the well-established correlation between increasing radiosurgical target volume and increasing incidence of radiation necrosis [36,45–47], the most important predictors of symptomatic radiation injury are lesion location and dose [24,43,48]. Radiation induced changes appear frequently (20% in the Pittsburgh series) on postradiosurgery MR images [49–51]. These changes tend to be asymptomatic if the lesion is located in a relatively "silent" brain area and symptomatic if the lesion is located in an "eloquent" brain area. This is further evidence that lesion location is an important consideration in radiosurgical treatment planning and dose selection [45].

6 CONCLUSIONS

Many reports indicate that approximately 80% of arteriovenous malformations in the "radiosurgery size range" will be angiographically obliterated 2 to 3 years after radiosurgical treatment. The likelihood of successful AVM obliteration decreases with increasing lesion volume and decreasing peripheral target dose. Accurate targeting is critical to successful AVM radiosurgery, and a three-dimensional image database (e.g., CT or MRI) is an indispensable element in the treatment planning process. Stereotactic angiography alone is inadequate.

The major drawback of this treatment method is that patients are unprotected against hemorrhage during the 2- to 3-year latent period after treatment. Radiosurgery does not significantly alter the natural rate of AVM hemorrhage until the lesion has completely thrombosed. Increasing AVM volume appears to be associated with a higher risk for hemorrhage, as are certain angiographic findings such as proximal aneurysms, venous outflow restriction, and periventricular location.

Radiation-induced neurological symptoms occur in 5% to 10% of patients, but the majority of these are transient, responding to steroid therapy. Permanent complications are rare (2% to 4%). The most significant predictors of radiation-induced complications are AVM volume, lesion location, and dose. Asymptomatic MRI changes are not uncommon.

REFERENCES

1. Brown RD, Wiebers DO, Forbes G. The natural history of unruptured intracranial arteriovenous malformations. J Neurosurg 68:352–357, 1988.
2. Crawford PM, West CR, Chadwick DW. Arteriovenous malformations of the brain: Natural history in unoperated patients. J Neurol Neurosurg Psychiatry 49:1–10, 1986.
3. Fults D, Kelly DL. Natural history of arteriovenous malformations of the brain: A clinical study. Neurosurgery 15:658–652, 1984.
4. Graf CJ, Perret GE. Torner JC. Bleeding from cerebral arteriovenous malformations as part of their natural history. J Neurosurg 58:331–337, 1983.
5. Ondra SL, Troupp H, George ED, Schwab K. The natural history of symptomatic arteriovenous malformations of the brain: A 24-year follow-up assessment. J Neurosurg 73:387–391, 1991.
6. Chang SD, Shuster DL, Steinberg GK, Levy RP, Frankel K. Stereotactic radiosurgery of arteriovenous malformations: Pathologic changes in resected tissue. Clin Neuropathol 16(2):111–116, 1997.
7. Ogilvy CS. Radiation therapy for arteriovenous malformations: A review. Neurosurgery 26:725–735, 1990.
8. Schneider BF, Eberhard DA, Steiner LE. Histopathology of arteriovenous malformations after gamma knife radiosurgery. J Neurosurg 87(3):352–357, 1997.
9. Szeifert GT, Kemeny AA, Timperley WR, Forster DM. The potential role of myofibroblasts in the obliteration of arteriovenous malformations after radiosurgery. Neurosurgery 40(1):61–65; discussion 65–66, 1997.
10. Yamamoto M, Jimbo M, Kobayashi M, Toyoda C, Ide M, Tanaka N, Lindquist C, Steiner L. Long-term results of radiosurgery for arteriovenous malformation: Neurodiagnostic imaging and histological studies of angiographically confirmed nidus obliteration. Surg Neurol 37:219–230, 1992.
11. Friedman WA, Buatti JM, Bova FJ, Mendenhall, WM. LINAC Radiosurgery —A Practical Guide. Berlin: Springer-Verlag, 1998.
12. Bova FJ, Friedman WA. Stereotactic angiography: An inadequate database for radiosurgery? Int J Radiat Oncol Biol Phys 20:891–895, 1991.
13. Spiegelmann R, Friedman WA, Bova FJ. Limitations of angiographic target localization in radiosurgical treatment planning. Neurosurgery 30:619–624, 1992.
14. Betti OO, Munari C, Rosler R. Stereotactic radiosurgery with the linear accelerator: Treatment of arteriovenous malformations. Neurosurgery 24:311–321, 1989.

15. Colombo F, Benedetti A, Pozza F, Marchetti C, Chierego G. Linear accelerator radiosurgery of cerebral arteriovenous malformations. Neurosurgery 24:833–840, 1989.
16. Colombo F, Pozza F, Chierego G, Casentini L, DeLuca G, Francescon P. Linear accelerator radiosurgery of cerebral arteriovenous malformations: An update. Neurosurgery 34:14–21, 1994.
17. Karlsson B, Lindquist C, Steiner L. Prediction of obliteration after gamma knife surgery for cerebral arteriovenous malformations. Neurosurgery 40(3): 425–430; discussion 430–431, 1997.
18. Kemeny AA, Dias PS, Forster DM. Results of stereotactic radiosurgery of arteriovenous malformations: An analysis of 52 cases. J Neurol Neurosurg Psychiatry 52:554–558, 1989.
19. Loeffler JS, Alexander EI, Siddon RL, Saunders WM, Coleman CN, Winston KR. Stereotactic radiosurgery for intracranial arteriovenous malformations using a standard linear accelerator. Int J Radiat Oncol Biol Phys 17:673–677, 1989.
20. Lunsford LD, Kondziolka D, Flickinger JC, Bissonette DJ, Jungreis CA, Maitz AH, Horton JA, Coffey RJ. Stereotactic radiosurgery for arteriovenous malformations of the brain J Neurosurg 75:512–524, 1991.
21. Pollock BE, Flickinger JC, Lunsford LD, Maitz A, Kondziolka D. Factors associated with successful arteriovenous malformation radiosurgery. Neurosurgery 42(6):1239–1244; discussion 1244–1247, 1998.
22. Pollock BE, Lunsford LD, Kondziolka D, Maitz A, Flickinger JC. Patient outcomes after stereotactic radiosurgery for "operable" arteriovenous malformations. Neurosurgery 35:1–8, 1994.
23. Souhami L, Olivier A, Podgorsak EB, Pla M, Pike GB. Radiosurgery of cerebral arteriovenous malformations with the dynamic stereotactic irradiation. Int J Radiat Oncol Biol Phys 19:775–782, 1990.
24. Steinberg GK, Fabrikant JI, Marks MP, Levy RP, Frankel KA, Phillips MH, Shuer LM, Silverberg GD. Stereotactic heavy-charged particle Bragg-peak radiation for intracranial arteriovenous malformations. N Engl J Med 323:96–101, 1990.
25. Steiner L. Treatment of arteriovenous malformations by radiosurgery. In: Wilson CB, Stein BM, eds. Intracranial Arteriovenous Malformations. Baltimore/London: Williams and Wilkins, 1984, pp 295–313.
26. Steiner L. Radiosurgery in cerebral arteriovenous malformations. In: Fein JM, Flamm ES, eds. Cerebrovascular Surgery. Vol. 4. Wien/New York: Springer-Verlag, 1985, pp 1161–1215.
27. Steiner L, Leksel L, Greitz T, Forster DM, Backlund EO. Stereotaxic radiosurgery for cerebral arteriovenous malformations. Report of a case. Acta Chir Scand 138:459–464, 1972.
28. Yamamoto M, Jimbo M, Hara M, Saito I, Mori K. Gamma knife radiosurgery for arteriovenous malformations: Long-term follow-up results focusing on complications occurring more than 5 years after irradiation. Neurosurgery 38: 906–914, 1996.

29. Yamamoto M, Jimbo M, Ide M, Tanaka N, Lindquist C, Steiner L. Long-term follow-up of radiosurgically treated arteriovenous malformations in children: Report of nine cases. Surg Neurol 38:95–100, 1992.

30. Ellis TL, Friedman WA, Bova FJ, Kubilis PS, Buatti JM. Analysis of treatment failure after radiosurgery for arteriovenous malformations. J Neurosurg 89(1): 104–110, 1998.

31. Flickinger JC, Pollock BE, Kondziolka D, Lunsford D. A dose-response analysis of arteriovenous malformation obliteration after radiosurgery. Int J Radiat Oncol Biol Phys 36:873–879, 1996.

32. Pollock BE, Kondziolka D, Lunsford LD, Bissonette D, Flickinger JC. Repeat stereotactic radiosurgery of arteriovenous malformations: Factors associated with incomplete obliteration. Neurosurgery 38(2):318–324, 1996.

33. Touboul E, Al Halabi A, Buffat L, Merienne L, Huart J, Schlienger M, Lefkopoulos D, Mammar H, Missir O, Meder JF, Laurent A, Housset M. Single-fraction stereotactic radiotherapy: A dose-response analysis of arteriovenous malformation obliteration. Int J Radiat Oncol Biol Phys 41(4):855–861, 1998.

34. Karlsson B, Lindquist C, Kihlstrom L, Steiner L. Gamma knife surgery for AVM offers partial protection from hemorrhage prior to obliteration. AANS Program Book 142, 1995 (Abstract).

35. Kjellberg RN. Stereotactic Bragg peak proton beam radiosurgery for cerebral arteriovenous malformations. Ann Clin Res 18(Suppl 47):17–19, 1986.

36. Kjellberg RN, Hanamura T, Davis KR, Lyons SL, Anans RD. Bragg-peak proton-beam therapy for arteriovenous malformations of the brain. N Engl J Med 309:269–274, 1983.

37. Seifert V, Stolke D, Mehdorn HM, Hoffman B. Clinical and radiological evaluation of long-term results of stereotactic proton beam radiosurgery in patients with cerebral arteriovenous malformations. J Neurosurg 81:683–689, 1994.

38. Steiner L, Lindquist C, Adler JR, Torner JC, Alves W, Stenner M. Clinical outcome of radiosurgery for cerebral arteriovenous malformations. J Neurosurg 77:2–8, 1992.

39. Friedman WA, Blatt DL, Bova FJ, Mendenhall WM, Kubilis PS, Bissonette DJ, Konzdziolka D. The risk of hemorrhage after radiosurgery for arteriovenous malformations. J Neurosurg 84:912–919, 1996.

40. Pollock BE, Flickinger JC, Lunsford LD, et al. Hemorrhage risk after stereotactic radiosurgery of cerebral arteriovenous malformations. Neurosurgery 38: 652–661, 1996.

41. Pollock BE, Flickinger JC, Lunsford LD, et al. Factors that predict the bleeding risk of cerebral arteriovenous malformations. Stroke 27:1–6, 1996.

42. Alexander EI, Siddon RL, Loeffler JS. The acute onset of nausea and vomiting following stereotactic radiosurgery: Correlation with total dose to area postrema. Surg Neurol 32:40–44, 1989.

43. Flickinger JC, Kondziolka D, Maitz AH, Lunsford LD. Analysis of neurological sequelae from radiosurgery of arteriovenous malformations: How location affects outcome. Int J Radiat Oncol Biol Phys 40(2):273–278, 1998.

44. Statham P, Macpherson P, Johnston R, Forster DM, Todd NY, Anam JH. Ce-

rebral radiation necrosis complicating stereotactic radiosurgery for arteriovenous malformation. J Neurol Neurosurg Psychiatry 53:476–479, 1990.
45. Flickinger JC. An integrated logistic formula for prediction of complications from radiosurgery. Int J Radiat Oncol Biol Phys 17:879–885, 1989.
46. Flickinger JC, Schell MC, Larson DA. Estimation of complications for linear accelerator radiosurgery with the integrated logistic formula. Int J Radiat Oncol Biol Phys 19:143–148, 1990.
47. Kjellberg RN, Abbe M. Stereotactic Bragg peak proton beam therapy. In: Lunsford LD, ed. Modern Stereotactic Neurosurgery. Ed 1. Boston: Martinus Nijhoff, 1988, pp 463–470.
48. Karlsson B, Lax I, Soderman M. Factors influencing the risk for complications following Gamma Knife radiosurgery of cerebral arteriovenous malformations. Radiother Oncol 43(3):275–280, 1997.
49. Flickinger JC, Kondziolka D, Pollock BE, Maitz AH, Lunsford LD. Complications from arteriovenous malformation radiosurgery: Multivariate analysis and risk modeling. Int J Radiat Oncol Biol Phys 38(3):485–490, 1997.
50. Kihlstrom L, Guo WY, Karlsson B, Lindquist C, Lindqvist M. Magnetic resonance imaging of obliterated arteriovenous malformations up to 23 years after radiosurgery [see comments]. J Neurosurg 86(4):589–593, 1997.
51. Marks MP, Delapaz RL, Fabrikant JI, Frankel KA, Philun MH, Levy RP, Enzmann DR. Intracranial vascular malformations: Imaging of charged-particle radiosurgery. Part I. Results of therapy. Radiology 168:447–455, 1988.

16

Stereotactic Radiosurgery with the Gamma Knife

Douglas Kondziolka and L. Dade Lunsford

The Center for Image-Guided Neurosurgery, University of Pittsburgh
School of Medicine, Pittsburgh, Pennsylvania, U.S.A.

Todd P. Thompson

Straub Clinic and Hospital, Honolulu, Hawaii, U.S.A.

1 STEREOTACTIC RADIOSURGERY

Surgeons use energy in many forms to cure disease. Scalpels, lasers, and
electrocautery were the initial tools of the neurosurgeon. Recent advances
in neuroimaging, computer science, and stereotactic dose planning allow
neurosurgeons to use sculpted radiation fields to alter the biology of disease.
Stereotactic radiosurgery is the mechanically precise delivery of a potentially
cytostatic, obliterative, or functionally incapacitating single dose of radiation
to an imaging-defined target volume while minimizing risk to surrounding
tissues. The goal of radiosurgery is to alter the molecular physiology to effect
a positive change on the disease process. Radiation transfers energy to its
target, initiating a cascade of high-energy electrons that interact with matter
ultimately to arrest tumor growth, alter the blood supply of tumors or vascular
malformations, or ablate undesirable nerve conduction. The unique design of
stereotactic radiosurgery systems allows small areas of the brain to be treated
with high doses of radiation. The sharp fall-off of radiation dose prevents
brain outside of the target area from receiving deleterious doses.

Radiosurgery is a "patient friendly" procedure that does not require open surgery and allows the patient to be discharged the day after surgery. This does not imply that radiosurgery is noninvasive or risk free. Successful radiosurgery requires a multidisciplinary team, including a neurosurgeon, a radiation oncologist, a medical physicist, a nurse, and an administrator. We review the current indications for Gamma Knife radiosurgery, treatment strategies, results, and complications for common neurosurgical indications.

The Gamma Knife design is a unique tool for the neurosurgeon. Two hundred and one sources of cobalt 60 radiation are directed to a focal point. The Leksell stereotactic frame allows patients to be positioned within the unit with 0.5-mm accuracy. Helmets with 201 collimators of 4, 8, 14, or 18 mm allow conformal shaping of the radiation field. The design is excellent for treating targets within the skull, down to the foramen magnum. The number of patients treated with the Gamma Knife has grown exponentially since its innovation in 1967. Currently, there are 51 Gamma Knife units in the United States, and 126 units worldwide. As of June 1999, more than 100,000 patients have been treated (Table 1).

2 FRAME APPLICATION AND IMAGING

The frame is applied in approximately 5 minutes in the stereotactic suite using local anesthesia, occasionally supplemented by intravenous sedation (midazolam and fentanyl). Children younger than age 12 generally undergo general anesthesia for stereotactic procedures. Patients are positioned supine on the stretcher with the head of the bed elevated 60°. The chest is supported with several pillows to flex the body 90 degrees at the waist, allowing greater access to the head. Ideally, two persons assist with frame placement. A nurse helps to stabilize the head while the surgeon and assistant attach the frame. After the head has been prepared with isopropyl alcohol and the patient is comfortably sedated, ear bars are placed into the external auditory canal with a 1-cm square foam pad on the end of the ear bar. The foam padding alleviates patient discomfort during frame application. The ear bars are intended to assist with symmetrical alignment and do not bear the weight of the frame. The surgeon supports the frame throughout the application.

The frame is shifted toward the side of the lesion to position the lesion as close as possible to the center of the frame and the collimator helmet. Lidocaine (0.5%) and bupivicaine (0.5%) buffered with sodium bicarbonate are injected into each pin site. The pin length is chosen to attach the frame bars with finger-tight torque and without pin protrusion beyond the frame. During imaging, a rigid frame adapter keeps the frame orthogonal to the imaging plane.

TABLE 1   Mean Marginal Doses and Results

Lesion	Marginal dose range	Maximum dose	Results
AVMs (<4 cm³)	18–25 Gy [10]		88% obliteration at 3 years
Acoustic neuromas	12–14 Gy		97% tumor control at 10 years
Meningiomas	16 Gy		93% tumor control at 5–10 years
Metastasis	10–27 Gy		86% local tumor control
Pituitary tumors	10–30 Gy		60%–90% tumor control
Trigeminal neuralgia*		80 Gy	80% pain relief
Tremor*		120–140 Gy	80% reduced tremor

*The dose used for trigeminal neuralgia and tremor represents the maximal dose within a single 4-mm isocenter.
AVM, Arteriovenous malfunction.

A sagittal localizing film is initially obtained. A contrast enhanced volume acquisition magnetic resonance imaging (MRI) scan is obtained with 1-mm slice thickness images, or 3-mm images for selected lesions. In imaging arteriovenous malformations (AVMs), contrast is given after the localizing sagittal image to assure a maximal contrast load during the axial image acquisition.

3   DOSE PLANNING

Gamma Knife dose planning uses one or more (sometimes many) small isocenters of radiation to create a conformal plan that encompasses the lesion and minimizes the dose received by surrounding structures. The Gamma Knife provides 4-, 8-, 14-, and 18-mm collimators. Similar conformal plans can be designed from one or more large isocenters or from the combination of a greater number of smaller isocenters. The plan created with the larger isocenters will deliver an equivalent dose of radiation, but in a shortened time because of the larger aperture of the collimator. Additionally, the radiation falloff into the surrounding tissues may not be as steep with larger collimators as compared with the smaller collimators. Conformal dose planning is particularly important when working near critical structures, such as the brainstem or optic nerves. Conformal radiosurgery is achieved through judicious selection of appropriate isocenters, proper interpretation of imaging, and dose selection.

The Gamma Knife provides the option of beam blocking as an additional tool for sculpting the fall-off pattern to protect surrounding structures, or to eliminate the passage of beams through important structures such as the ocular lens. Each of the 201 collimator ports on the helmet can be blocked. Blocking a group of beams requires that a greater dose of radiation be passed through the remaining beams to achieve the same target dose. As a consequence, the fall-off is shifted along the axis of the remaining beams. For example, blocking the entrance of beams entering from the left and right, the fall-off is diminished in the left-right axis, and shifted to the rostro-caudal, or antero-posterior axis. A limitless variety of blocking combinations is possible to achieve the best result. The effect of various blocking patterns is quickly evaluated on the planning software, before implementing the plan. We most often use blocking patterns to protect the ocular lens optic apparatus.

4   ARTERIOVENOUS MALFORMATIONS

The best AVM for radiosurgery is not necessarily the same AVM that is treated by conventional surgery. The ideal candidate for radiosurgery is a patient with a small, deep-seated AVM, not a patient with a larger AVM who was considered unsuitable for microsurgery. In evaluating AVMs for radiosurgery, the Spetzler-Martin scale may not apply, as it is not sensitive to smaller volumes. The success of radiosurgery is not as limited as microsurgery by critical locations or the venous drainage. The major shortcoming of radiosurgery for AVMs is the persistent risk of hemorrhage until the AVM is obliterated. Before treatment, the risk of hemorrhage is estimated to be 2% to 4% per year. The risk of hemorrhage is not increased by radiosurgery.

Proper imaging of the vascular malformation is required for successful radiosurgery. Imaging of AVMs includes a volume acquisition MRI as well as conventional angiography. Both modalities are needed to distinguish the nidus from draining veins and nearby critical structures. Embolization has been evaluated in conjunction with radiosurgery and shown to have a 12.8% morbidity, 1.6% mortality, and 11.8% 1-year recanalization rate [1]. Given the morbidity and sometimes limited efficacy, we do not routinely advocate embolization before radiosurgery.

The radiosurgical dose given to AVMs is a function of the volume, location, and risk assessment. Giving a higher dose increases the probability of AVM obliteration, but may increase the risk of side effects. University investigators reviewed the histology of AVMs that were resected after radiosurgery and found that a dose of more than 20 Gy was necessary for the desired histological effects (endothelial injury, hyperplasia, and thrombosis). After 4 years, there was not much additional effect. In our own experience, AVMs that have not occluded within 3 years of radiosurgery require additional treatment. The probability of AVM obliteration is approximately 98% for volumes treated with a minimum dose of 25 Gy, and 90% with a minimum dose of 20 Gy. Arteriovenous malformations that are larger than 10 cm to 15 cm^3 may require irradiation in staged volumes with a 3- to 6-month interval between procedures (Fig. 1).

5 ACOUSTIC NEUROMAS

The goals of acoustic neuroma management include tumor control (radiosurgery) or complete removal (microsurgery), preservation of facial nerve function, and maintenance of "useful" hearing in appropriate patients. A comparison of microsurgery and radiosurgery from 1990 to 1992 revealed that hearing was preserved in 14% of microsurgery procedures and 75% of Gamma Knife procedures [2]. Normal facial function was achieved in 63% of microsurgical procedures and 83% of Gamma Knife procedures. Since then, radiosurgery results have improved significantly.

Radiosurgery is performed with an axial volume acquisition contrast-enhanced MRI. The treatment of acoustic neuromas at our institution has evolved over the past 10 years. Initially, the tumor margin was treated with approximately 18 Gy to 20 Gy, with the center of the tumor receiving up to 40 Gy. The marginal dose has been gradually reduced to 12 Gy to 14 Gy, allowing a significant reduction in complications and continued tumor control. We usually treat the tumor margin with 50% of the maximal dose. For patients between 1987 and 1992, the 10-year tumor control rate was 98% with normal facial function in 79% and normal facial sensation in 73% of patients [3]. For patients managed between 1992 and 1997, the control rate was 99%, and the facial nerve morbidity was 1%. More than 60% of patients had a reduction in the volume of their tumor. We have treated 10 patients with intracanalicular acoustic neuromas with 14 Gy or less to the margin and preserved hearing for all patients (Fig. 2) [4].

6 MENINGIOMAS

Meningiomas of the falx, convexity, olfactory groove, and lateral spenoid wing can be treated with radiosurgery, but they can also be resected with low morbidity. Meningiomas that are not as easily resected, such as those along the petrous apex and clivus or extending into cavernous sinus, are often optimal radiosurgical cases. The steep fall-off of radiosurgical dose

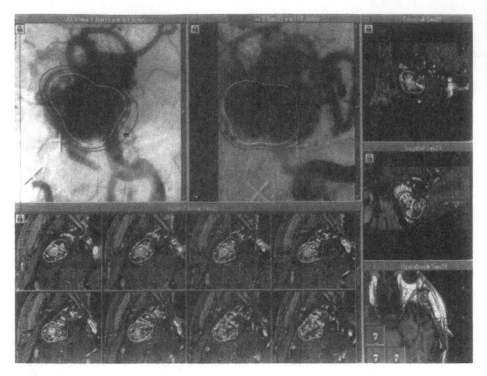

Figure 1 A 45-year-old man with a right temporal arteriovenous malformation declined operative resection. The radiosurgery plan demonstrates the use of both magnetic resonance imaging and angiography for dose planning. The combined imaging allows more precise planning and exclusion of the large anterior superior draining vein. A maximal dose of 36 Gy and marginal dose of 18 Gy were used.

planning allows these difficult tumors to be treated with marginal doses of 13 Gy to 16 Gy, with a low risk of injury to the associated cranial nerves, pituitary gland, or optic nerve. As for other indications, we generally prescribe a marginal tumor dose that is 50% of the maximal dose.

Using an average marginal dose of 16 Gy, we have achieved long-term tumor control in 93% of meningiomas, more than half of which had been previously resected. Neurological deficits occurred in only 5%. Overall, 96% of patients surveyed believed that radiosurgery provided a satisfactory outcome for their meningioma [5]. We believe that planned judicious microsurgery, when indicated, followed by radiosurgery may improve overall clinical outcomes (Fig. 3).

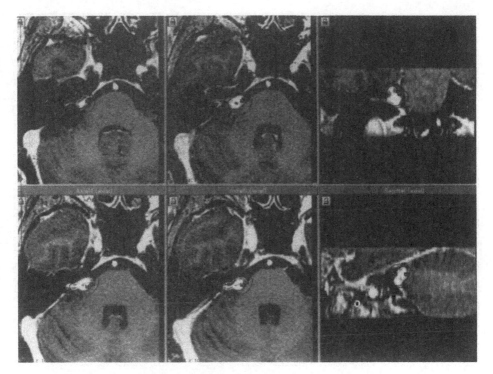

FIGURE 2 This 64-year-old woman had a gross total resection of a right acoustic neuroma 8 years earlier. The recurrent tumor was treated a maximal dose of 26 Gy, with a marginal dose of 13 Gy. The conformal plan included seven 4-mm isocenters.

7 PITUITARY TUMORS

Microsurgery remains the procedure of choice for the rapid treatment of pituitary tumors that are causing mass effect or secreting adrenocorticotropic hormone or growth hormone. Stereotactic radiosurgery is an effective alternative for patients who do not require decompressive surgery, rapid normalization of endocrine abnormalities, or who suffer from recurrent tumors despite medical and surgical intervention. The treatment goals for pituitary tumors are control of tumor growth, cessation of abnormal hormone secretion, and avoidance of neurological injury. We have achieved tumor control in 94% of tumors [6]. In our series, cortisol secretion was normalized or reduced in 62.5% of patients. Growth hormone levels were normalized in 67% of patients and significantly improved in most of the remaining patients. None of our patients developed pituitary insufficiency as a consequence of radiosurgery.

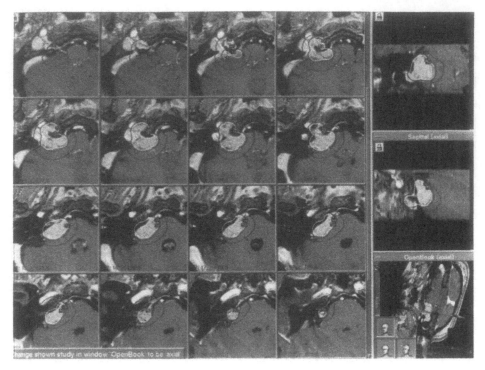

FIGURE 3 A petroclival meningioma in a 61-year-old woman who had diminished hearing and dysequilibrium. The conformal plan with a maximal dose of 28 Gy and marginal dose of 14 Gy used one 14-mm isocenter, six 8-mm isocenters, and one 4-mm isocenter.

The greatest risk in treating pituitary lesions with radiosurgery is damage to the optic nerves and optic chiasm. We recommend radiosurgery only for those tumors that are at least 1 mm to 2 mm away from the optic nerve. The steep fall-off of radiosurgery units allows pituitary lesions to be treated with 40 Gy to 50 Gy maximal doses (20–25 Gy marginal doses) while exposing the optic nerve to less than 8 Gy. Lesions in the sellar area provide an excellent demonstration of the unique radiation fall-off pattern for the different Gamma Knife units. The "B" unit has a steeper fall-off in the rostral–caudal dimension, whereas the earlier "U" or "A" unit has a steeper fall-off in the left–right dimension. This differential can be exploited, depending on the configuration of the tumor and the surrounding structures. Additionally, some of the collimators on the helmets can be blocked to alter the fall-off pattern.

8 BRAIN METASTASES

More than 100,000 patients are diagnosed with brain metastasis annually. The management of brain metastasis patients remains a challenge for oncologists, radiation oncologists, and neurosurgeons. Traditional therapy of single metastasis has been either resection or whole brain radiation (WBRT), with a boost to the affected region, or combined surgery with whole brain radiation. The surgical resection of solitary metastasis with WBRT has been shown to improve survival compared to WBRT alone [7]. The complications of whole brain fractionated radiation include memory loss, alopecia, dementia, and radiation necrosis.

Stereotactic radiosurgery is changing the long-standing management of brain metastasis. Radiosurgery can achieve many of the same goals as resection, (tumor control, reduced mass effect), one of the goals of fractionated radiation therapy (the treatment of multiple lesions), and effectively treat deeply located tumors that are not considered for resection. For patients with solitary metastasis, radiosurgery may allow the avoidance of WBRT and its potential complications. In conjunction with WBRT, radiosurgery can provide rapid improvement in peritumoral edema, local tumor control, and prolonged survival compared with WBRT alone [8]. Radiosurgery provides nearly equivalent tumor control rates for breast, lung, and renal cell carcinoma, as well as melanoma. With control of brain metastasis, the management of systemic disease becomes the survival limiting factor. Radiosurgery has the additional benefits of 1- to 2-day hospital stays and low costs (Fig. 4).

9 OTHER LESIONS

Stereotactic radiosurgery can be used to manage effectively other intracranial lesions, such as chordomas, chondrosarcomas, gliomas, and cavernous malformations (CM). Stereotactic radiosurgery is an adjuvant therapy, providing a radiation boost to the enhancing component of malignant glial neoplasms. We have also obtained good results in the treatment of juvenile pilocytic astrocytomas in children. Cavernous malformations are treated with radiosurgery after a second symptomatic hemorrhage using the same dose algorithm applied to AVMs. The baseline risk of hemorrhage for CMs is approximately 1% annually; however, the natural history of CMs suggests that those with a second symptomatic hemorrhage have an increased tendency toward hemorrhage (> 30% annually).

10 FUNCTIONAL RADIOSURGERY

Lars Leksell originally designed the Gamma Knife in 1967 to create functional lesions for the treatment of psychiatric disorders. Today, radiosurgery

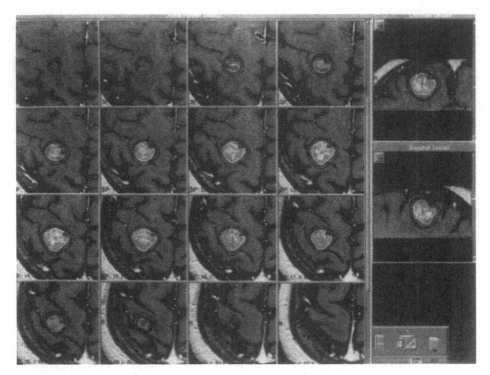

FIGURE 4   A 56-year-old woman presented with this solitary metastasis, 2 years after a mastectomy for breast cancer. The dose plan was created with two 14-mm isocenters and three 8-mm isocenters. The maximal dose was 32 Gy. The marginal dose was 16 Gy.

is used to treat trigeminal neuralgia, essential tremor, parkinsonian tremor, and selected psychiatric or epileptic disorders. In trigeminal neuralgia, a maximum dose of 80 Gy is targeted to the proximal trigeminal nerve just anterior to the pons, using a single 4-mm isocenter. Radiosurgical thalamotomy (ventral intermediolateral thalamic nucleus) is performed with anatomical MRI localization. Tremor is improved in most patients after a latency interval of 2 to 6 months.

11   CRITICISMS OF RADIOSURGERY

Radiosurgery was initially viewed as a competitor to traditional neurosurgical techniques. Common criticisms of radiosurgery included the following: (1) The tumor is not removed; (2) There is no rapid reduction in mass effect; (3) Future surgery will be more difficult; (4) Additionally, patients may have a false sense of cure. It is true that the tumors often are not eliminated, but the goal of radiosurgery is tumor control, not extirpation. A rapid reduction in mass effect is often not required, and edema is often significantly reduced after radiosurgery. It is unlikely that radiosurgery complicates future operations. One study of arteriovenous malformations that were resected after radiosurgery found they were less vascular and easier to remove. One microsurgeon has noted that three of four tumors that he resected after radiosurgery were no more difficult to remove compared with the average tumor. Finally, patient misconceptions are addressed with education and long-term follow-up. We obtain MRI scans at 6, 12, 24, 48 and 96 months after treatment of benign lesions, and every 3 years or so thereafter. We obtain more frequent follow-up for patients with malignant diseases.

12 COMPLICATIONS OF RADIOSURGERY

It is true that there are almost no immediate complications of radiosurgery, but complications do occur. Such problems include small patches of alopecia for tumors adjacent to the scalp, brain edema, radiation necrosis, neurological deficits, and failure to achieve the intended goal. The risk of complications is a function of the tissue volume being treated, the dose delivered, the location, and prior radiation treatments.

There is no absolute maximal tolerated dose that important neuroanatomical structures, such as the optic nerve, can tolerate, but our general guidelines are included in Table 2. The maximum volume treated also depends on the location, the radiosurgical indication, and prior therapies. Large volumes are more easily treated in the frontal lobe, as compared with the brainstem. In general, treating volumes larger than 10 cm^3 increase the risk of complications. A study by Flickinger et al. found that complications after

TABLE 2 Potential Complication Limits

Location	Dose
Scalp—temporary epilation	3 Gy
Scalp—main erythema	6 Gy
Scalp—permanent epilation	7 Gy
Scalp—desquamation/atrophy	> 10 Gy
Scalp—ulceration/necrosis	> 15 Gy
Ocular lens	0.08 Gy
Optic nerve	8 Gy
Brainstem	14 Gy

AVM radiosurgery varied dramatically with location and the volume of tissue receiving greater than 12 Gy [9]. Locations in order of increasing risk for radiosurgery complications were frontal, temporal, intraventricular, parietal, cerebellar, corpus callosum, occipital, medulla, thalamus, basal ganglia, and pons/midbrain. Oncologic indications may dictate the use of higher doses, accepting higher risk, than nononcological indications.

The risk-benefit ratio weighs heavily in favor of radiosurgery. In our experience treating more than 3500 cases with the Gamma Knife, the risk of significant morbidity is approximately 3%. The chance of successful tumor control is more than 90% for most lesions. Long-term results now demonstrate that radiosurgery is an important therapeutic alternative for patients who are ineligible for surgery because of deep-seated lesions or serious medical conditions, or for patients who would like to avoid the risks of microsurgery.

REFERENCES

1. Gobin YP, Laurent A, Merienne L, Schlienger M, Aymard A, Houdart E, Casasco A, Lefkopoulos D, George B, Merland JJ. Treatment of brain arteriovenous malformations by embolization and radiosurgery. J Neurosurg 85(1):19–28, 1996.
2. Pollock BE, Lunsford LD, Kondziolka D, Flickinger JC, Bissonette DJ, Kelsey SF, Jannetta PJ. Outcome analysis of acoustic neuroma management: A comparison of microsurgery and stereotactic radiosurgery [published erratum appears in Neurosurgery 1995 Feb; 36(2):427]. Neurosurgery 36(1):215–224; discussion 224–229, 1995.
3. Kondziolka D, Lunsford LD, McLaughlin MR, Flickinger JC. Long-term outcomes after radiosurgery for acoustic neuromas. N Engl J Med 339(20):1426–1433, 1998.
4. Niranjan A, Lunsford LD, Flickinger JC, Maitz A, Kondziolka DK. Dose reduction improves hearing preservation rates after intracanalicular acoustic tumor radiosurgery. Neurosurgery 45(4):753–762, 1999.
5. Kondziolka D, Levy EI, Niranjan A, Flickinger JC, Lunsford LD. Long-term outcomes after meningioma radiosurgery: Physician and patient perspectives. J Neurosurg 91:44–50, 1999.
6. Witt TC, Kondziolka D, Flickinger JC, Lunsford LD. Stereotactic radiosurgery for pituitary tumors. In Kondziolka D, ed. Radiosurgery. Vol 1. Basal, Switzerland: Karger, pp 55–65, 1996.
7. Mintz AH, Kestle, J, Rathbone MP, Gaspar L, Hugenholtz H, Fisher B. A randomized trial to assess the efficacy of surgery in addition to radiotherapy in patients with a single cerebral metastasis. Cancer 78:1470–1476, 1996.
8. Auchter RM, Lamond JP, Alexander E, Buatti JM, Chappell R, Friedman WA, Kinsella TJ, Levin AB, Noyes WR, Schultz CJ, Loeffler JS, Mehta MP. A multiinstitutional outcome and prognostic factor analysis of radiosurgery for

resectable single brain metastasis. Int J Radiat Oncol Biol Phys 35(1):27–35, 1996.

9. Flickinger JC, Kondziolka D, Maitz AH, Lunsford LD. Analysis of neurological sequelae from radiosurgery of arteriovenous malformations: How location affects outcome. Int J Radiat Oncol Biol Phys 40:273–278, 1997.

10. Flickinger JC, Pollock BE, Kondziolka D, Lunsford LD. A dose-response analysis of arteriovenous malformation obliteration after radiosurgery. Intl J Radiat Biol Phys 36(4):873–879, 1996.

17

Stereotactic Radiosurgery with the X-Knife System

David W. Andrews and M. Beverly Downes
Thomas Jefferson University, Philadelphia, Pennsylvania, U.S.A.

1 INTRODUCTION

Linear acceleration (LINAC)-based stereotactic radiosurgery became feasible because of the pioneering efforts in the 1980s of Betti in South America [1], Colombo in Italy [2], Barcia-Saloria in Spain [3], and in the United States, Winston and Lutz at the Joint Center for Radiation Therapy in Boston [4] and Friedman at the University of Florida at Gainesville [5]. These early series reported the successful treatment of patients with intracranial lesions on modified linear accelerators. In all such cases, the configuration of retrofitted LINACs and the software necessary to plan and treat patients was unique to each institution, and, as a result, the accuracy, precision, and efficiency of these early units varied widely.

This chapter will be devoted to the development and refinements of X-Knife, the first commercially available treatment planning software for LINAC-based radiosurgery, so named to reflect focused X-ray photon radiation just as Gamma Knife reflects focused gamma-ray photon irradiation. The original work of Winston and Lutz at the Joint Center provided one of the first systematic approaches to a LINAC-based radiosurgery technique, which was refined using software developed and named X-Knife by Kooy [6]. Soon thereafter, the X-Knife software was commercially launched through the collaborative efforts of the Radionics Corporation. In its initial version, it represented a robust and versatile treatment planning software capable of providing a user-friendly interactive three-dimensional environment in which precise and complex stereotactic radiosurgery dose computations could be performed. The introduction of X-Knife immediately increased the range of treatment-planning capabilities and the treatment variables, such as a larger range of collimator aperture sizes for the treatment of larger lesions, thus broadening the application and standardizing the practice of LINAC-based radiosurgery. With the advent of a noninvasive, relocatable frame introduced by Gill [7,8] and commercially developed by Radionics, later versions of X-Knife supported fractionated stereotactic radiosurgery treatments, or what is now referred to as fractionated stereotactic radiotherapy (SRT). A further advance in LINAC radiosurgery was achieved when the first LINAC designed for and dedicated to stereotactic radiosurgery was developed at the Joint Center in collaboration with the Varian Corporation [9]. This LINAC was engineered to include more precise couch and gantry rotational axes, minimal gantry sag with a fixed, lighter primary and secondary collimation system, and perhaps most importantly, a couch-mount system in which to immobilize the patient's head. This feature allowed, for the first time, 360° of gantry rotation around the head to optimize noncoplanar arc beam configurations that conformed to the shape of the intracranial target. These developments have provided a LINAC-based treatment-planning platform unsurpassed in its versatility, which allows clinicians to treat a broad array of intracranial lesions safely and effectively.

2 THE PRACTICE OF X-KNIFE STEREOTACTIC RADIOSURGERY AND FRACTIONATED STEREOTACTIC RADIOTHERAPY

Patient selection for radiosurgery treatment is of utmost importance, and one must always judge whether a radiosurgical intervention better serves a patient when compared with microneurosurgery. As with any proposed treatment of a patient with a brain tumor or arteriovenous malformation (AVM), a thorough understanding of intracranial lesions, the contiguous central nervous system tissue, and the response of both to a particular intervention must be mastered and the array of risks and benefits discussed with the patient. In the case of radiosurgery using X-Knife, mastery of radiobiological principles must precede the practice of radiosurgery, as any one of an array of techniques ranging from single fraction stereotactic radiosurgery (SRS) to conventional fraction SRT might be best suited for an intracranial lesion. Because radiobiological models, for example, ascribe a direct relationship between late normal tissue damage and dose per treatment delivered to these tissues [10,11], recent published series from a growing number of institutions, including our own, have explored the use of LINAC-based SRT for the treatment of benign tumors, such as acoustic tumors. Although this experience is smaller and more recent, SRT data reflect comparable tumor control rates, and higher rates of cranial nerve preservation, most notably hearing preservation [12–14].

At our institution, we have established a stereotactic radiosurgery program that includes the use of a LINAC designed for and dedicated to SRS and SRT, the Varian 600SR [15]. Recognizing that most institutions have general-purpose LINACS, we will describe our experience using both techniques, which should be generally applicable to the typical practice of SRS and SRT, and will include case treatments as examples of each.

2.1 General Principles and Procedures

As with any stereotactic technique, the cranium must be rigidly fixed with a frame that associates a reference coordinate system to an intracranial target, providing an accurate localization of the target using only computed tomography (CT) or, additionally, either magnetic resonance imaging (MRI) or angiographic data. All imaging data are either digitized first (angiographic data) or directly electronically transferred to the treatment planning workstation. We are currently using a Hewlett-Packard Visualize C3000 treatment planning workstation. Either the Brown-Roberts-Wells (BRW) stereotactic headring (with or without the MRI-compatible adaptor) or the Gill-Thomas-Cosman (GTC) relocatable frame is used for rigid head fixation. The X-Knife software always uses CT data as a primary imaging modality because of its high spatial fidelity, and the BRW localizer is used for the CT scan. Magnetic resonance imaging data, obtained before or after CT and without the frame, can be fused to CT data using an image fusion algorithm developed by Radionics [16]. Fused images have the advantage of both high spatial fidelity and anatomical detail. Angiographic data are obtained with the angiographic localizer, and treatment planning for AVMs is primarily based on digitized biplanar stereotactic angiographic data, although we are currently exploring the use of MR angiography as an additional image data file that promises to remove ambiguities created with two-dimensional angiographic images.

The case of interest is selected as a folder, which must include CT data and additional fused or angiographic data sets, if obtained. Treatment planning commences with the default CT file or, in the case of an AVM, the digitized stereotactic angiogram. In the CT-based cases—typically tumors —the nine fiducial rod coordinates are first manually identified in one axial partial-screen CT image and subsequently autodetected throughout the axial

CT file and reconstructed as a three-dimensional reformatted image in "X-Knife space," the three-dimensional treatment-planning workspace also featured as a larger partial-screen image. If treatment planning involves an AVM, the fiducial coordinates in the angiographic localizer are identified. For CT-based cases, if fusion data are desired for treatment planning, one axial fused image slice is featured and the same nine fiducial rod coordinates are again manually identified, autodetected throughout the remainder of the axial slice file, reconstructed, and integrated into the pre-existing image established from the CT file. The lesion is then identified by the neurosurgeon in either CT or fused axial slices, as are any critical dose-limiting normal structures or "anatomes," and all contoured structures are reformatted, each color-coded, as three-dimensional structures in X-Knife space. At our institution, AVMs are identified and manually contoured on the cut film with a wax pencil by the neurosurgeon before digitization so the transferred images feature the nidus in each plane. Because of the constraints imposed by two-dimensional stereotactic angiography, other institutions have based AVM treatment planning on either CT or MRI data.

Treatment planning then commences. This task is customarily performed by the medical physicist but may include the neurosurgeon, the radiation oncologist, or both. Treatment planning is constrained by the relationship between the volume of the lesion and the safe dose considered effective in the treatment of the lesion. This relationship was originally established by Kjellberg and serves as a fundmental treatment planning principle in radiosurgery. The ideal treatment plan involves a dose that is perfectly configured to the target (dose conformality) and homogeneous (dose homogeneity), although dose inhomogeneity remains a variable suggested but not unambiguously related to treatment-related morbidity. Recent measurements have been set forth by the Radiation Therapy Oncology Group (RTOG), which serve to assess dose conformality and homogeneity. These include the ratio of the prescription isodose volume to target volume as a reflection of conformality (the PITV ratio), and the ratio of maximum dose to prescribed dose ratio as a reflection of homogeneity (the MDPD ratio). Neither of these objectives (ideally, in each case, a ratio of 1) can be practically achieved because of the comparatively small collimator sizes and the limitations of circular collimators, particularly when used for the treatment of large irregularly shaped lesions such as skull base meningiomas or large AVMs, examples of which are discussed below. A more formal and detailed description of target volumes and dose distributions within them can be found in a recent report furnished by the International Commission of Radiation Units and Measurements [17].

Tools provided by the X-Knife software maximize the likelihood of optimizing these important treatment planning objectives, thereby maximizing the therapeutic outcome and minimizing any treatment-related morbidities. As illustrations, we will provide examples of simple and complex treatment plans. A more detailed account of LINAC radiosurgery dosimetry can be found in a recent chapter by Kooy and colleagues [18].

2.2 Simple Treatment Plan: Acoustic Schwannoma

Typically, an X-Knife radiosurgery system will include 12 to 14 collimators ranging in size from 5 to 50 mm in bore diameter. An acoustic schwannoma represents a typical spherical or near-spherical target and, therefore, is a lesion requiring a simple, usually single isocenter treatment plan. An acoustic tumor and typical treatment plan are featured in Figures 1 and 2. After the lesion is contoured and reformatted in X-Knife space, X-Knife will, at the designation of the treatment planner, autoposition a default target isocenter in the geometric center of the lesion. A collimator size is chosen from a pop-up menu based on its depiction in X-Knife space as the smallest sphere that covers the broadest diameter of the lesion (Fig. 1A). The treatment planner must then designate a family of noncoplanar and nonoverlapping arcs of radiation that intersect a target in a way that creates a highly conformal plan. An arc is a single angular sweep of the LINAC gantry through space at a fixed couch angle. Different couch angles for each arc creates a

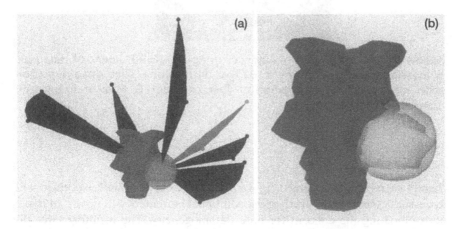

FIGURE 1 Simple treatment plan for an acoustic schwannoma. **A**, Three-dimensional depiction of collimation sphere and noncoplanar arcs converging on target in X-Knife space. **B**, Three-dimensional depiction of volume dose covering target.

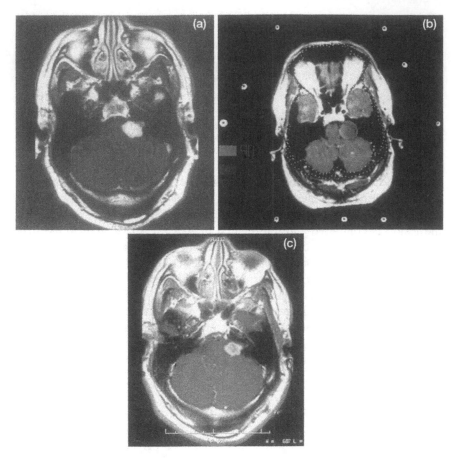

Figure 2 **A,** Magnetic resonance imaging (MRI) scan of acoustic schwannoma at pretreatment. **B,** Two-dimensional slice dose depiction with color wash representation of dose gradient. **C,** Posttreatment MRI scan at 18 months.

family of noncoplanar arcs (Fig 1A). Because only a single isocenter will be used, hotspots from overlapping additional isocenters will not be an issue, thus obviating the concern for dose inhomogeneity. The resulting three-dimensional dose is featured as a translucent "dose cloud," as featured in Figure 1B. If the target is near a dose-limiting structure, such as the optic apparatus, arc beams should be placed to avoid passage through these structures. X-Knife provides a means of visualizing the radiation path through the brain with a tool called "beam's eye view" (BEV), which allows the treatment planner an efficient means of avoiding dose-limiting structures with the appropriate gantry start and stop angles for each arc. As an efficient starting point, the treatment planner may also elect to start a plan with an X-Knife option called "autoplan," which automatically configures a family of arcs to optimize dose to target yet minimize dose to contiguous critical structures using parameters designated by the treatment planner. These tools increase the efficiency of the treatment planning process and allow the radiosurgery team time to refine the plan with adjustments to each arc.

2.3 Complex Treatment Plan: Skull Base Meningioma

With the exception of brain metastases, the shapes of many intracranial targets are infrequently spherical and often not even elliptical, and target size often exceeds the range of collimators available. Target size and shape, therefore, often require multiple isocenter treatments. A common strategy involves multiple isocenters that create a composite dose distribution approximating the target's shape and size. This strategy maximizes conformality but minimizes dose homogeneity. With techniques that include arc beam shaping and differential beam weighting, fewer isocenters can be used for complex shapes and sizes while maintaining a high degree of conformality. Skull base meningiomas often represent complex three-dimensional targets that require complex treatment plans. Unlike the single shot treatment discussed above, hotspots from overlapping additional isocenters will now be a concern, thus requiring an effort to minimize dose inhomogeneity, which can be achieved by weighting isocenters as well as converging arcs differently. In the interactive three-dimensional X-Knife environment, the evolving treatment plan can be continually assessed with three-dimensional or two-dimensional depictions either in graphic form (dose-volume histograms), or in tabular form (dose-volume summaries with average dose, minimum dose, and maximum dose reported for each anatome).

2.4 SRS Technique

X-Knife technique involves application of the BRW stereotactic headframe with an attempt to center the lesion as much as possible in stereotactic space. We routinely use a fused data set, so before frame application, patients are usually scanned in the MRI unit then sedated with Ativan, and the scalp is anesthetized with 0.5% Sensorcaine (9 parts Sensorcaine: 1 part sodium bicarbonate to minimize sting) for BRW frame application. After CT, patients are discharged to a room where they rest in the frame during treatment planning.

Treatment planning proceeds as described above and when completed, the LINAC is prepared and each isocenter qualified before patient treatment according to the printed treatment plan protocol. Qualification of the LINAC begins as a routine before any patient treatments with verification of mechanical isocenter. Because we use a couch-mount system, a device referred to as a mechanical isocenter standard (MIS) is placed in a floor housing and allows assessment of the alignment of four independent aiming lasers (Fig. 3A). Any drift that may have occurred over a 24-hour period is corrected and the MIS is then removed. The appropriate collimator is installed and the couch mount microdrives are adjusted, guided by the aiming lasers, to the first isocenter position, using the rectilinear phantom pointer (RLPP, the same device used as a phantom in CRW-based stereotactic surgery, Fig. 3B,C), which is inserted in the couch mount and calibrated to isocenter coordinates by one technologist. To verify isocenter colinearity and stability, we replace the RLPP target pointer with a spherical tungsten ball and, with a film holder attached to the collimator housing unit, expose a film strip at three different gantry positions (Fig. 3C). Each developed film strip, therefore, represents a survey of gantry rotational stability at a particular isocenter, and a variation less than 0.8 mm between the ball center and radiation field center in all three exposures is considered acceptable. As a redundant check of isocenter coordinates, a second device called the laser target localizing frame (LTLF, Fig. 3D) which is calibrated by a second technologist, is placed on the RLPP. This device has engraved brass burnishments and an arcing steel burnishment, all of which align with the aiming lasers when at isocenter. When placed on the RLPP, correct alignment at isocenter is once again confirmed and the couch mount is cleared of these devices.

When these quality assurance checks are complete, the patient is brought to the LINAC suite and placed on the couch with the BRW headring immobilized in the couch mount apparatus calibrated at isocenter. Isocenter is once again verified with the patient in position with the LTLF, which is now applied to BRW headring. We also verify that the BRW headring has not moved from initial frame application by reassessing scalp marks alignment made at frame application using a device called the depth confirmation helmet which is discussed below. The patient is now ready for treatment.

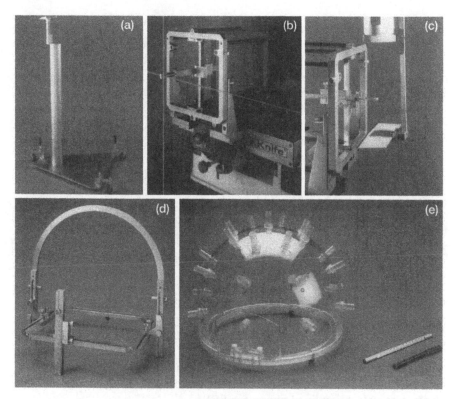

FIGURE 3 Array of quality assurance devices for the X-Knife system. **A**, Mechanical isocenter standard (MIS). **B**, Rectilinear phantom pointer (RLPP) in couch mount apparatus. **C**, RLPP in couch mount apparatus with film holder off tertiary collimator for tungsten ball film test. **D**, Laser target localizer frame (LTLF). **E**, Depth confirmation helmet.

2.5 SRT Technique

Our SRT technique involve fractionation protocols based on radiobiology of the lesion and associated dose-limiting structures. Historically, before the installation of a dedicated Varian 600SR LINAC, we designed hypofrac-tionation schemes involving 4 Gy fractions delivered twice a week, typically Monday/Thursday or Tuesday/Friday, over 5 weeks for a total dose of 36 Gy. This fractionation method was designed to maximize tumor control and minimize the risk of cranial neuropathy and radiation necrosis associated with single fraction treatments. Without the logistical constraints of a ret-rofitted LINAC, we additionally created a conventional fraction treatment scheme designed to preserve special sensory cranial nerves in patients with tumors involving or near these critical structures [12]. This paradigm involved the use of 1.8 Gy fractions delivered daily to a cumulative dose of 50 to 54 Gy over 5 weeks.

Imaging data include both CT and MRI data sets that are fused for treatment planning and treatment. We use the Gill-Thomas-Cosman relocatable frame with Reprosil® to fashion a customized site-block for each patient. Single isocenters, infrequently two, and rarely three, are used and high conformality is once again established with noncoplanar arc beam-shaping and differential beam weighting.

For SRT treatment, we have developed a quality assurance program, as previously described [12]. The accurate reproduceability of GTC frame application is verified by assessing the relationship of the frame to the skull contour through a device called a depth conformation helmet. This device, designed by the Radionics Corporation, is a lucite spherical helmet which attaches to the GTC frame. Its design includes 26 tube portals arrayed equidistantly at right angles to the sphere over its outer surface, which allows the technologist to assess the distance from the top of each tube to the scalp with a probe calibrated in millimeters (Fig. 3E). Each time the frame is applied, serial measurements for each tube portal should agree within a millimeter of previous measurements obtained before CT data acquisition. We have successfully treated more than 600 patients with accuracy and precision with this technique on the Varian 600SR.

All other quality assurance procedures for SRT treatments follow the same protocols as outlined above for SRS.

3 FUTURE DIRECTIONS OF X-KNIFE TECHNOLOGY

This chapter has emphasized the open architecture of the LINAC-based X-Knife treatment platform for both SRS and SRT. As this technology evolves in its response to ineluctably broader applications, new refinements promise to provide more effective treatments for challenging intracranial targets. As examples, optic nerve sheath meningiomas were originally considered inoperable and untreatable, but our initial experience with conventional fraction SRT has suggested promising tumor control with preservation of vision in the affected optic nerve. Similarly, large AVMs with complex three-dimensional shapes including difficult concave and convex facets were originally thought to be untreatable, but we have initiated a hypofractionation SRT technique that has achieved high obliteration rates at a threshold fraction dose of 6 to 7 Gy. All such lesions represent awkward spatial targets perhaps better served by noncircular collimation techniques such as miniature multileaf collimation couples with static-field/multiple subfield microintensity-modulated radiation therapy, techniques that are currently being incorporated into the latest version of X-Knife. As this treatment planning platform evolves with an increasing array of tools, we as treating clinicians should be able to move seamlessly between different focused radiation treatment strategies to arrive at optimal treatment plans for a variety of intracranial targets.

REFERENCES

1. Betti OO, Galmarini D, Derechinsky V. Radiosurgery with a linear accelerator. Methodological aspects. Stereotact Funct Neurosurg 1991;57:87–98.
2. Colombo F, Benedetti A, Pozza F, et al. Radiosurgery using a 4MV linear accelerator. Technique and radiobiologic implications. Acta Radiol Suppl 1986; 369:603–607.
3. Barcia-Salorio JL, Roldan P, Lopez-Gomez L. Radiosurgery of central pain. Acta Neurochir Suppl 1987;39:159–162.
4. Winston KR, Lutz W. Linear accelerator as a neurosurgical tool for stereotactic radiosurgery. Neurosurgery 1988;22:454–464.
5. Friedman WA, Bova FJ, Spiegelmann R. Linear accelerator radiosurgery at the University of Florida. Neurosurg Clin N Am 1992;3:141–166.
6. Kooy HM, Nedzi LA, Loeffler JS, et al. Treatment planning for stereotactic radiosurgery of intra-cranial lesions. Int J Radiat Oncol Biol Phys 1991;21: 683–693.
7. Gill SS, Thomas DG, Warrington AP, Brada M. Relocatable frame for stereotactic external beam therapy. Int J Radiat Oncol Biol Phys 1991;20:599–603.
8. Kooy HM, Dunbar SF, Tarbell NJ, et al. Adaptation and verification of the relocatable Gill-Thomas-Cosman frame in stereotactic radiotherapy. Int J Radiat Oncol Biol Phys 1994;30:685–691.
9. Dunbar SF, Tarbell NJ, Kooy HM, et al. Stereotactic radiotherapy for pediatric and adult brain tumors: Preliminary report [see comments]. Int J Radiat Oncol Biol Phys 1994;30:531–539.
10. Larson DA, Flickinger JC, Loeffler JS. The radiobiology of radiosurgery [editorial; comment]. Int J Radiat Oncol Biol Phys 1993;25:557–561.
11. Marks LB, Spencer DP. The influence of volume on the tolerance of the brain to radiosurgery [published erratum appears in J Neurosurg 1992 Feb;76(2): 343] [see comments]. J Neurosurg 1991;75:177–180.
12. Andrews DW, Silverman CL, Glass J, et al. Preservation of cranial nerve function after treatment of acoustic neurinomas with fractionated stereotactic radiotherapy. Preliminary observations in 26 patients. Stereotact Funct Neurosurg 1995;64:165–182.
13. Hoban PW, Jones LC, Clark BG. Modeling late effects in hypofractionated stereotactic radiotherapy. Int J Radiat Oncol Biol Phys 1999;43:199–210.
14. Kagei K, Shirato H, Suzuki K, et al. Small-field fractionated radiotherapy with or without stereotactic boost for vestibular schwannoma. Radiother Oncol 1999;50:341–347.

15. Das I, Downes MB, Corn BW, Curran WJ, Werner-Wasik M, Andrews DW. Characteristics of a dedicated linear accelerator-based stereotactic radiosurgery-radiotherapy unit. Radiother Oncol 1996;38:61–68.
16. Kooy HM, van Herk M, Barnes PD, et al. Image fusion for stereotactic radiotherapy and radiosurgery treatment planning. Int J Radiat Oncol Biol Phys 1994;28:1229–1234.
17. New ICRU dose specification report for external beam radiotherapy: Technical report 50. Bethesda, MD: International Commission of Radiation Units and Measurements (ICRU), 1993.
18. Kooy HM, Bellerive MR, Loeffler JS. Technical concepts of linac radiosurgery dosimetry. In: Tasker PGaR, ed. Textbook of Functional and Stereotactic Neurosurgery. New York: McGraw-Hill; 1998, pp 687–704.

18

Stereotactic Radiosurgery with the Linac Scalpel

Sanford L. Meeks, John M. Buatti, and Edward C. Pennington
University of Iowa Health Care,
Iowa City, Iowa, U.S.A.

Francis J. Bova, William A. Friedman, and Thomas H. Wagner
University of Florida Brain Institute,
Gainesville, Florida, U.S.A.

1 INTRODUCTION

Since Lars Leksell's conception of stereotactic radiosurgery [1], the technology has proliferated, and this treatment technique is widely available through both the Gamma Knife and modified linear accelerators (linacs). One of the early linac radiosurgery groups was based at the University of Florida [2]. The system they developed, the Linac Scalpel, included state of the art dose planning software and a linear accelerator modification that increases the accuracy of the linac to that of the Gamma Knife. This precise delivery of radiation has remained the hallmark of Linac Scalpel radiosurgery, but recent developments in computer hardware and software have tremendously improved Linac Scalpel dose planning. Over the past decade, radiosurgery dose planning has evolved from a little understood art into a well understood process that can be described mathematically and efficiently applied either manually [3–5] or automatically [6,7]. This new understanding in dose planning has provided dramatic increases in dose conformality to the target volume which, in turn, has translated into improvements in clinical outcomes [8,9].

Rather than offer an extensive review of radiosurgery literature or developments, our purpose is to provide a guide to the current practice of stereotactic radiosurgery using the Linac Scalpel system. The primary steps in the process include imaging, dose planning, and dose delivery. The following sections present these steps in their order of execution during a radiosurgery session.

2   STEREOTACTIC IMAGING AND LOCALIZATION

Imaging is one of the most important aspects in radiosurgery. The accuracy achieved with stereotactic head rings and the Linac Scalpel treatment delivery system leaves the imaging modality used as the only uncertainty. Poor imaging techniques increase this uncertainty and nullify efforts to improve accuracy in treatment planning and delivery. Therefore, it is important to understand stereotactic imaging techniques, the increased quality assurance demands that are placed on the diagnostic imaging apparatus used, and the limitations associated with each modality. Following are brief explanations of the stereotactic imaging techniques used with the Linac Scalpel: computed tomography (CT), angiography, and magnetic resonance imaging (MRI).

2.1   Computed Tomography

Computed tomography is the most reliable imaging modality for radiosurgery treatment planning. Computed tomography numbers correspond directly to electron density. This is important, because the knowledge of electron density within tissue is necessary for correctly calculating the X-ray beam attenuation characteristics. Computed tomography also provides an accurate spatial database that introduces little image distortion and provides an accurate representation of the patient's external contour and internal anatomy. Stereotactic CT images are obtained with a Brown-Roberts-Wells (BRW) compatible CT localizer attached to the stereotactic head ring. Because the geometry of the localizer is known relative to the head ring, stereotactic coordinates may be accurately calculated based on the CT scan of the localizer. The characteristic N shape allows for a scanner-independent calculation of stereotactic coordinates. In other words, the x,y,z coordinates of any point in space can be mathematically determined relative to the head ring rather than relying on the CT coordinates. This method provides more accurate spatial localization, and minimizes the CT scanner quality assurance requirements [10].

To minimize the inaccuracies associated with the stereotactic imaging, it is important to obtain all imaging studies with the best available spatial resolution. With a BRW localizer, CT images must be obtained using a minimum 34.5 cm field of view, which is just large enough to image all the stereotactic fiducials. Using a 512 × 512 matrix with this field of view results in an in-plane pixel, or picture element, dimension of 0.67 mm. The vertical resolution of the image set, and thus the accuracy of determining the axial coordinate of a pixel, is determined by the slice thickness. Again, it is imperative to minimize the uncertainty associated with the vertical resolution, and we obtain 1-mm thick CT slices through the region of interest.

2.2 Magnetic Resonance Imaging

Magnetic resonance imaging often provides superior tumor visualization, but MRI alone does not necessarily present a sufficient database from radiotherapy treatment planning calculations, as the pixel intensity values are not correlated with electron density. Furthermore, main magnetic field nonuniformity and patient-specific artifacts can introduce significant geometric image distortions that affect the accuracy of treatment plans generated by MRI alone. Introducing a stereotactic frame and localizer into the system further perturbs the magnetic field, worsening the inherent field nonuniformity, patient-specific artifacts, and image distortion. These image distortions have been shown to be on the order of 0.7 to 4 mm in each orthogonal plane (axial, sagittal, coronal) of a stereotactic MRI [11–13]. Further complicating stereotactic MRI localization is the size of the stereotactic head frame and its compatibility with the MRI head coil. The standard BRW frame, for example, is too large to place in a standard MRI head coil. Use of a larger MRI coil, such as the standard body imaging coil, degrades the image quality by reducing the signal-to-noise-ratio.

We use an image correlation technique to avoid these problems. A three-dimensional volumetric MR scan is acquired before head ring placement. For T1-weighted images, we typically use a spoiled gradient recall fast pulse sequence using a General Electric 1.5 Tesla MR scanner. This sequence allows us to acquire 1.5-mm thick slices throughout the entire head in less than 15 minutes. After acquiring the stereotactic CT scan, this non-stereotactic MRI dataset is mapped onto the CT image space. Anatomical landmarks are selected in both the CT and MR image sets, and the MR images are digitally manipulated to match the CT image coordinates. During treatment planning, the dose distribution may be displayed on either the MRI or CT images, but dosimetry calculations are always performed on the underlying CT database. This way, diagnostic information may be obtained from the MRI database, but geometric and dosimetric information is obtained from the CT database. The ability to obtain nonstereotactic MRI removes one potential source of geometric distortion, namely perturbation of the magnetic field by the stereotactic head ring and localizer. Furthermore, because the images are acquired through the standard diagnostic head coil, a high resolution image set is obtained. Careful review of the MRI and its agreement with the CT database is essential, especially as all currently available image correlation routines consider the MR images as rigid bodies and do not remove local image distortions that can exist in the MR data. This comparison should focus on internal anatomy such as the ventricles, tentorium, sulci, among others. Basing the image correlation on external anatomy leads to unavoidable errors, as the external contour can be shifted 3 to 4 mm on MR. This shift, known as the fat shift, is caused by the difference in the resonant frequency of protons in fat relative to their resonant frequency in water.

2.3 Angiography

Angiography is clearly the gold standard for diagnosis and anatomic characterization of cerebral arteriovenous malformations (AVMs). Anteroposterior (AP) and lateral films are obtained with contrast injected rapidly at the point of interest, allowing excellent visualization of fine vasculature. Stereotactic angiography uses 16 radiopaque fiducials imbedded in a localizer that attaches to the stereotactic ring. Eight of these fiducials appear in both the AP and lateral films. Because the geometry of these fiducials is known relative to the head ring, the stereotactic coordinates of any point within the localizer may be calculated very accurately. However, the use of stereotactic angiography as the sole localization method for treatment planning leads to unavoidable errors in determining the shape, size, and location of the AVM nidus [14–16]. Angiography provides two-dimensional projections of a three-dimensional object. These two-dimensional projections represent the maximum target dimensions for that view. For a truly spherical nidus, its shape and size may be correctly determined from these biplane projections. As the target deviates from spherical geometry, however, these projections provide insufficient information to reconstruct the actual three-dimensional shape of the target volume. Further complicating the use of angiography for treatment planning is that overlapping structures, such as feeding or draining blood vessels, may obscure the view of the AVM. Including these blood vessels as part of the targeted AVM results in unnecessary irradiation of normal tissue.

Given angiography's limitations, radiosurgery treatment planning requires the use of a three-dimensional image base in addition to, or in replacement of, stereotactic angiography. Because CT provides geometrically sound three-dimensional information, it is the logical supplement to stereotactic angiography. A high-resolution CT scan is obtained with simultaneous infusion of intravenous contrast. One-millimeter thick slices are obtained through the region of interest while contrast is injected at a rate of 1 cc/sec. The resultant CT images provide a three-dimensional description of the AVM nidus, along with the feeding and draining vessels.

3 RADIOSURGERY TREATMENT PLANNING

Subsequent to localizing the target volume from a three-dimensional stereotactic database, these images are used to develop a radiosurgery dose plan. Our philosophy is to design treatment plans in which the isodose shell is tightly conformal to the target volume, while all normal tissue is excluded from the high-dose region. Because radiosurgery is used to treat benign lesions and as a boost for malignant disease, no margin is added to the gross target volume to irradiate microscopic disease. Furthermore, every effort has been made to remove all possible sources of error from our treatment delivery system, and no margin is added to account for setup uncertainty.

Linac Scalpel radiosurgery treatment planning and delivery uses noncoplanar arc therapy delivered through circular collimators. The intersection of multiple beams, each with unique entry and exit pathways, results in a peaked dose at the isocenter and a very steep dose gradient outside of the target volume. The use of noncoplanar arc therapy results in a dose fall-off from the prescription isodose shell to half the prescription dose in approximately 2 to 4 mm.

Radiosurgery treatment planning using the Linac Scalpel typically begins with a standard nine arc set [3–5]. Each arc is 90° to 100° in length, and the arcs are separated from one another by a 20° table rotation. The 80% isodose shell (normalized to the maximum dose in three-dimensional space) is chosen for prescription because it achieves a steep dose gradient outside of the target volume. When a spherical target is encountered, this nine arc set is sufficient to produce a conformal treatment plan. Figure 1 demonstrates a nominally spherical meningioma that was treated using these 9 standard arcs. By carefully choosing the appropriate collimator, the 80% isodose shell tightly conforms to the shape of the lesion, and the dose gradient outside the target volume is very steep.

As the target shape deviates from spherical geometry, the treatment planning parameters must be modified to generate a treatment plan that

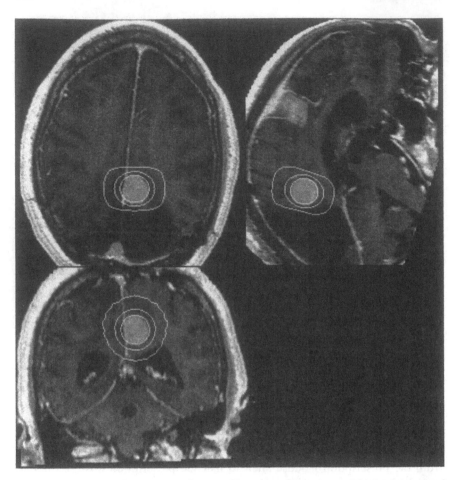

FIGURE 1 Using the appropriate collimator diameter with the standard nine-arc set results in a highly conformal dose distribution. The 80%, 40%, and 16% of maximum isodose lines are shown on three orthogonal MRI slices through the center of a nominally spherical meningioma.

conforms to the shape of the target. Linac radiosurgery provides several treatment planning parameters that allow production of nonspherical treatment plans. Arc weighting, collimator size, and arc length may all be altered to produce ellipsoidal dose distributions while maintaining a single isocenter plan. More irregular targets require multiple isocenter planning.

Linac radiosurgery treatment planning is a difficult skill to master. The University of Florida radiosurgery planning algorithm, shown in Figure 2

University of Florida
Treatment Planning Algorithm for Optimization

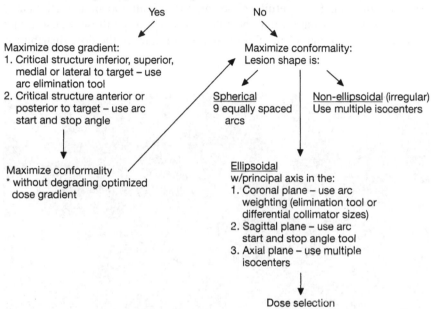

FIGURE 2 The University of Florida Treatment Planning Algorithm is a decision tree that helps guide the radiosurgery treatment planner through the planning process.

[3,4], provides the basis for use of the treatment planning methods outlined in this section. This algorithm organizes the tools available to the radiosurgery planner to efficiently generate conformal radiosurgery plans that provide appropriate sparing of non-target tissues. The first step of the algorithm is to determine whether the targeted lesion is adjacent to a radiosensitive structure. If so, single isocenter arc parameters (presented in a later section) are adjusted to steepen the dose gradient in the direction of the radiosensitive structure, if possible. If the lesion is very irregular in shape or is an ellipsoid with the major axis aligned along the anterior-posterior direction, multiple isocenters are used to conform the dose distribution to the shape of the lesion. Each of the tools encountered in the treatment planning algorithm is explained in more detail in the following sections.

3.1 Arc Elimination

Eliminating arcs from the standard nine-arc set elongates the dose distribution in the direction of the remaining arcs, thus producing an ellipsoidal dose distribution. By carefully choosing the orientation of the eliminated arcs, the dose distribution may be tilted to match any ellipse whose major axis lies in the coronal plane. For example, in Figure 3, the dose distribution

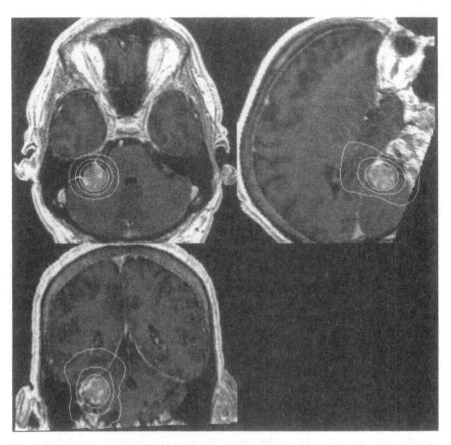

FIGURE 3   In the case of acoustic neuromas, the target volume is directly lateral to the brainstem. To steepen the dose gradient in the direction of the brainstem, the most lateral arcs are removed from the nine-arc set. In this example, the two most lateral arcs are removed, providing a steep dose gradient in the lateral direction and a slight elongation of the dose distribution in the superior-inferior direction. This improves the conformality to the targeted lesion.

is elongated in the superior-inferior direction by eliminating the two most lateral arcs. The resultant dose distribution is ellipsoidal, as it is elongated in the direction of the remaining arcs. When nine symmetric arcs overlap at isocenter, the intersection of all nine arcs results in a spherical dose distribution. If the contribution from the most lateral arcs is removed, the intersection of the more vertically oriented arcs is in a more superior-inferior direction. For the acoustic schwannoma shown in Figure 3, this elongation results in a highly conformal dose distribution.

A second consequence of arc elimination is that it improves the dose gradient in the direction of the eliminated arcs while reducing the dose gradient in the direction of the remaining arcs. Thus, arc elimination is often used not for dose conformality to a lesion, but rather as a means of avoiding critical neural structures in close proximity to the target. When treating acoustic schwannomas, as in Figure 3, the most lateral arcs are often eliminated to minimize the dose to the medially located brainstem. This removes the arcs that enter or exit through the brainstem, thus improving the dose gradient in the direction of the brainstem. Because the remaining arcs are more vertically oriented, the dose gradient in the superior-inferior direction is worsened. This is typically acceptable, as it forces the low isodose lines to bulge to a portion of the brain in which fewer radiosensitive neural structures are located. Similarly, arc elimination may be used to improve the dose gradient in the direction of any critical structure located medial, lateral, superior, or inferior to the target volume.

3.2 Differential Collimators

Choosing the collimator diameter separately for each arc within an isocenter may be done in conjunction with, or as an alternative to, arc elimination to produce a variety of ellipsoidal dose distributions. The general idea is to select the collimator for each arc, such that the collimator diameter closely matches the "beam's-eye-view" (BEV) projection of the target in each arcing plane. The superior-inferior dimension of the dose distribution (the "height") is determined primarily by the collimator diameter chosen from the lateral arcs, whereas the lateral dimension of the dose distribution (the "width") is affected primarily by the diameter of the most vertical arcs. As demonstrated in Figure 4, reducing the collimator diameter on the most lateral arcs reduces the height of the dose distribution and results in an ellipsoidal distribution that tightly matches an ellipsoidal metastasis.

Conversely, reducing the collimator diameter for the most vertical arcs narrows the width of the distribution. The use of differential collimator sizes within a single isocenter dose not result in as extreme an elongation of the dose distribution as does arc elimination, and is generally used as a fine-

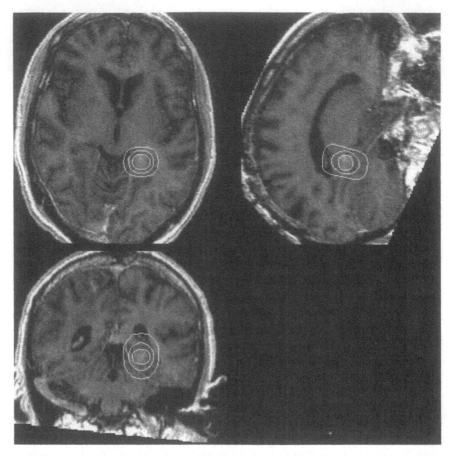

FIGURE 4 Choosing smaller collimator diameters for the more lateral arcs results in a highly conformal plan for this slightly ellipsoidal target metastasis. Again the 80%, 40%, and 16% of maximum isodose shells are superimposed on the MRI cuts through isocenter.

tuning mechanism. Furthermore, differential collimator sizes do not affect the dose gradient as much as arc elimination and, therefore, are not useful for avoiding critical structures.

3.3 Arc Start/Stop Angles

As can be seen in the previous figures, the standard arc configuration results in a slight AP tilt of the dose distribution. This tilt is simply the result of the geometry of irradiation; the sagittal arc is rotated 10° anteriorly, resulting in a 10° AP tilt in the low isodose lines. Often, the lesion has a different AP orientation in the sagittal plane. The tilted dose distribution may be rotated to more closely match the lesion orientation by altering the arc start and stop angles.

More often, however, manipulation of the arc lengths is used to avoid a critical structure that is directly anterior or posterior to a target. Removing the anterior or posterior portion of the arcs improves the dose gradient in the AP direction and worsens the dose gradient in the superior-inferior direction. Similar to arc elimination, altering the length of the arc span is used to eliminate beams that intersect a radiosensitive neural structure that is anterior or posterior to the target, and to improve the dose gradient in that direction.

3.4 Multiple Isocenter Planning

As the previous sections illustrate, manipulating the arcs within a single isocenter can be used to conform the dose distribution to all spherical and most ellipsoidal target volumes. Most of the targets encountered in radiosurgery are neither spherical nor ellipsoidal, however, and multiple isocenters must be used to conform the dose distribution to any target that deviates from ellipsoidal geometry. Multiple isocenter planning requires packing small spherical dose distributions within the target volume. Any arbitrary shape may be achieved if these spherical dose distributions are placed correctly within the volume. In contrast to other radiosurgery modalities, linac radiosurgery has the added ability to produce ellipsoidal dose distributions by altering the previously discussed parameters. Therefore, both spherical and ellipsoidal dose distributions may be placed within the target to minimize the number of isocenters while still producing a conformal dose distribution.

3.4.1 Isocenter Selection and Placement

To use multiple isocenters, the three-dimensional shape of the target must first be ascertained. This is accomplished by viewing sequential axial CT or MR images from the top to the bottom of the lesion. Alternatively, a three-dimensional viewing window can simplify this task if the lesion has been manually contoured. If the lesion is generally cylindrical, two isocenters are used. If it is generally triangular, three isocenters are used. If it is shaped like a rectangular solid, four isocenters are used. Occasionally, more isocenters are necessary to conform to a lesion of very irregular shape.

Once the three-dimensional shape of the lesion and the number of isocenters needed are determined, the isocenters must be positioned. For multiple isocenter planning, a standardized, equally spaced *five-arc set* with a spherical dose distribution is used for each isocenter. The isocenters are roughly positioned in the appropriate orientation and an appropriate collimator size is selected for each.

3.4.2 Isocenter Spacing

Placing these isocenters such that the prescription isodose tightly conforms to the surface of the lesion is important; it is also critical that the isocenters are spaced correctly relative to one another, because insufficient interisocenter spacing results in a large dose inhomogeneity, possibly increasing the risk of permanent complications [17]. Overlap of the dose distributions introduces some additional dose inhomogeneity, and multiple isocenter plans are typically prescribed to the 70% isodose shell, normalized to maximum. All dose distributions within this report are normalized to the point of maximum dose, as consistent normalization is important in the assessment of the overall dose inhomogeneity. If dose distributions are normalized to isocenter, 200% hot spots can easily result and are often undetected. The inhomogeneity can be minimized by allowing adequate spacing between the isocenters, but excessive interisocenter distance will force the isodose distribution to assume a characteristic dumbbell appearance with a significant waist between the two isocenters. Thus, the optimal spacing between isocenters minimizes the additional dose inhomogeneity introduced, minimizes the waist between the isocenters, and preserves the steep dose gradient outside of the target volume.

The effects of isocenter spacing on the overall dose distribution may be seen in Figure 5, which shows 50% and 70% isodose curves in an axial plane for two equally weighted isocenters at several interisocenter spacings, each with a standard five arc set delivered with a 30-mm collimator. For this discussion, it is helpful to consider each isocenter as a solid, 30-mm sphere, corresponding approximately to the 70% isodose surface of a five arc set. As a first approximation, one would expect a sphere separation of about 30 mm (the sum of the radii of each sphere) to be correct. As will be shown, this is approximately correct, but slightly more separation is optimal.

The 70% volume in the dose distributions shown in Figure 5 correspond approximately to the geometrical coverage of a 30-mm diameter sphere placed at each isocenter. At an isocenter spacing of 40 mm, the 70% volume is slightly greater than the sum of two 30-mm spheres, and the 50% volume (outer isodose line) is slightly larger. The "waist" between the 70% isodose lines is so pronounced that the 70% isodose shells are actually separated from one another. As the isocenters are moved closer together, the 70% isodose shell more strongly resembles two 30-mm diameter spheres. At approximately 32 to 33-mm interisocenter spacing, the isodose distributions are near ideal. As the isocenters are moved closer to one another for

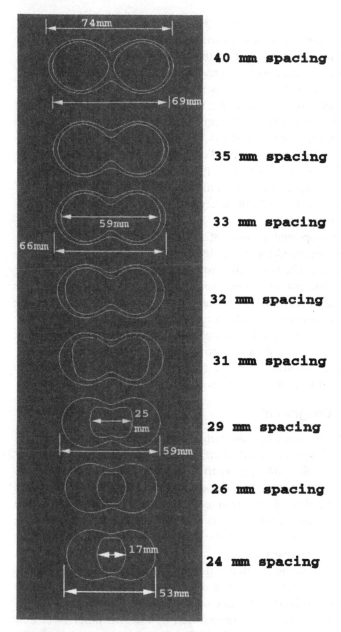

FIGURE 5 Effects of isocenter spacing on the multiple isocenter dose distribution. The 70% and 50% isodose lines are shown in a transaxial plane for two equally weighted 30-mm isocenters, each with a five arc set.

distances less than about 32 mm, the 70% isodose volume contracts dramatically. This is because each dose distribution is renormalized to 100% at the point of maximum dose, so that as the hotspot where the two spheres overlap one another becomes more intense, the volume covered by 70% of this increasing maximum dose becomes smaller and smaller. This can be seen by the rapid decrease in size of the middle 70% isodose region, from 59 mm across with a spacing of 33 mm, down to a region only 17 mm across when the interisocenter spacing is reduced to 24 mm. The 70% isodose region shrinks to less than one third of its initial size, whereas the 50% isodose region shrinks much more gradually from 66 mm to 53 mm (a 20% decrease). For this example of two 30-mm isocenters, the 70% isodose shell may be approximated as two 30-mm spheres, if an interisocenter spacing of at least 32 mm is maintained.

To achieve this optimal spacing of the isocenters relative to one another, we use a computerized lookup table of predetermined values for each collimator combination. The two collimator sizes are entered into the spacing table, and the table returns an optimal spacing for the two isocenters. The positions of the isocenters relative to one another are fine-tuned with the help of an *isocenter moving tool*, which can be used to automatically move one isocenter relative to another. In clinical application, the optimal isocenter spacing from the table is used as a starting point for isocenter placement, but iterative spacing adjustments are commonly required to optimize the dose distribution conformality to a given target volume.

3.4.3 Isocenter Weighting

Conceptually, multiple isocenter planning is a simple sphere packing arrangement, with each sphere size corresponding to the available collimator diameters. In this simple paradigm, each radiosurgery isocenter would be weighted equally (with respect to dose at its isocenter). However, when attempting to obtain a dose distribution as uniform as possible throughout a region containing several isocenters, it is usually beneficial to consider the dose contribution to an isocenter from neighboring isocenters when selecting an isocenter's weight (intensity of dose).

Consider the following example of four 14-mm diameter isocenters spaced equally in a line along the lateral direction, shown in Figure 6. Each isocenter is equally weighted, such that each isocenter contributes 1.0 relative units of dose at its center. However, each of the two inner isocenters receives a greater dose contribution from the other isocenters than do the two outer isocenters, resulting in an uneven dose distribution. As shown by the total dose curve in Figure 6, when the isocenters *deliver* equal doses, they *receive* unequal doses; the two inner isocenters receive about 1.4 rel-

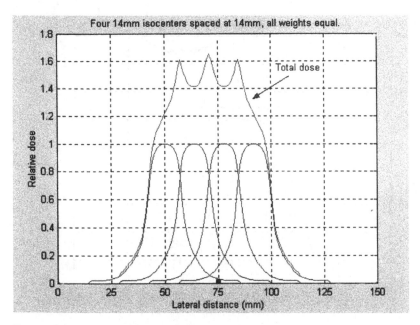

FIGURE 6 Dose profile through four optimally spaced 14-mm isocenters, each with an equally weighted five arc set. The dose profile for each isocenter and the total combined dose profile are shown.

ative units of dose, whereas the outer isocenters receive about 1.2 relative dose units.

Figure 7 shows the individual and total dose distribution after the isocenter dose weighting has been adjusted to 1.17:0.94:0.94:1.17. Peripherally weighting the isocenters in this fashion results in a uniform dose received by each of the four isocenters. Although the total dose distribution is still somewhat heterogeneous, it is more homogeneous than the total dose distribution in Figure 6. This is illustrated more clearly in Figure 8, which shows the total dose distribution for both situations. The overall dose distribution after adjusting the weights is more homogeneous, in that the volume of the 70% isodose surface has been increased, and the "hot" volume (hotspot) receiving more than 90% of maximum dose has been reduced. Also, note that the prescription to half-prescription isodose gradient is steeper for the adjusted weights distribution. The 35% isodose shell is almost identical between the two plans, but because the 70% isodose shell is larger for the adjusted weights plan, it is closer to the 35% isodose shell and offers a steeper dose fall off. In most radiosurgery planning situations, the same advantage holds for adjusting the isocenter weights to improve the dose

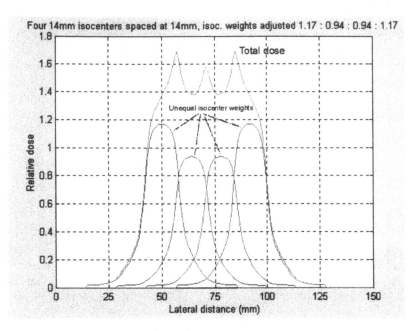

FIGURE 7   Dose profile through four optimally spaced 14-mm isocenters, each weighted to achieve equal total doses at each of the four isocenters. The dose profile for each isocenter and the total combined dose profile are shown.

homogeneity and gradient around the target volume. An automatic weighting tool to perform this task has been implemented in the Linac Scalpel treatment planning system. This tool iteratively adjusts the arc weights associated with each isocenter to achieve a uniform dose to each isocenter.

In addition to automated isocenter weight optimization, this tool can be used manually to fine tune the dose distribution. At times, it is desired to have more or less contribution to the dose distribution from a particular isocenter. The isocenter weighting tool can be used to adjust the weight delivered to a particular isocenter while maintaining a constant weight delivered to all of the other isocenters in the treatment plan.

3.4.4   Limited Arc Isocenters

During the final stages of multi-isocenter treatment planning, it is common to arrive at a prescription isodose contour that conforms closely to the target lesion with the exception of very small volumes where the target protrudes outside the prescription isodose. If the volume of target outside the prescription isodose surface is small and is underdosed by not more than 5% to

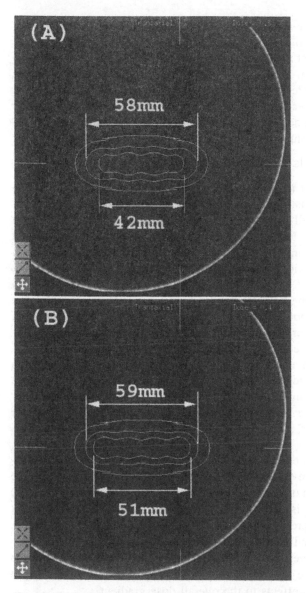

FIGURE 8   Axial plane dose distribution (70%, 35%, and 14% isodose lines shown) for four 14 mm isocenters. **(A)** All weights equal, **(B)** Weights adjusted to obtain equal isocenter doses.

10%, a single arc can be directed at a new isocenter near the periphery of the volume that needs to be covered [18]. This results in "dose painting" that provides a small yet adequate expansion of the prescription surface to cover the exposed target. It is important to select the orientation of this arc such that it provides the least possible contribution to the existing isocenters. If this orientation is selected properly, a limited arc isocenter will provide the desired target coverage without affecting the conformality of the remainder of the target volume.

3.4.5 Clinical Multi-Isocenter Planning

The general sequence of multiple isocenter treatment planning is illustrated on an irregular metastasis shown in Figure 9. The general shape of the target volume is assessed in all three dimensions. A standard five-arc set is then placed, and the isocenter location and collimator diameter are chosen to treat the largest possible volume of the target while not irradiating any normal tissue. The dose distribution is then calculated for this single isocenter plan, as shown in Figure 9. A second five-arc set is then placed, as shown in Figure 10. Even with the correct spacing between the two isocenters, the dose distribution may not be optimal because of dose contributions from one isocenter to the other. This is particularly true when the collimator diameter used on one isocenter is substantially larger than the diameter used on another isocenter in the same plan. In Figure 10, for example, even though the doses delivered by each isocenter are the same, the actual dose received by isocenter number 2 is 20% higher than the dose received by isocenter number 1. The isocenter weighting tool is then used to equalize the two isocenter doses, resulting in the dose distribution shown in Figure 11.

Subsequent isocenters are then placed and weighted in a similar fashion until a plan is achieved that closely corresponds to the target volume with minimal irradiation of normal tissue outside of the target volume. Often, a very conformal plan is achieved that has very small regions of target volume outside of the prescription isodose shell, as shown in Figure 12. A single arc can be directed near the periphery of this target region to provide just enough dose to cover the underdosed region. After adding this single arc, as shown in Figure 13, the dose distribution conforms to the target volume without adverse effects to the overall dose gradient.

Using this systematic approach to multiple isocenter planning, a conformal treatment plan can be generated for any target volume. Clearly, a great deal of expertise and practice are required to generate conformal plans for highly complex target volumes. Therefore, an automated algorithm that follows this systematic approach to multiple isocenter planning has been developed [7].

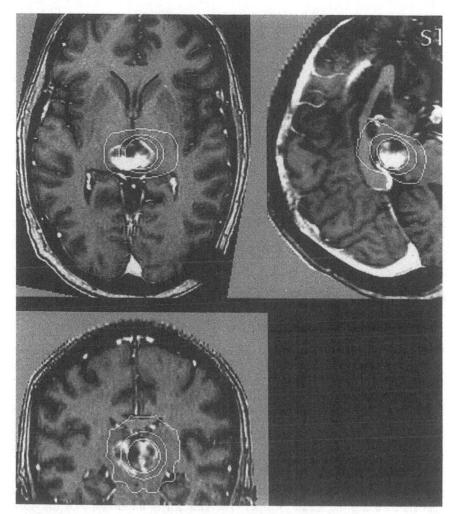

FIGURE 9   A five-arc delivered through a 20-mm diameter collimator treats the largest possible target volume without unnecessary irradiation of normal tissue. This isocenter serves as the starting point for a multiple isocenter plan. In this and all subsequent figures, the 70%, 35%, and 14% of maximum isodose are shown on the MRI scan.

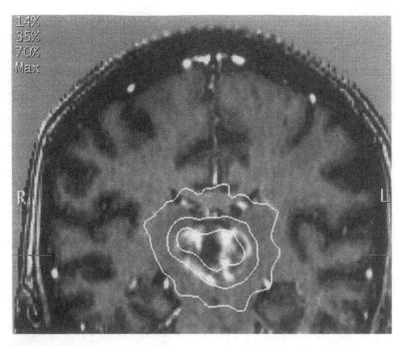

FIGURE 10 A second isocenter, delivered through a 10-mm diameter collimator is placed in the target volume. Even though the isocenters are
spaced properly relative to one another, dose communication between
the two isocenters causes a suboptimal dose distribution.

4 TREATMENT DELIVERY

As the preceding section demonstrates, highly conformal dose plans can be
generated using the Linac Scalpel. Therefore, it is important that the dose
delivery system is capable of accurately delivering these conformal plans.
Unfortunately, a standard radiotherapy linac is not necessarily capable of
achieving such accuracy; the basic acceptance criteria for a radiotherapy
linac requires that the gantry maintain a radiation focus about isocenter to
an accuracy of ±1 mm. In other words, the gantry radiation isocenter must
remain confined to a 2-mm sphere. The generally accepted tolerance for
patient support rotation about isocenter is also ±1 mm. It is generally assumed that the rotation of the patient support system's axis coincides with
that of the gantry. It is, however, possible that the centers of the two 2-mm
spheres will differ and that the combined tolerance will be greater than either
of the individual 2-mm tolerances. Therefore, care should be taken to prop-

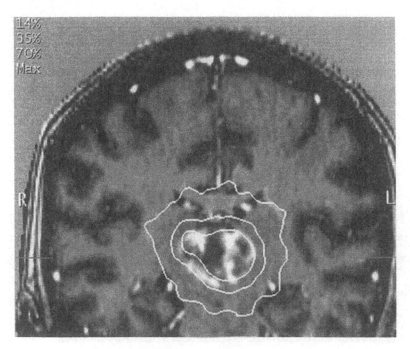

FIGURE 11 Using the isocenter weighting tool to equalize the doses delivered to isocenter results in a more homogeneous distribution for the two isocenter plan.

erly evaluate the accuracy of any linac to be used as part of a radiosurgery system.

The linac scalpel uses a special modification to the linac that enables a treatment accuracy of 0.2 ± 0.1 mm for rotation of both gantry and patient about isocenter. This modification, known as a floor stand, uses a system of bearings that allow the beam to stay focused on isocenter, effectively eliminating isocentric inaccuracies caused by the patient support system and gantry sag [2].

4.1 Testing Procedure

Testing the linac radiosurgery system requires a local standard, known as the phantom base. It is very important to test not only the center of the stereotactic reference system but to also test points throughout the entire stereotactic space that can be used for routine treatment. Our testing procedure is similar to that designed by Winston and Lutz [19,20]. In this test, a coordinate is set on the phantom base and by means of mechanical transfer,

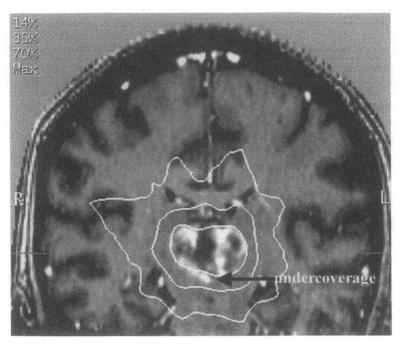

FIGURE 12 After 11 isocenters have been placed in the target volume, a very conformal dose distribution is achieved with the exception of a small region at the inferior portion of the tumor.

a target sphere is placed on the linac. In our system, the phantom base has been redesigned to eliminate the mechanical transfer, and the target sphere may be placed directly on the linac. Films are obtained of the target with the linac set at various gantry and patient support unit rotations. These films are analyzed to establish the overall system accuracy. The system accuracy may be ascertained by measuring the target's displacement from the center of the radiation field through all of the linac's rotations. Most often, the displacement is measured using a set of concentric circles in conjunction with a 10X magnifier with internal 0.1-mm scale. The outer circle is 24 mm in diameter, which corresponds to the collimator diameter used to expose the films. The inner circle is 8 mm in diameter, which corresponds to the target sphere diameter. These two circles are concentric to within 0.01 mm. The outer circle is first aligned with the image of the collimator on the film. If the target is perfectly centered in the radiation beam, the image of the target will align perfectly with the inner circle. If there is a misalignment, this is measured using the magnifier's internal scale.

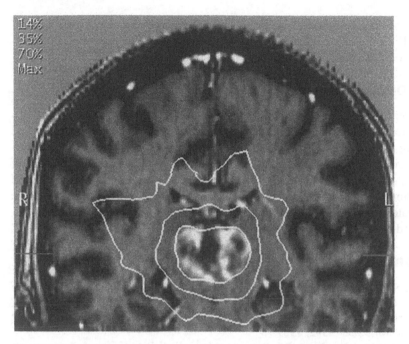

FIGURE 13 Adding a single arc to isocenter number 12 covers the small region of target and completes the very conformal plan.

For daily treatment, the preceding quality assurance procedure is followed for each patient. This daily test is used to verify the stereotactic coordinates rather than to test the system accuracy. This is important, as studies have shown that errors are often made in setting the stereotactic coordinates [21]. The isocentric coordinates obtained from the treatment planning computer are set on the phantom base by one individual, and independently set on the patient support system by another. The phantom target is transferred to the patient support system and a film is exposed. The film is visually inspected to assure its quality. It has been our experience that by inspection, any error greater than 0.5 mm is obvious to a trained observed. Because this is a test to ensure that the target has been setup without error, we feel that measuring each individual target film is not necessary.

Subsequent to coordinate verification, the patient is treated following a detailed checklist generated by the treatment planning computer. Following such a list prevents errors in treatment execution. If a second isocenter is required, the new isocenter coordinates are set on the isocentric subsystem.

After the new coordinates are set, a blind read is conducted by two individuals. If all readings agree, then the second isocenter is treated. This procedure is repeated for all subsequent isocenters on that patient.

5 CONCLUSIONS

Stereotactic radiosurgery is a complex process that is most successful when executed by a knowledgeable multidisciplinary team from neurosurgery and radiation oncology. It is important that neurosurgeons involved in radiosurgery understand the entire treatment process, including diagnostic imaging, stereotactic localization, treatment planning, and radiation delivery. Careful attention to each of these details results in better target visualization, more accurate target localization, more conformal treatment planning, and decreased overall uncertainty in radiation delivery.

REFERENCES

1. Leksell L. The stereotaxic method and radiosurgery of the brain. Acta Chir Scand 102:316–319, 1951.
2. Friedman WA, Bova FJ. The University of Florida radiosurgery system. Surg Neurol 32:334–342, 1989.
3. Friedman WA, Buatti JM, Bova FJ, Mendenhall WM. Linac radiosurgery: A practical guide. New York, Springer Verlag, 1998.
4. Meeks SL, Buatti JM, Bova FJ, Friedman WA, Mendenhall WM. Treatment planning optimization for linear accelerator radiosurgery. Int J Radiat Oncol Biol Phys 41(1):183–197, 1998.
5. Foote KD, Friedman WA, Meeks SL, Buatti JM, Bova FJ. Fundamentals of stereotactic radiosurgery: Software and dose planning. In: Radiosurgery, AANS, 2000, in press.
6. Meeks SL, Bova FJ, Buatti JM, Friedman WA, Eyster B, Kendrick LA. Analytic characterization of radiosurgery dose distributions for fast optimization. Phys Med Biol 44(11):2777–2787, 1999.
7. Wagner TH, Yi T, Meeks SL, Bova FJ, Brechner BL, Chen Y, Foote KD, Bouchet LG, Friedman WA, Buatti JM. A geometrically based method for automated radiosurgery planning. Int J Radiat Oncol Biol Phys, 48(5):1591–1603, 2000.
8. Foote KD, Buatti JM, Friedman WA, Meeks SL, Bova FJ. An analysis of risk factors in radiosurgery for vestibular schwannoma, (abstract). Neurosurgery 45(3):724, 1999.
9. Meeks SL, Buatti JM, Foote KD, Friedman WA, Bova FJ. Calculation of cranial nerve complication probability for acoustic neuroma radiosurgery. Int J Radiat Oncol Biol Phys 47(3), 2000.
10. Bova FJ, Meeks SL, Friedman WA. Linac Radiosurgery: System requirements, procedures and testing. In: Khan FM, Potish RA, editors. Treatment Planning in Radiation Oncology. Baltimore: Williams and Wilkins, 1997, pp 215–241.

11. Burcheil KJ, Nguyen TT, Commbs BD, Szumoski J. MRI distortion and stereotactic neurosurgery using the Cosman-Roberts-Wells and Leksell frames. Stereotact Funct Neurosurg 66:123–136, 1996.
12. Huh SN. Incorporation of magnetic resonance imaging and digital angiography in the application of stereotactic radiosurgery. [Dissertation] Gainesville, FL, University of Florida, 1994.
13. Kitchen ND, Lemieux K, Thomas DG. Accuracy in frame-based and frameless stereotaxy. Stereotact Funct Neurosurg 61:195–206, 1993.
14. Blatt DR, Friedman WA, Bova FJ. Modifications based on computed tomographic imaging in planning the radiosurgical treatment of arteriovenous malformations. Neurosurgery 33(4):588–596, 1993.
15. Bova FJ, Friedman W. Stereotactic angiography: An inadequate database for radiosurgery? Int J Radiat Oncol Biol Phys 20:891–895, 1991.
16. Spiegelmann R, Friedman WA, Bova FJ. Limitations of angiographic target localization in planning radiosurgical treatment. Neurosurgery 30(4):619–624, 1992.
17. Nedzi LA, Kooy H, Alexander E, Gelman RS, Loeffler JS. Variables associated with the development of complications from radiosurgery of intracranial tumors. Int J Radiat Oncol Biol Phys 21:591–599, 1991.
18. Schulder M, Narra V, Cathcart C, Halpern J. Limited arc radiosurgery. In: International Stereotactic Radiosurgery Society (ISRS) 3rd Congress, Madrid, 1997, pp 90.
19. Lutz W, Winston KR, Maleki NM. A system for stereotactic radiosurgery with a linear accelerator. Int J Radiat Oncol Biol Phys 14:373–381, 1988.
20. Winston KR, Lutz W. Linear accelerator as a neurosurgical tool for stereotactic radiosurgery. Neurosurgery 22(3):454–464, 1988.
21. Flickenger JC, Lunsford LD, Kondziolka D, Maitz A. Potential human error in setting stereotactic coordinates for radiosurgery: Implications for quality assurance. Int J Radiat Oncol Biol Phys 27:397–401, 1993.

19

Stereotactic Radiosurgery with the BrainLab System

M. Raphael Pfeffer and Roberto Spiegelmann

The Chaim Sheba Medical Center, Tel Hashomer, Israel and
The Sackler School of Medicine, Tel Aviv University,
Tel Aviv, Israel

1   INTRODUCTION

The BrainLab stereotactic irradiation software, BrainScan, includes modules
for planning stereotactic irradiation (SRS) using dynamic noncoplanar arcs
or fixed conformal beams when the linear accelerator is equipped with a
beam-shaping tool, either a mini multileaf collimator (mMLC) or cylindrical
cerrobend collimators. We have been using BrainScan version 5.0 for the
last year. Our system includes both conventional circular collimators and a
computerized mMLC, allowing us the choice of either delivering traditional
radiosurgery (noncoplanar arcs) or conformal (fixed shaped beams combined
with an mMLC) stereotactic radiation, depending on the size and shape of
the lesion. We will describe here the basic principles and stages of planning
and delivery of both techniques, including the benefits and drawbacks of the
two methods. We will also highlight the strong and weak points of the
BrainLab radiosurgery system.

2 DISPLAY

The BrainLab stereotactic planning system runs on Windows NT, and most of the functions can easily be controlled from the computer mouse. In all modes, the display consists of a main window and up to five smaller windows. The initial (default) main window after loading the patient's file is a single axial image from the first data set [either computed tomography (CT) or magnetic resonance imaging (MRI)]. This can be changed to show 4, 9, or 16 consecutive axial slices of a predefined area of interest (usually the target region). Buttons on the right of the main screen are used for zooming in or out of the region of interest. Scrolling between images is achieved either with a prior/next button or a scroll bar for rapid scrolling through many images with a couple of mouse clicks. Alternatively, the main window can show a three-dimensional display of the patient's head that can be zoomed or rotated in any axis. Beneath the main window are two smaller windows that display both sagittal and coronal reconstructions or multiple coplanar sets of CT and MR images. The multiple sets are useful for checking the quality of the image fusion (see later) and for comparing structures seen on both MRI and CT. On the left of the main window, there are three more small windows for sketches, which assist in visualizing the treatment planning. These displays differ depending on whether the stereotactic or conformal modes are used, and are described later in the planning section.

3 IMAGE ACQUISITION

Magnetic resonance imaging and CT are obtained for all patients (except for patients for whom MR imaging is contraindicated). The MRI is performed before placing the stereotactic head ring. For convenience, we perform the MRI one to several days before the planned radiosurgery, although it could be done on the same day as the radiosurgery before head-ring fixation. Magnetic resonance imaging data can be acquired and transferred to the planning system in axial, coronal, and sagittal planes, although in usual practice axial MR images are obtained in 2-mm slices. When performing the MRI, it is important to note that oblique (tilted) planes are not recognized by the BrainScan software.

The BrainScan planning system can accommodate several commercially available head ring localizers, including a proprietary BrainLab frame. Computed tomography is carried out after fixing the head ring in place. The appropriate localizer is attached and locked firmly to the head ring during acquisition of the CT. We use the fixed BRW stereotactic frame for all our single fraction treatments, and the relocatable BrainLab frame for fractionated stereotactic irradiation.

4   DATA TRANSFER

Datasets from the MRI and CT are transferred via network to the BrainScan planning computer. A backup system of data transfer by optical disc or tape is available in case online communication breaks down. Tape or disc data transfer can be used by medical centers where direct data transfer is not available. After transferring the MRI and CT data, the first planning step is the identification and localization of the fiducial rods of the CT localizer. The software requires manual identification of the fiducial rods on the first CT slice, after which it proceeds with automatic recognition of the fiducials' position on the remaining slices. The CT and appropriate MRI image sets for each patient are stored in a single file and are now ready for contour outlining in preparation for image fusion and treatment planning. The software allows digitization of data from standard analog angiographic images for planning radiosurgery of arteriovenous malformations (AVMs). Our institution has digital angiography equipment only (which cannot be used for stereotactic localization because of inherent spatial inaccuracies), and we use MRI and high-dose contrast-enhanced CT for all our patients, including those with AVM.

5   STRUCTURE CONTOURING TOOLS

Contours of objects are drawn in the two-dimensional axial CT or MR images displayed in the main window, whereas coronal and sagittal reconstructions of the objects are simultaneously displayed in the smaller windows below. Each completed object (defined in CT or MRI) is transferred to the three-dimensional database. The target is defined on both CT and MRI. The main drawing tool takes advantage of the three mouse buttons and consists of a circular cursor that can be used as a brush either for drawing or for erasing. The left mouse button is used for outlining and the right for erasing. The middle button is used to accept the completed outline. Additional tools are available in the Autocontour function and include a spherical contour tool for outlining the eyes. This is positioned at the center of the eye on the axial, sagittal, and coronal images. The size of the sphere is adjusted with the mouse to match the size of the eye. An autocontour tool for automatic outlining of volumes with a common density threshold is also available. Only the first and list slices of the object need to be outlined manually (the threshold can be adjusted to improve identification of the structure to aid in outlining). This tool is useful for those who use the entire ventricles for image fusion (see below), but in our experience, image fusion with the entire ventricles is too laborious to achieve a good fit.

The completed objects are transferred to the three-dimensional database, which lists all contoured objects (CT and MRI) in the patient file. All these images can be displayed on either CT or MRI slices such that a target defined on MRI can be superimposed onto a CT image set for planning purposes. One object from the three-dimensional database (usually either MRI target or CT target) is designated as the planning target volume (PTV). Several objects can be defined as organs at risk (RO). The isocenter cannot be placed in an RO. In the planning stage, the three-dimensional database is used to define which objects will be visible in the various planning windows.

6 IMAGE FUSION

Image fusion on BrainLab version 5.0 is automatic. To shorten the process time for the fusion, the CT and MR images are manually overlaid for a very approximate match before automatic fusion. Automatic fusion then takes a couple of minutes. A check of the fusion is carried out with the multiple sets tool, in which a small rectangular window showing part of the comparable reconstructed MR image is superimposed over part of the CT image. This rectangular MR window can be moved around the CT image for final verification of the alignment of the CT and fused MR image. After the automatic fusion, minor manual adjustments are sometimes required to obtain a perfect match.

7 PLANNING

7.1 Conventional Stereotactic Arc Radiosurgery

The radiosurgery module is opened and the desired target (as defined on either the CT or MR image) is selected. The RO to be displayed during radiosurgery planning are selected from the three-dimensional database. Either CT or MR images of the target area are chosen for the main screen display, and the number of consecutive images that shows the entire target (usually 9 or 16 slices) is selected. Coronal and sagittal reconstructions are displayed below the main window and planning sketches, including an axial arc collision map, a coronal sketch of arc planes in relation to the isocenter and ROs, and a three-dimensional overview are shown in the left-sided windows.

The first isocenter is added and automatically placed at the center of the defined target. A pop-up window allows selection of the number and range of treatment arcs. The default is five arcs with a range of table positions of 160° and a range of gantry start/stop angles from 30° to 130°. The isocenter can be moved with the mouse by drag and drop on the axial, coronal, and sagittal views and on the three-dimensional overview. Alternatively the isocenter can be moved at 1-mm intervals at the click of a button. Smaller increments are possible by typing the coordinates of the isocenter position in the appropriate windows. The position of the isocenter is confirmed with the middle button. A collision warning prevents selection of incompatible arc-planes and table angles. A circle representing approximately the 80% isodose of the individual beam is displayed on each image in the main window and is useful in positioning the isocenter and selecting the ideal collimator diameter for each arc. For each isocenter, individual arcs can be removed or added, and the table and gantry positions of each arc can be modified by clicking on the axial arc sketch screen or using the arc plane table on the left of the screen.

The main screen can be switched to a beam's eye view (BEV), which displays 16 consecutive images of the BEV of the arc at $10°$ intervals and can be zoomed to improve clarity. The BEV includes sketches of the organs at risk and enables alteration of the range of the arc to avoid the beam passing through the ROs. It is possible to plan and deliver split arcs that skip over the area of the RO, in such cases each portion gets half of the original dose of the arc. The PTV can be made transparent to better visualize the ROs.

The results of the initial planning are now reviewed. The isodose settings have a limited color scheme. For single isocenter treatment, we usually plan to treat to the 80% isodose, and we display the 80%, 40%, and 16% isodose lines in planning. For multiple isocenters, a 55% to 70% isodose line is usually selected. The two-dimensional axial planes throughout the lesion and the sagittal and coronal reconstructions are examined to ensure that the prescription isodose line covers the entire target. For elliptically shaped targets, the table angles and arc ranges are modified so that the prescription (80%) isodose line covers the entire target with minimal extra tissue, allowing treatment with a single isocenter. Planning of a single isocenter takes 15 to 30 minutes.

For irregular targets, additional isocenters can be added and positioned manually with the mouse drag and drop using all three planes or by keying in exact coordinates. Positioning and weighting of isocenters in multiple isocenter plans requires experience and patience. Changing the weighting or arc angles of one isocenter will affect the weighting of the other isocenter(s). We try to avoid similar table angles for arcs of different isocenters to prevent high-dose areas outside of the target caused by the coincident entry of several beams.

After a plan is approved, the prescription dose is entered into the dose-setting window. Planning and treatment of irregular targets is much simpler with fixed conformal mMLC fields (see below) than with stereotactic arcs; therefore, we rarely plan treatments with multiple isocenters, particularly as the use of several isocenters requires many manual modifications of the treatment plan. The isodose lines that are displayed on the screen, even after minor modifications in the treatment plan, are relevant to the total dose before the change in the plan. To see the actual dosimetry relevant to the modified plan, it is necessary to perform two functions to normalize the dose, and this can take several minutes for treatments involving multiple isocenters. The first step requires setting the normalization point within the target volume. After recalibrating to the normalization point, the second step is to enter the dose prescribed to the 100% point. The system recalculates the isodoses for the new prescription dose, preserving the relative weights of the individual beams. The isodoses can now be re-evaluated and if satisfactory, the plan is saved and printed for the actual treatment. The normalization sometimes results in an unexpected change in isodose lines, as it is not possible to immediately see the true change in prescription isodoses on the screen images, requiring further manipulation of the beams or downward adjustment of the prescription isodose to cover the entire target, and then repeating the two-step normalization process. This is a major drawback of the present BrainLab dosimetry software.

We usually plan multiple isocenters only if several targets are to be treated (e.g., for a patient with several brain metastases). The isodose settings of each target must be checked at completion of the plan to ensure that the beams of the later targets did not interfere with the dosimetry of the earlier targets.

A final check of the treatment plan is carried out by examining the dose volume histogram. This reports the target volume and the volume of normal brain within the prescription isodose and is useful to ensure that the entire target is within the prescription isodose. The conformity index (CI) of the plan is defined as the ratio between the total volume treated to the prescription isodose and the target volume. Thus, any measure greater than 1 refers to normal brain within the prescription isodose. The ideal CI = 1, although in practice the CI usually ranges from 1.5 to 2. This means that the volume of normal tissue included in the prescription isodose is between 50% and 100% of the volume of the target. In cases with a large target volume or a high CI, we will lower the prescription dose to reduce the risk of complications.

7.2 Multiple-Shaped Fixed Beams

For irregularly shaped fields, we use the conformal radiosurgery module together with the BrainLab mMLC. The mMLC is based on the Varian 52 leaf multileaf collimator. There are 26 leaves on each side, which cover an area of up to 10 × 10 cm, with leaves 3-mm wide in the center of the field and 5.5-mm wide at the edges.

The main screen display for the conformal module is similar to the display for conventional radiosurgery. As with the conventional stereotactic arc module, the number of slices (usually 9 or 16) needed to show the entire target is selected. The sketches show a spherical overview of the arc positions and a room's eye view of the beam directions. A treatment target is selected and the isocenter is placed automatically on its center. Beams are added on the treatment plan and positioned with the mouse using the axial sketches. The mMLC leaves are automatically adjusted to cover the target area in the BEV. A predetermined margin can be used and is automatically included in the BEV. For malignant lesions, we sometimes add a 1-mm to 2-mm margin, depending on the planning isodoses. The target and selected ROs are displayed in the BEV in the planning sketches. We usually select 10 to 12 beams covering a wide range of angles, taking care to avoid beam angles that cross ROs.

The isodose display is now examined on the axial CT or MRI slices in the main window and on the coronal and sagittal reconstructions. With conformal beams, the 80% prescription dose will adequately cover the target as the target is included in the BEV of each field. When the target has a highly irregular shape, the prescription isodose may include a significant amount of normal brain tissue, which is in the path of several beams toward the target or within the folds of the target, resulting in a large conformity index (> 2). In such cases, we manually adjust the mMLC leaves to reduce the normal tissue within the prescription volume without compromising the target dose. This is achieved by outlining the area of normal tissue within the prescription isodose on the CT or MRI images, and then moving them to the three-dimensional database as "areas of regret," which are made visible in the sketches windows. The target is made transparent to be able to see the areas of regret clearly. All the beams are now examined. Beams that show the area of regret at the edge of the target are selected, and the mMLC leaves of these beams are manually modified to block off part of the area of regret. Usually 3 to 4 beams are modified to significantly reduce the dose in the area of regret. The plan is then re-examined. There may be remaining areas of regret after the initial manipulation, or there may be areas of geographical miss beneath the manually adjusted leaves. The areas of geographical miss are now drawn on the CT slices in the main window and transferred to the three-dimensional database. The mMLC leaves are readjusted to cover the areas of geographical miss. We usually carry out 2 to 4 iterations of the procedure of manually adjusting the mMLC leaves to reduce the dose in the area of regret and to increase the dose in the areas of geographical miss until a satisfactory plan is achieved. Each iteration adds 5 to 10 minutes to the planning time. The entire manual dose optimization takes 20 to 45 minutes. The planning time of a simple conformal plan without manual optimization is around 15 minutes. The volume of normal tissue included in the prescription isodose is reduced by up to 50% by this manual dose optimization.

Different plans for each patient can be prepared and compared side by side to select the best plan. This is most often useful when we are in doubt whether the noncoplanar arcs plan is preferable to the fixed beam conformal plan. After deciding on a treatment plant, the prescription is printed, together with the target positioning films for aligning the patient on the treatment couch.

7.3 Stereotactic Treatment Delivery

Stereotactic treatment is carried out on a Varian 2100 C linear accelerator using a couch-mounted head fixation device. The couch-mount slides onto the siderails of the treatment couch. The couch is equipped with stabilizers to prevent couch displacement and vibration during treatment. Stereotactic arc treatment is delivered using round collimators ranging from 10 cm to 40 cm in 2.5-cm intervals. These collimators are inserted into a collimator mount fixed to the linear accelerator head. For conformal fixed beam treatments, we use the BrainLab mMLC, which weighs 31 kg and is stored on a mobile trolley until use. Before beginning a session of stereotactic conformal radiotherapy the mMLC is mounted underneath the linear accelerator head. To mount the mMLC, the linear accelerator head is placed at the 180° position and the mMLC slides from the trolley onto the accelerator head and is secured in place. It requires about 30 minutes to insert and initialize the mMLC.

Patient positioning for stereotactic treatment is achieved with three sets of cross-haired lasers placed laterally at 90° and 270° and on the ceiling above the patient at 360°. Before each session of stereotactic treatments, the couch-mount attachment is fixed to the treatment couch and a phantom isocenter pointer is attached to the couch-mount. The system is calibrated by placing the phantom isocenter pointer at the point of coincidence of the three sets of lasers. The position of the phantom is checked with the couch at 0°, and the gantry at 0°, 90°, and 270°, and then with the couch at 90° and the gantry at 0° and 90°. Fine adjustments of the couchmount are carried out with a set of four screws for fine tuning of linear displacement in the lateral, vertical, and superior/inferior directions. The couch stabilizers are now fixed into place.

The target positioner is a perspex box that attaches to the stereotactic frame and fits over the patient's head. Target positioning films showing the isocenter and incident beam positions are printed out for each stereotactic treatment. They are carefully aligned on all four sides and at the top of the target positioner box. Before treatment, the target positioner box is attached to the couch mount and the couch is positioned and fixed in place so that the lasers pass through the isocenter marker on each film with the couch at 0°, and the gantry at 0°, 90°, and 270°, and then with the couch at 90° and the gantry at 0° and 90°. Fine adjustment of the couch position is obtained with the tuning screws. The target positioner is removed and the patient is placed on the couch and the head ring is attached to the couch-mount. The target positioner is attached to the head ring, and alignment is checked in all directions. There is usually a slight sag in the target positioner from the weight of the patient's head, but this does not usually affect the position of the isocenter.

For stereotactic arc treatments, the appropriate diameter collimator is inserted into the collimator mount and the table is positioned at the appropriate angle for the specific arc. The arc range and requisite monitor units are keyed into the treatment console and then delivered. Between each arc, the technicians enter the treatment room to reposition the couch and gantry to the appropriate angle for the next arc and to change the collimator if necessary.

The leaf positions for fixed beam mMLC treatments are downloaded from the stereotactic planning system and the data are transferred by diskette to the computer controlling the mMLC so that for each field, the leaves are adjusted automatically. In addition to the isocenter positioning described above, the target positioner films show the shadow of each beam as it passes the positioner film and we check the position and shape of the first beam before beginning treatment. Between each beam, the technicians enter the room to change the couch and gantry positions and to ensure that there is no collision between the couch and gantry. For treatments with multiple isocenters, the target positioner is replaced over the patient's head and the couch is fixed for each additional isocenter and accurately positioned with the screw mounts without moving the patient.

8 CONCLUSIONS AND FUTURE DEVELOPMENTS

The BrainLab stereotactic planning system is versatile and can plan radiosurgery with dynamic noncoplanar arcs or with conformal fixed beams. To be able to plan and treat all kinds of lesions efficiently, it is necessary to have the means of delivering both classic arcs and fixed conformal beams. Most of the drawbacks of previous versions of the BrainLab planning system have been corrected or improved in the present version, particularly the image fusion process, which is now reported to be completely automatic. The screen view with the MRI reconstruction overlying the CT image is included in the fusion module, and it is no longer necessary to go back and forth between the treatment module and the fusion module for final approval of the image fusion. It is still necessary to carry out a two-step dose normalization after each modification of the treatment plan. Dynamic conformal arc software and intensity modulated radiotherapy software are now available and these will increase the dose conformity and ease of planning stereotactic treatments with the BrainLab system.

20

Stereotactic Radiosurgery and Intensity Modulation Radiotherapy

Antonio A. F. De Salles and Timothy Solberg
UCLA School of Medicine, Los Angeles, California, U.S.A.

1 INTRODUCTION

Stereotactic radiosurgery (SRS) is a well-accepted treatment for a large number of neurosurgical pathologies, including arteriovenous malformations, primary and metastatic brain tumors, several skull base tumors, and selected chronic pain syndromes [Alexander et al, 1993; De Salles et al, 1993; Friedman et al, 1993; Kondziolka et al, 1991; Lunsford et al, 1992; Mehta et al, 1997; Selch et al, 2000; Solberg et al, 2001; Steiner et al, 1992]. During the last 50 years and mainly during the last two decades, SRS has given neurosurgeons and radiation oncologists the ability to maximize the dose of radiation to the tumor with physical sparing of the normal brain. Most recently, radiobiological sparing is also being explored in the form of stereotactic radiation therapy [Selch et al, 2000]. Despite the enormous development on the techniques of conformal radiation, including multiple isocenters [Goetch et al, 1993; Kondziolka et al, 1991], shaped beam [Solberg et al, 2001], and pencil beam approaches [Chenery et al, 1999], afforded by computerized imaging and three-dimensional treatment planning software, the need to further improve the normal tissue sparing and enhance dose of radiation to the pathologies remains important [Lax and Karlsson

1996; Pollock et al, 1996]. This can be determined by the less than optimal results of SRS when treating several pathologies [Flickinger et al, 1992; Flickinger et al, 1998; Mehta et al, 1997; Selch et al, 2000].

The radiation dose response of solid tumors and arteriovenous malformations has been demonstrated repeatedly [Betti et al, 1989; Colombo et al, 1994; De Salles et al, 1996; Karlsson et al, 1997; Lunsford et al, 1992; Steiner et al, 1992; Voges et al, 1996]. The delivery of higher doses of radiation is associated with a higher probability of tumor and arteriovenous malformation (AVM) control and cure, although accompanied by increased risk of normal tissue complications [De Salles et al, 1999; Ellis et al, 1998; Karlsson et al, 1997]. Intensity Modulated Radiotherapy (IMRT) offers a potential solution to enhance significantly the efficacy of radiation delivery, allowing higher control and cure rates in solid tumors or AVMs while simultaneously reducing morbidity. Although clinically in use with university and commercially available platforms [Yu et al, 1996], IMRT has not been developed fully for fine intracranial applications [Verhey, 1999]. The developed IMRT treatment system dedicated for intracranial applications promises to improve efficiency in planning and delivery of the treatment [Cardinale et al, 1998]. These advantages depend on enhanced integrations of treatment planning software and radiation delivery systems capable of handling manipulation of beam intensity.

2   INTENSITY MODULATED RADIOTHERAPY

The term "intensity modulated radiotherapy" is relatively new, although the concept of deliberately creating a non-uniform radiation beam to achieve a superior dose distribution is not. Modulation of heavy particle beam with a variable column of water or Lucite model in the beam pathway has allowed the placement of the Bragg Peak in tumors and vascular malformations since the early 1950s [Kjellberg et al, 1964; Koehler et al, 1977; Tobias et al, 1956]. These techniques are not effective, however, in modulating photon beams.

Several techniques have been proposed and used to improve the distribution of radiation dose within a patient when a photon beam is used [Grant and Cain, 1998; Khoo et al, 1999]. Physical compensators have been used in limited fashion over the past four decades [Ellis, 1959; Hall et al, 1961; Khan et al, 1968]. Physical wedges are still used routinely in most radiotherapy centers. Although these techniques can provide a more uniform target dose, they in no way provide the optimal solution that IMRT can with respect to avoiding important normal structures that cannot otherwise be excluded from a radiation field. Anders Brahme first described the modern IMRT concepts. He proposed in 1988 that the conventional trial-and-error paradigm for treatment planning be reversed, and that one derive the optimum beam intensities from the desired dose distribution using deterministic techniques [Brahme, 1988]. Since that time, several methods have been developed to both plan and deliver technology that allows the optimal intensity to be determined and delivered. The basic IMRT paradigm is shown in Figure 1.

With the advent of micromultileaf collimators (MLCs), an effective mechanism now exists for the application of IMRT techniques to targets within the brain, that is, intensity modulated radiosurgery (IMRS). The success of IMRS hinges on the development and implementation of three key components: (1) inverse planning—the calculation of optimal beam profiles, given physical or biological constraints to a target and organs at risk; (2) leaf sequencing—conversion of the beam profiles calculated by the inverse algorithm into a series of leaf positions and corresponding monitor units that are physically deliverable; (3) delivery—the administration of the IMRT treatment delivered by a tightly integrated accelerator and MLC. In this chapter, we present our efforts in each of these areas and discuss the clinical implementation for cranial neoplasms. Some discussion of underlying theory is necessary in this developing field.

2.1   Inverse Planning Techniques

The task of inverse planning is an optimization process whereby one specifies a desired dose distribution and searches for the beam intensity distribution that will satisfy the request. This is generally found in the form of an objective function that is subsequently minimized through a mathematical operation. In theory and practice, there are a number of functions, both physically and biologically based, that can be used as the objective function. This process is shown diagrammatically in Figure 2.

Inverse planning solutions fall into three general classes. Several investigators have proposed the use of iterative techniques similar to methods used in the reconstruction of tomographic images [Bortfeld et al, 1990; Bortfeld et al, 1995; Holmes et al, 1993]. Although these solutions do produce the desired dose distribution, the calculated intensity profiles can contain negative beam weights. This is a major drawback, in that the delivery of negative beams is not physically realizable. Several attempts have been made to overcome this shortcoming. For example, negative beam weights can be truncated to zero with the hope that the resulting distribution does not suffer significantly.

The second class of solutions can be thought of as random-walk approaches. Simulated annealing, first applied to radiotherapy optimization by Steve Webb in 1989, is such an approach [Webb, 1989]. With simulated

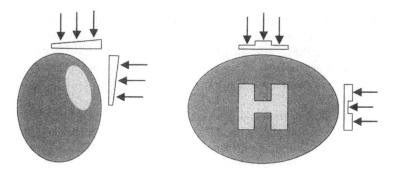

FIGURE 1   The principles of intensity modulated radiotherapy (IMRT) are illustrated in the two diagrams above. Wedge filters (**left**) can correct for surface curvature and produce a uniform dose distribution within a target. Individually designed compensating filters (**right**) can correct for organ shape as well as surface curvature. Intensity modulated radiotherapy extends these concepts by providing a generalized way to achieve the *optimal* dose distribution with respect to both target and normal tissue.

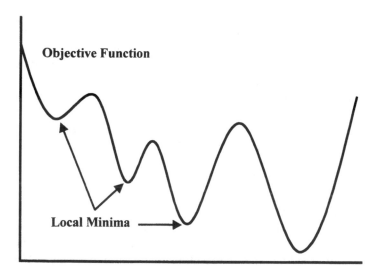

FIGURE 2   Example of an objective function that can be minimized through a mathematical operation. In theory and practice, there are a number of functions, both physically and biologically based, that can be used as the objective function.

annealing, one seeks a global minimum through a series of pseudo-random walks that seek to minimize the difference between a present value (distribution) and that desired. Those paths that result in a smaller difference are preferred, although to prevent the solution from finding a local minimum, other paths may be selected. Simulated annealing has gained some popularity within the radiotherapy field and was the first algorithm used in a commercial system capable of inverse planning [Carol, 1995]. However, it suffers from two major drawbacks, which subsequent methods have improved upon. First, simulated annealing requires a dose calculation at each iteration. Thus the implementation of a sophisticated dose algorithm that considers scatter, divergence, and the effect of tissue heterogeneities—all in a three-dimensional fashion—yields an inverse procedure that is extremely time consuming. Second, because of the random nature of the optimization process, simulated annealing results are very sensitive to optimization parameters. Without careful selection of the parameters, the process can easily converge to a local minimum, which may be a significantly poorer solution than the true optimum.

A third class of inverse planning solutions are the so-called gradient techniques. In a standard gradient approach, the solution space is searched along a path of steepest descent. The optimal solution, then, is one in which the gradient no longer decreases. This approach, however, is also prone to being trapped within local minima. An enhancement to the standard gradient approach was proposed by Spirou and Chui [1998]. The conjugate gradient method alternates between a steepest descent direction and a direction orthogonal (or conjugate) to the steepest descent. This allows an escape route when local minima are encountered, although the size of the conjugate step must be carefully chosen.

Most recently, a new approach based on the maximum likelihood estimator (MLE) used in imaging was proposed as a possible solution to the inverse problem [Llacer, 1997]. In the basic MLE as follows, the likelihood that a set of beamlets with energy fluency a (Fa) will produce a prescribed dose distribution D is given by:

$$P(D|a) = \sum_i \sum_j \left\{ e^{-F_{ij}a_j} \frac{(F_{ij}a_j)^{d_i}}{d_i!} \right\}$$

where D is assumed to have elements that a Poisson distributed with a mean of $F_i a_j$. F_{ij} is the matrix element that defines the dose delivered to anatomy voxel i from beamlet j, and d^i is the desired (prescribed) dose in anatomy voxel i. The inverse process is to maximize the likelihood function P to find the beamlet fluences that will produce the desired dose distribution. Jorge Llacer proposed the addition of a penalization term, which changes dynamically, in an attempt to drive the dose to the organs at risk (e.g., brainstem) as low as possible while maintaining the constraints on the target volume [Llacer, 1997]. The MLE with dynamic penalization [also known as the dynamically penalized maximum likelihood (DPL) algorithm] has recently been integrated into the commercial treatment planning system for inverse planning of intracranial targets.

A key strength of the DPL approach is the ability to compute a number of inverse plans simultaneously. This allows, for example, varying levels of emphasis to be placed on the target and risk organs, with the clinician selecting the appropriate plan for the individual tumor site and patient. As an example, two plans for an ependymoma, abutting the inferior portion of the brainstem, are shown in Figure 3. The plans, representing two extremes of target coverage/brainstem avoidance, were calculated simultaneously along with several others using the DPL algorithm. The accompanying dose-volume histograms show the trade-offs involved when choosing brainstem sparing over target coverage.

2.2 Leaf Sequencing

Recently, algorithms for translation of intensity profiles determined during inverse planning into physical multileaf segments that a treatment device can deliver have been described (Bortfeld et al, 1994; Bortfeld and Boyer, 1995; Mackie et al, 1993]. Essentially the continuous intensity profiles are segmented into discrete profiles, which can be defined by two opposed leaves, the so-called *leading* and *trailing* leaves. To make the process efficient, it is desirable to have the leaves proceed in one direction only and not to backtrack. This is generally referred to as the *sliding window* technique. To accomplish this, the discrete profiles can be re-binned as a function of time rather than position.

Another important consideration in the sequencing code involves the resolution of the desired intensity profiles. If an intensity distribution has significant structure, the delivery must obviously be broken into finer steps (i.e., more segments). Rather than specifying the number of segments desired, it is preferable to specify an RMS error between the calculated and delivered profile. The translation algorithm will then determine the number and size of steps necessary to achieve this.

Leaf sequencing algorithms must also consider a number of machine-specific parameters. These include leaf speed, leaf transmission and leakage, dose rate, delivery method [static multileaf collimator (SMLC) versus dynamic multileaf collimator (DMLC)] and tongue-and-groove effect. In general, the number of monitor units required for an IMRT treatment is approximately two to three times greater than that for an equivalent open field treatment. As a result, a significant portion of the delivered dose can come

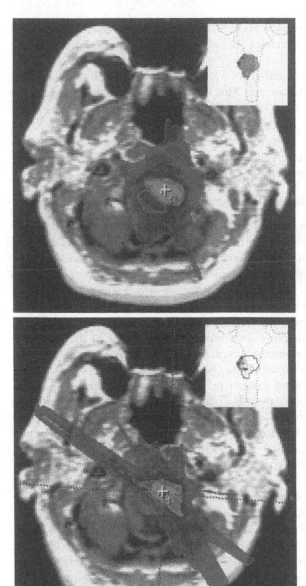

FIGURE 3 Two inverse plans for a patient with a spinal cord ependymoma. The plan on top emphasizes target dose homogeneity whereas the bottom plan emphasizes sparing of the brainstem. The inset figures show the intensity profile for a single beam superimposed over an outline of the anatomy. Clearly, the intensity of that portion of the beam passing through the brainstem has been reduced in the bottom plan.

from leakage and transmission sources, making it necessary to account for and minimize radiation leakage between and transmission through the leaves.

Similarly, the tongue-and-groove effect comes as a result of the manner in which the MLC is constructed. This construction is meant to reduce the leakage between neighboring leaves. However, when part or all of a neighboring leaf is retracted, the tongue portion of a leaf can provide added attenuation of the beam in regions where it is not anticipated. This can, in turn, cause small regions of underdosing of as much as 15% to 20%. By synchronizing the leaf motion, these effects can be minimized.

2.3 Intensity Modulation Delivery

As with inverse planning, several techniques have been proposed with regard to radiation delivery of IMRT. The most common approach to IMRT delivery is through the use of multileaf collimators. This can be performed in either a static or dynamic fashion, as explained in Figure 4. The most simple to implement and verify is the static technique, in which a treatment port is divided into a number of smaller overlapping segments [De Neve et al, 1996; Bortfeld et al, 1994; Boyer, 1997]. This type of approach is now referred to as static MLC (SMLC) delivery. One shortcoming with the SMLC approach is that in order to obtain a good representation of the desired intensity profile, a large number (> 10) of segments may be required. This makes static IMRT delivery with even a modest number of ports fairly inefficient. A more efficient approach is to allow the MLC leaves to move while the radiation beam is on. This is referred to as dynamic MLC delivery (DMLC). Dynamic MLC delivery presents several challenges that can make accurate implementation difficult [Boyer and Yu, 1999]. Multileaf collimator leaf speed may not be adequate to deliver the intended profile, allowing more radiation to be delivered in regions where it was not intended. In addition, dosimetric verification and the accompanying quality assurance procedures are significantly more complex with dynamic delivery.

Three techniques for IMRT delivery have been developed in which the radiation source rotates about the patient while simultaneously modulating the intensity with the leaves. The first is called intensity modulated arc therapy (IMAT), proposed by Cedric Yu at the William Beaumont Hospital in Detroit [Yu, 1995; Yu et al, 1995]. In IMAT, the conventional multileaf is used to shape and modulate the beam as the linear accelerator rotates about the patient. This presents the ultimate in treatment flexibility and efficiency but also in complexity. Three-dimensional dosimetric verification is an absolute prerequisite.

A similar approach is that taken by the one commercial IMRT system currently being marketed. The Mimic™ (Nomos Corporation, Sewickley,

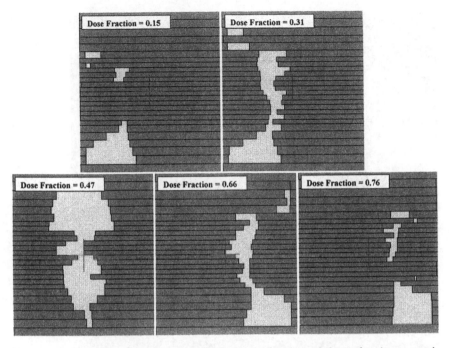

FIGURE 4 The five diagrams demonstrate the principles of using a multileaf collimator (MLC) for intensity modulated radiotherapy (IMRT) delivery. A predetermined amount of radiation is delivered at each segment (leaf pattern) of a single portal. Associated with each segment is a fraction of monitor units reflecting the relative amount of dose to be delivered by each particular pattern. In static MLC (SMLC) delivery, the beam is off as the leaves move between segments. In dynamic MLC (DMLC) delivery, the leaves move continuously between segments while the beam is on.

PA) is a device that attaches to conventional radiotherapy accelerators [Carol, 1995]. It consists of two banks of 1 cm × 1 cm "leaves" and is a binary device in the sense that its leaves can only provide collimation that is either fully open or fully closed. The leaves are controlled by a compressed air supply. It drives the leaves in and out of the field in less than 150 ms. The device is operated in a rotational fashion, but because it is capable of treating only 2 cm at a time, the patient must be translated after each of many rotations. This field-matching problem adds to the complexity as well as the time required for treatment [Carol, 1996].

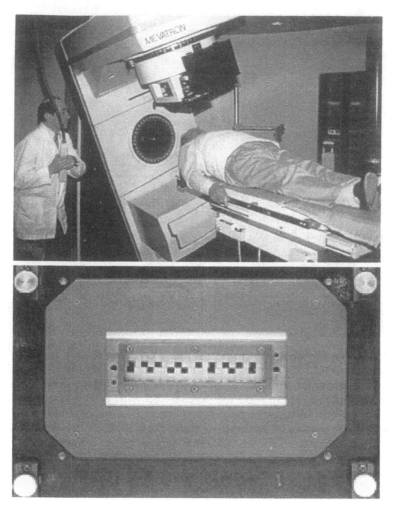

FIGURE 5 The Mimic collimator (Nomos Corporation) mounted to a conventional linear acclerator (**top**). The Mimic leaves produce individual 1 × 1 cm² or 1 × 2 cm² openings and are driven pneumatically.

The third rotational approach to IMRT delivery has been termed "tomotherapy" or "helical tomotherapy" to distinguish it from the Mimic™ form of delivery. Rock Mackie and his colleagues at the University of Wisconsin [Mackie, 1993] proposed helical tomotherapy. A prototype device is currently under construction. Like the Mimic™, radiation is delivered in a

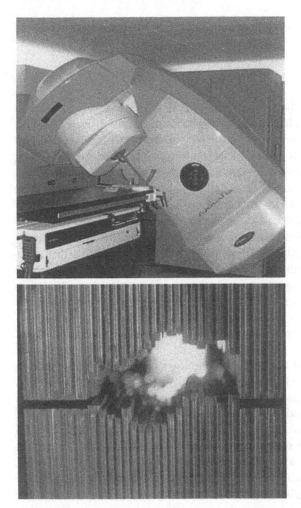

FIGURE 6   The Novalis accelerator (BrainLAB GmbH) is capable of static multileaf collimation (SMLC) and dynamic MLC (DMLC) IMRT. A close up of the integrated MLC, with leaves projecting between 3.0 and 5.5 mm, is shown in the bottom frame.

"strip" fashion, approximately 1 cm at a time, with a binary MLC in place to provide the beam modulation. The helical tomotherapy technique has several unique capabilities. It is built in a ring gantry configuration and the patient is translated through the opening in a continuous fashion. Because of this, the field-matching problem is eliminated. In addition, by incorporating a bank of detectors, tomographic imaging can be performed while the patient is treated.

3 DISCUSSION

Consider two examples. The first is an extremely aggressive primary malignancy of the brain called glioblastoma [or glioblastoma multiforme (GBM)]. A diagnosis of GBM nearly always results in death within a matter of months. Those tumors that can be removed through surgical means almost always recur. Chemotherapy is of limited benefit because of the inability to penetrate the blood-brain barrier. The delivery of an effective radiation dose via conventional external beam arrangements is limited by the tolerance of the surrounding normal brain. Brachytherapy, the use of implanted radioactive materials, is a common approach to delivering higher doses in a localized fashion, and several investigations have demonstrated that the delivery of higher doses of radiation can have a significant impact on patients with GBM. In the largest study to date, Sneed et al reported on 102 glioblastoma patients who received an implant boost using I-125 after standard external beam radiotherapy [Sneed et al, 1996]. Their results demonstrated a strong correlation between a longer freedom from local failure (FFLF) and higher brachytherapy dose. In a smaller group of patients, Halligan et al observed a 1-year survival rate of 59% from the time of implant in patients presenting with recurrent GBM [Halligan et al, 1996]. The conclusion that the use of 125-I brachytherapy results in improved survival compared with historical controls is shared by a number of investigators [Fernandez et al, 1995; Halligan et al, 1996; Sneed et al, 1996]. Radiosurgery can make a tremendous impact on the management of intracranial malignancy based on its ability to increase the dose tumor/brain ratio.

The second example in which the delivery of a highly localized radiation dose results in superior outcome is in carcinoma of the prostate. The extension of stereotactic techniques developed by neurosurgeons into other fields of medicine is natural and now becoming common. Examples are the use of stereotactic techniques for breast and liver tumors biopsy. This allows bringing outside of the intracranial arena the radiosurgical approach. Although prostate cancer is less aggressive and more easily controlled, it is much more common than primary brain tumors, and whereas the consequences of improper treatment can result in mortality, most often the patient is left with complications involving the adjacent organs at risk, namely the bladder and rectum, and sexual impotency. Pollack and Zagars [1998] reported on a series of 643 patients with early stage (T1/T2) prostate cancer treated with external beam radiotherapy [Pollack and Zagars, 1998]. That study demonstrated a significantly higher freedom from failure rate (87% to

67%; $P < 0.0001$) in patients treated with radiation doses greater than 67 Gy. After a study of 232 patients treated with 3D conformal external beam irradiation, Hanks et al [1998] have gone so far as to suggest that future clinical trials use doses of 76 to 80 Gy.

Because radiation doses of more than 67 Gy delivered through conventional field arrangements carry probabilities for acute and chronic complication that are not insignificant, brachytherapy using temporary or permanent implants has been seen as a way to further enhance the target dose while minimizing normal tissue complications. This approach is following the same historical course as the treatment of brain tumors with brachytherapy in the early 1990s, when radiosurgery took the place of brachytherapy for escalation of dose to tumors [Alexander et al, 1993; Selch et al, 2000].

Prostate implants have become widely used within the past 5 years. In a study of 212 patients with localized (T1–T3) prostate cancer treated with 125-I implantation, Zeitlin et al. [1998] estimated a 5-year biochemical [prostate specific antigen (PSA)] regress rate of 91%. Stokes et al. [1997] observed 2 and 5-year disease free survival rates of 90 and 76 percent respectively in 142 patients treated with 125-I implantation. In the largest reported experience to date, Ragde et al [1997] observed an actuarial freedom from biochemical failure of 80% at 7 years in patients receiving implant only and 65% at 8 years in a higher risk subgroup receiving implant plus external beam irradiation. Wallner et al. [1996] have reported a 63% rate of freedom from PSA recurrences at 4 years.

One issue with the use of radioactive implants is that the resulting distribution of dose within the target is highly nonuniform. In the case of brain tumor patients treated with brachytherapy, "hot spots," that is, regions of dose greater than the peripheral target dose, may result in localized areas of necrosis that can be life threatening. These hot spots have been shown to increase the complication rate when using stereotactic radiosurgery [Nedzi et al, 1991]. Similar problems occur when implanting carcinoma of the prostate. Zeitlin et al [1998] reported significant instances of impotence and proctitis, 38% and 21.4% of patients respectively, as well as other complications, such as urinary incontinence and rectal wall breakdown. Other authors also observed similar complications with similar frequencies, including asymptomatic rectal bleeding or ulceration in 47% of patients and nocturia in 45% of patients 12 months or more after implant.

It is important to re-emphasize the focal nature of the radiation dose that is delivered through implant techniques. Only through the exclusion of the normal tissues can higher and potentially more curable doses be safely administered. The ideal focal radiation paradigm then would be to exploit the localization properties of stereotactic radiosurgery in a manner that produces a uniform dose within the target volume. Stereotactic radiosurgery that uses multiple isocenters and small-diameter collimators suffers limitations similar to the brachytherapy approach. Stereotactic intensity modulation radiosurgery and radiotherapy promise to overcome this problem [Kramer et al, 1998].

4 CONCLUSIONS

A bright future is ahead for the use of stereotactic external beam radiation for treatment of pathologies of the central nervous system or elsewhere in the body. Stereotactic techniques associated with intensity modulation paradigms and radiobiological sparing promise an increase in therapeutic ratio of radiation.

REFERENCES

1. Alexander III EB, Black PM, Wen PY, Fine H, Loeffler JS. Results of radiosurgery versus brachytherapy for malignant gliomas. In: AAF De Salles and SJ Goetch (eds). Stereotactic Surgery and Radiosurgery. Madison, Wisconsin: Medical Physics Press, 1993, pp 455–461.
2. Betti OO, Munari C, Rosler R. Stereotactic radiosurgery with the linear accelerator: Treatment of arteriovenous malformations. Neurosurgery 24:311–321, 1989.
3. Bortfeld T, Burkelbach J, Boesecke R, Schlegel W. Methods of image reconstruction from projections applied to conformation therapy. Physics Med Biol 35:1423–1434, 1990.
4. Bortfeld TR, Kahler DL, Waldron TJ, Boyer AL. X-ray field compensation with multileaf collimators. Int J Radiat Oncol Biol Phys 28:723–730, 1994.
5. Bortfeld TR, Boyer AL. The exponential radon transform and projection filtering in radiotherapy planning. Int J Imaging Syst Technol 6:62–70, 1995.
6. Boyer AL, Geis P, Grant W, Carol M. Modulated beam conformal therapy for head and neck tumors. Int J Radiat Oncol Biol Phys 39(1):227–236, 1997.
7. Boyer AL, Yu CX. Intensity-modulated radiation therapy with dynamic multileaf collimators. Sem Rad Oncol 9(1):48–59, 1999.
8. Brahme A. Optimization of stationary and moving beam radiation therapy techniques. Radiother Oncol 12:129–140, 1988.
9. Carol MP. Peacock: A system for planning and rotational delivery of intensity-modulated fields. Int J Imaging Syst Technol 6:56–61, 1995.
10. Cardinale RM, Benedict SH, Wu Q, Zwicker RD, Gaballa HE, Mohan R. Comparison of three stereotactic radiotherapy techniques, Arcs vs. noncoplanar fixed fields vs. intensity modulation. Int J Radiat Oncol Biol Phys 2:431–436, 1998.
11. Carol MP, Grant WH, Bleier AR, Kania AA, Targovnik HS, Butler EB, Woo SY. The field matching problem as it applies to the Peacock 3-D conformal

system for intensity modulation. Int J Radiat Oncol Biol Phys 34(1):183–187, 1996.

12. Chenery SG, Massoudi F, De Salles AAF, Davis DM, Chehabi HH, Adler JD. Clinical experience with the Cyberknife at Newport Radiosurgery Center. Radiosurgery 3:34–40, 1999.

13. Colombo F, Pozza F, Chierego G, Casentini L, Deluca G, Francescon, P. Linear accelerator radiosurgery of cerebral arteriovenous malformations: An update. Neurosurgery 34:14–21, 1994.

14. De Neve W, De Wagter C, De Jaeger K, Thienpont M, Colle C, Derycke S, Schelfhout J. Planning and delivering high doses to targets surrounding the spinal cord at the lower neck and upper mediastinal levels: Static beam-segmentation technique executed with a multileaf collimator. Radiother Oncol 40(3):271–279, 1979.

15. De Salles AAF, Solberg TD, Michel P, Massoud TF, Plasencia A, Goetsch S, De Souza E, Vinuela F. Arteriovenous malformation animal model for radiosurgery: The rete mirabile. Am J Neuroradiol 17:1451–1458, 1996.

16. Ellis TL, Friedman WA, Bova FJ, Kubilis PS, Buatti JM. Analysis of treatment failure after radiosurgery for arteriovenous malformations. J Neurosurg 89: 104–110.

17. Ellis F, Hall EJ, Oliver R. A compensator for variations in tissue thickness for high energy beams. Br J Radiol 32:421–422, 1959.

18. Fernandez PM, Zamorano L, Yakar D, Gaspar L, Warmelink C. Permanent iodine-125 implants in the up-front treatment of malignant gliomas. Neurosurgery 36(3):467–473, 1995.

19. Flickinger JC, Lunsford LK, Kondziolka D, Maitz AH, Epstein AH, Simons SR, Wu A. Radiosurgery and brain tolerance: An analysis of neurodiagnostic imaging changes after Gamma Knife radiosurgery for arteriovenous malformations. Int J Radiat Oncol Biol Phys 23:19–26, 1992.

20. Flickinger JC, Kondziolka D, Maitz AH, Lunsford LK. Analysis of neurological sequelae from radiosurgery of arteriovenous malformations: How location affects outcome. Int J Radiat Oncol Biol Phys 40:273–278, 1998.

21. Friedman W, Bova F. LINAC radiosurgery for cerebral vascular malformations. In: Alexander E III, Loeffler JS, Lundsford LD (eds). Stereotactic Radiosurgery. New York: McGraw-Hill Inc., 1993, pp 147–156.

22. Goetch SJ, De Salles AAF, Solberg T, Holly FH, Selch MT, Bajada C. Treatment planning for stereotactic radiosurgery. In: AAF De Salles, SJ Goetch (eds). Stereotactic Surgery and Radiosurgery. Madison, Wisconsin: Medical Physics Press, 1993, pp 227–292.

23. Grant W 3rd, Cain RB. Intensity modulated conformal therapy for intracranial lesions. Medical Dosimetry 23(3):237–241, 1998.

24. Hall EJ, Oliver R. The use of standard isodose distributions with high energy radiation beams—the accuracy of a compensator technique in correcting for body contours. Br J Radiol 34:43, 1961.

25. Halligan JB, Stelzer KJ, Rostomily RC, Spence AM, Griffin TW, Berger MS. Operation and permanent low activity 125I brachytherapy for recurrent high-grade astrocytomas. Int J Radiat Oncol Biol Phys 35(3):541–547, 1996.

26. Hanks GE, Hanlon AL, Schultheiss TE, Pinover WH, Movsas B, Epstein BE, Hunt MA. Dose escalation with 3D conformal treatment: Five year outcomes, treatment optimization, and future directions. Int J Radiat Oncol Biol Phys 41(3):501–510, 1998.
27. Holmes T, Mackie TR. A filtered backprojection dose calculation method useful for inverse treatment planning. Med Phys 21:303–313, 1993.
28. Karlsson, B, Lax I, Soderman M. Factors influencing the risk for complications following Gamma Knife radiosurgery of cerebral arteriovenous malformations. Radiother Oncol 43:275–280, 1997.
29. Khan FM, Moore VC, Burns DJ. An apparatus for the construction of irregular surface compensators for use in radiotherapy. Radiology 90:593, 1968.
30. Khoo VS, Oldham M, Admans EJ, Bedford JL, Webb S, Brada M. Comparison of intensity-modulated romotherapy with stereotactic guided conformal radiotherapy for brain tumors. Int J Radiat Oncol Biol Phys 2:425–425, 1999.
31. Koehler AM, Schneider RJ, Sisterson J. Flattening or proton dose distributions for large-field radiotherapy. Med Phys 4:297–301, 1977
32. Kondziolka D, Lunsford LD, Coffey RJ, Flickinger JC. Stereotactic radiosurgery of meningiomas. J Neurosurg 74:552–559, 1991.
33. Kjellberg RN, Koehler AM, Preston WM. Intracranial lesions made by bragg peak of a proton beam. In: TJ Haley, RS Snider (eds). Response of the Nervous System to Ionizing Irradiation. Boston: Little, Brown and Company, 1964, pp 36–53.
34. Kramer BA, Wazer DE, Engler MJ, Tsai JS, Ling MN. Dosimetric comparison of stereotactic radiosurgery to intensity modulated radiotherapy. Radiat Oncol Investig 6:18–25, 1998.
35. Lax I, Karlsson B. Prediction of complications in Gamma Knife radiosurgery of arteriovenous malformations. Acta Oncolog 35:49–55, 1996.
36. Llacer J. Inverse radiation treatment planning using the dynamically penalized likelihood method. Med Phys 24(11):1751–1764, 1997.
37. Lunsford LD, Kondziolka D, Flickinger JC, Bissonette DJ, Jungreis CA, Martz AH, Horton JA, Coffey RJ. Stereotactic radiosurgery for arteriovenous malformations of the brain. J Neurosurg 75:512–524, 1992.
38. Mackie TR, Holmes T, Swerdloff S, Reckwerdt P, Deasy JO, Yang J, Paliwal B, Kinsella T. Tomotherapy: A new concept for the delivery of dynamic conformal radiotherapy. Med Phys 20(6):1709–1719, 1993.
39. Mehta MP. Radiosurgery of malignant brain tumors. In: A De Salles, R Lufkin. Minimally Invasive Therapy of the Brain. New York: Thieme, 1997, pp 213–224.
40. Nedzi LA, Kooy H, Alexander E 3rd, Gelman RS, Loeffler RS. Variables associated with the development of complications from radiosurgery of intracranial tumors. Int J Radiat Oncol Biol Phys 21:591–599, 1991.
41. Pollock BE, Kondziolka D, Lunsford LD, Bissonette D, Flickinger JC. Repeat stereotactic radiosurgery of arteriovenous malformations: Factors associated with incomplete obliteration. Neurosurgery 38:318–324, 1996.
42. Pollack A, Zagars GK. External beam radiotherapy for stage T1/T2 prostate cancer: How does it stack up? Urology 51(2):258–264, 1998.

43. Ragde H, Blasko JC, Grimm PD, Kenny GM, Sylvester J, Hoak DC, Cavanagh W, Landin K. Brachytherapy for clinically localized prostate cancer: Results at 7- and 8-year follow-up. Sem Surg Oncol 13(6):438–443, 1997.

44. Selch MT, Der Salles AAF, Solberg TD, Wallace RE, Do TM, Ford J, Cabatan-Awang C, Withers HR. Hypofractionated stereotactic radiotherapy for recurrent malignant gliomas. J Radiosurg 3:3–12, 2000.

45. Sneed PK, Lamborn KR Larson DA, Prados MD, Malec MK, McDermott MW, Weaver KA, Phillips TL, Wara WM, Gutin PH. Demonstration of brachytherapy boost dose-response relationships in glioblastoma multiforme. Int J Radiat Oncol Biol Phys 35(1):37–44, 1996.

46. Solberg TD, Boedeker KL, Fogg R, Selch MT, De Salles AAF. Dynamic arc radiosurgery field shaping: A comparison with static field conformal and non-coplanar circular arcs. Int J Radiat Oncol Biol Phys 2001, (in press).

47. Solberg TD, Arellano AR, Agazaryan N, Paul TJ, Chetty IC, DeMarco JJ, Selch MT, De Salles AAF. A program for inverse planning and intensity modulated radiosurgery. Radiosurgery 3:53–63, 1999.

48. Spirou SV, Chui CS. A gradient inverse planning algorithm with dose-volume constraints. Med Phys 25(3):321–333, 1998.

49. Stokes SH, Real JD, Adams PW, Clements JC, Wuertzer S, San W. Transperineal ultrasound-guided radioactive seed implantation for organ-confined carcinoma of the prostate. Int J Radiat Oncol Biol Phys 37(2):337–341, 1997.

50. Steiner L, Leksell L, Greitz T, Forster DMC, Backlund EO. Stereotactic radiosurgery for cerebral arteriovenous malformations: Report of a case. Acta Chir Scand 138:459–462, 1972.

51. Tobias CA, Roberts JE, Lowrence JH, et al. Irradiation hypophysectomy and related studies using 340-MeV protons and 190 MeV deuterons. Proceedings of the International Conference on the Peaceful Uses of Atomic Energy, Vol 10. United Nations Publications, 1956, pp 95–106.

52. Verhey LJ. Comparison of three-dimensional conformal radiation therapy and intensity-modulated radiation therapy systems. Sem Radiat Oncol 9(1):78–98, 1999.

53. Voges J, Treuer H, Sturm V, Buchner C, Lehrke R, Kocher M, Staar S, Kuchta J, Muller RP. Risk analysis of linear accelerator radiosurgery. IJROBP 36: 1055–1063, 1996.

54. Wallner K, Roy J, Harrison L. Tumor control and morbidity following transperineal iodine 125 implantation for stage T1/T2 prostatic carcinoma. J Clin Oncol 14(2):449–453, 1996.

55. Webb S. Optimization of conformal radiotherapy dose distributions using simulated annealing. Phys Med Biol 34:1349–1369, 1989.

56. Yu CX. Intensity-modulated arc therapy with dynamic multileaf collimation: An alternative to tomotherapy. Phys Med Biol 40:1435–1449, 1995.

57. Yu CX, Symons MJ, Du MN, Martinez AA, Wong JW. A method for implementing dynamic photon beam intensity modulation using independent jaws and a multileaf collimator. Phys Med Biol 40:769–787, 1995.

58. Zeitlin SI, Sherman J, Raboy A, Lederman G, Albert P. High dose combination radiotherapy for the treatment of localized prostate cancer. J Urol 160(1):91–95, 1998.

21

Stereotactic Radiosurgery with the Cyberknife

Steven D. Chang, David P. Martin, and John R. Adler, Jr.
Stanford University School of Medicine,
Stanford, California, U.S.A.

1   INTRODUCTION

Stereotactic radiosurgery combines stereotactic localization with multiple cross-fired beams from a highly collimated radiation source. This noninvasive method has proven to be an effective alternative to conventional neurosurgery, cranial irradiation, and brachytherapy for selected small cranial tumors and arteriovenous malformations. Current stereotactic techniques rely on a rigid frame fixed to a patient's skull for head immobilization and target localization. However, such a frame-based system results in numerous limitations to treatment options, including: (1) existing cranial fixation systems only allow treatment of intracranial or, at most, high cervical lesions, (2) a fixed frame limits the treatment degrees of freedom, whereas the metal components of current frames produce imaging artifacts on computed tomography (CT) and magnetic resonance imaging (MRI) scans, and (3) the discomfort associated with skeletal fixation makes treatment of children difficult and fractionation cumbersome.

A fixed isocenter, where all beams converge on a well-defined point, is the basis for standard radiosurgery instruments, such as the Gamma Knife and conventional linear accelerators. This concept works well with spherical targets but is not ideal for complex or irregular shapes. To treat complex-shaped tumors, these radiosurgery methods rely on multiple overlapping spherical dose volumes, a method that results in target dose heterogeneity and proportionately longer treatment times. A system that achieves shape matching without significantly compromising dose homogeneity could improve the treatment of many intracranial lesions. Furthermore, a frameless stereotactic radiosurgery system with increased degrees of freedom would allow treatment of extracranial (and even nonneural) tumors.

The Cyberknife (Fig. 1), developed by Accuray, Inc. (Sunnyvale, Calif., USA), uses noninvasive image-guided localization, a lightweight high

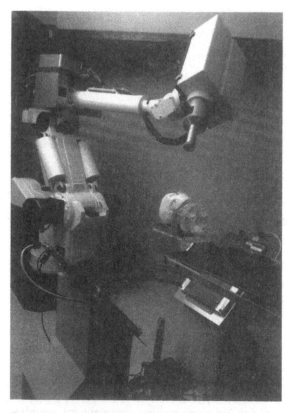

FIGURE 1 A picture of the Cyberknife showing the linear accelerator, the robotic arm, the treatment couch, and the amorphous silicon x-ray cameras (mounted on the floor). Reprinted with permission from Adler JR, Murphy MJ, Chang SD, Hancock SL. Image-guided robotic radiosurgery. Neurosurgery 44:1299–1307, 1999.

energy radiation source, and a robotic delivery system, to address these limitations [1]. This radiosurgical system has been used to treat intracranial tumors and arteriovenous malformations (AVMs), as well as extracranial targets within the spine and abdomen.

1.1 Image-Guided Radiosurgery

The present design of the Cyberknife derives from the original concept of a frameless alternative to conventional intracranial radiosurgery. The system presumes a fixed relationship between the target and the skull, as with other forms of stereotaxy. A compact 130 kg, 6 MV X-ray LINAC is accurately positioned by a robotic arm that can move and point the LINAC with 6° of freedom. Two X-ray imaging devices (amorphous silicon detectors) are positioned on either side of the patient's anatomy and acquire real-time digital radiographs of the skull at repeated intervals during treatment. The images are automatically registered to digitally reconstructed radiographs (DRRs) derived from the treatment planning CT. This registration process allows the position of the skull (and thus the treatment site) to be translated to the coordinate frame of the LINAC. A control loop between the imaging system and the robotic arm adjusts the pointing of the LINAC therapeutic beam to the observed position of the treatment anatomy (target). If the patient moves, the change is detected during the next imaging cycle and the beam is adjusted and realigned with the target.

The Cyberknife delivery treatment follows a sequential format. Once the patient is on the treatment table, the imaging system acquires a pair of alignment radiographs and determines the initial location of the treatment site within the robotic coordinate system. This information allows initial positioning of the LINAC. The robotic arm then moves the LINAC through a sequence of preset points surrounding the patient. At each point the LINAC stops and a new pair of images is acquired, from which the position of the target is redetermined. The position of the target is delivered to the robotic arm, which adapts beam pointing to compensate for a small amount of patient movement. The LINAC then delivers the preplanned dose of radiation for that direction. The complete process is repeated at each point, for a total of approximately 100 points.

1.1.1 Robotic Manipulator

A standard gantry-mounted LINAC moves in a planar arc and always points at a fixed isocenter. In contrast, the Cyberknife can position and point the LINAC anywhere in space. Because of this increased maneuverability, consideration of the robotic arm's "workspace," defined as the total volume within which the robot can maneuver without contacting any other object or interfering with any lines of sight for the imaging instrumentation, is necessary during treatment planning and delivery. The workspace is defined by a three-dimensional computer model of all the objects within the robotic manipulator's reach, including floor, ceiling, walls, and the patient. The robotic arm avoids collisions while in motion by continually comparing its position to the computer model.

The robot workspace for cranial radiosurgery occupies a hemispherical volume centered on a coronal plane through the patient's head. Portions of this hemisphere are excluded by the lines-of-sight between the X-ray sources and cameras and by the floor directly below the patient resulting in a geometric coverage of about 1.6π steridians for the beam directions. When moving from point to point, the robot follows planned trajectories, and thus it is important not to reconfigure the workspace without updating the computer model.

1.2 Targeting Precision of the Cyberknife

The principal innovation used by the Cyberknife is the use of radiographic images of internal anatomical features or implanted fiducials to align the treatment beam with the target volume. This advancement eliminates the need for a stereotactic frame. The Cyberknife has several sources of dose placement uncertainty comparable to conventional frame-based radiosurgery, beginning with the process of treatment planning.

The Cyberknife requires DRRs generated from computed tomography, so CT or CT/MR coregistration is the necessary basis for treatment planning. A standard CT slice thickness of 1.25 mm introduces an uncertainty of approximately 0.625 mm in the inferior/superior coordinate of the treatment volume. Radiographic technical limitations, including edge softening from attenuation of the diagnostic X-rays and blurring from the reconstruction result in an uncertainty of about 0.5 to 1.0 mm in the other two planning coordinates. However, this error is comparable to frame-based radiosurgery [2].

The mechanical accuracy of the robotic arm also introduces some error. The LINAC beam is pointed by the robotic arm at an isocenter from each of about 100 different beam positions. The individual beams miss the isocenter with errors that are randomly distributed around a zero mean for each coordinate axis, with a net root mean square (rms) radial error of 0.7 mm [3]. For a treatment that uses all beams, the effect of this source of error is to blur rather than offset the dose distribution. This rms radial pointing error of the Cyberknife is comparable to the deviation in the arc motion of a LINAC moving along a gantry path, which has been reported to be approximately 0.6 mm [4].

Digital image-to-image correlation results in an additional small margin of error. The location of the patient's anatomy within the coordinate frame of the camera relative to the position in the CT coordinate frame is measured by the image guidance system. This is accomplished by registering a pair of digital radiographs acquired by the camera system with DRRs, which are calculated from prior CT data in an exact emulation of the camera perspectives. Differences in the position and orientation of the anatomical images within the radiographs correspond to differences in the three-dimensional position and orientation of the anatomy between the camera and CT coordinate frames. Once this measurement is complete, a lesion visualized on the treatment planning CT can be located within the workspace of the robot, and the beam directed at this target. The precision of this registration is analogous to the mechanical precision, stability, and stiffness of a stereotactic frame [5]. The imaging process currently used in the Cyberknife measures the three translational degrees of position with an rms precision of 0.3 to 0.6 mm per axis [3].

The above errors combine to produce a net radial offset of the delivered dose from the targeted site. If the individual sources of error contributed randomly and independently, then the rms overall radial error is approximately 2.0 mm. A series of trials using a dosimetric phantom suitable for radiographic imaging has shown an observed rms radial error of 1.8 mm. This clearly demonstrates that the Cyberknife dose distribution is placed with the same accuracy as a typical stereotactic frame-based radiosurgical system [6].

1.2.1 Patient Movement

Because frameless radiosurgery allows some motion, it introduces a fifth factor in the precision of dose placement. In the Cyberknife, patient position is measured before delivering each dose, typically at approximately 20- to 40-second intervals. If the patient moves while the beam is on, that portion of the dose will be misdirected. The patient's changed position will be detected and compensated for at the beginning of the next treatment point. With more than 100 points, a single patient movement affects no more than about 1% of the total administered dose in a single-fraction treatment. Clinical experience with the Cyberknife has shown that in the vast majority of patients, movements are few in number and small in magnitude.

1.2.2 Practical Considerations

Because the Cyberknife relies on DRRs a CT of the patient is required prior to treatment, and provides the image basis for treatment planning. If MRI is to be used for planning, then such images must be coregistered with the CT. Furthermore, the system acquires a pair of positioning images 100 or more times in the course of a typical radiosurgical treatment, each exposing the patient to X-rays. The imaging system is currently limited to an exposure of less than about 5 rads during a treatment, or 25 mrads per image. This is not a significant issue for cranial treatments, in which the skull silhouette can be clearly imaged with an exposure of 1.5 mrads, but can become a limiting factor when the system is to be used to locate extracranial sites.

1.2.3 Treatment Planning

The Cyberknife can be programmed to administer either spherical single or overlapping multiple-isocenter doses. However, as with other radiosurgical devices, the treatment of irregular tumor volumes with multiple isocenters becomes time-consuming. The treatment planning system of the Cyberknife exploits the robot's six-degrees-of-freedom maneuverability, and allows an array of overlapping beams to be superimposed without an isocenter. An inverse planning procedure optimizes the set of beam directions and dose to be used on lesions of arbitrary shape, and had been demonstrated to deliver homogenous dose distributions (Figs. 2 and 3) that closely conform to even highly irregular volumes [7,8].

The Cyberknife corrects for changes in patient position by preserving the pattern in which both the beams traverse patient anatomy and intersect within the target. If the patient's treatment position in the camera coordinate system is exactly the same as in the CT study, then the image-guidance system makes no positioning correction and the robot moves the LINAC to the original workspace nodes specified by the treatment plan. If the patient moves during treatment or is displaced relative to the CT coordinates at initial setup, then the robot adjusts the spatial position and orientation of the nodal hemisphere in a way that keeps the position of the beams fixed with respect to the targeting feature (bone or fiducials), thereby ensuring that all beams not only continue to point at the planned target, but also pass through the patient anatomy as prescribed.

1.3 Amorphous Silicon Detectors

The Cyberknife localization method can, in principle, be used wherever radio-opaque features are associated with an anatomical target, a concept that would allow the extension of radiosurgical technique to extracranial sites. The Cyberknife has already been used to treat sites within the spine [9–11], lung, and pancreas.

1.3.1 Limitations of Previous Cameras

There are multiple shortcomings to the prior imaging system used by the Cyberknife. As previously configured, the X-ray sources used with the Cy-

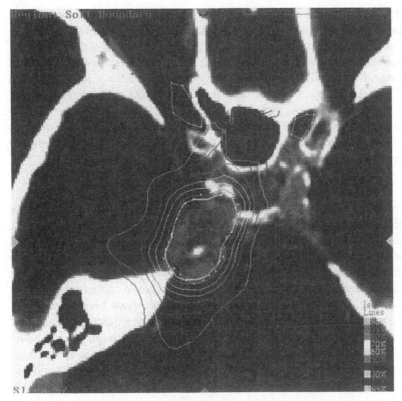

FIGURE 2 A graph showing a typical Cyberknife treatment plan for a mesial petrous ridge meningioma.

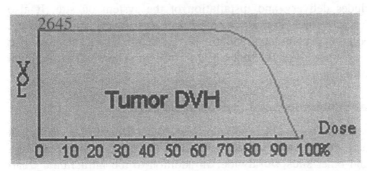

FIGURE 3 The dose volume histogram for the tumor shown in the above treatment plan showing excellent dose homogeneity throughout the majority of the target.

berknife are positioned 365 cm from the cameras to allow the robot a large workspace. Because this is approximately three times the conventional distance for diagnostic imaging, there is a resulting ninefold reduction in X-ray level at the patient's head. The prior X-ray cameras were fluoroscopes consisting of a gadolinium oxysulfide screen viewed by a light-amplified video CCD. Lens optics require that the CCD be 60 cm from the screen, which results in (1) poor signal-to-noise at low exposure levels, (2) low contrast, and (3) significant veiling glare. This design has made it difficult to obtain good quality images of the skeletal anatomy within and around the thorax and abdomen.

1.3.2 Advantages of the Amorphous Silicon Detectors

To overcome the above limitations, the previous cameras in the Cyberknife have been replaced with flat-panel amorphous silicon X-ray cameras (dpiX, Palo Alto, CA) [12,13]. These devices have a pixel pitch of 0.125 mm and acquire flat images that avoid distortions inherent to lensed or X-ray image intensifier techniques. When images from these sensors are processed by the new 6D registration software, a tenfold improvement in spatial resolution is achieved. The new imaging software and hardware have been specifically designed to provide variable fields of view and magnification ranges that can be adapted to multiple anatomical locations. For example, amorphous-silicon X-ray sensors create a high-quality image of the lumbar spine using the typical Cyberknife imaging geometry [10 mAs, 75 kV X-ray exposure [12]. Such an exposure corresponds to a dose per image of approximately 25 mrads.

1.4 Cost of the Cyberknife System

The total cost for a Cyberknife radiosurgical system is $3.5 million U.S. This fee includes delivery and installation of the system on site. It also includes a 1-year service contract with respect to software and hardware, with extended service contracts available for purchase. The total price also includes the software upgrade necessary for the treatment of extracranial radiosurgical targets.

1.5 Clinical Experience with Intracranial Lesions

As of August 2002, more than 3000 patients with benign and malignant intracranial tumors have been treated with the Cyberknife at Stanford Medical Center and other sites worldwide. In addition to the intracranial treatments, spinal lesions, including intramedullary spinal cord tumors or vascular malformations have been treated at Stanford. Radiosurgery of the spine has been performed by using the vertebral bodies as points of radiographic reference and spatial location. To date, the outcome for all lesions, as defined clinically and radiographically, appear to mirror that achieved with standard radiosurgery.

1.6 Clinical Experience with Extracranial Lesions

A primary objective behind the development of image-guided radiosurgery was the ability to treat extracranial lesions. With the implementation of an amorphous silicon camera system, achieving this goal has become feasible. Because most extracranial lesions within the thorax and abdomen typically move with respiration, that is, are not fixed with respect to bony structures, a system for target localization has been developed that relies on implanted fiducials, respiratory gating, and target tracing using infrared transduced chest and abdominal wall respiratory movement.

1.6.1 Targeting with Fiducials

Several metal implantable fiducials have been identified with the requisite characteristics to be readily imaged by the Cyberknife. For example, gold spheres 2 to 3 mm in diameter can be successfully sutured to soft tissue within the abdomen, allowing the targeting of abdominal cancers. Alternatively, smaller gold balls can be implanted with a 14-gauge needle [14], or gold wires (1 mm diameter) have also been used [15]. For spine fiducials, small bone screws can be anchored to the spine through stab incisions and provide an acceptable level of contrast relative to bone. Fiducials fixed to bone can be assumed to maintain their relative position, but it is unclear whether, and if so over what time interval, markers attached to soft tissue can migrate. Studies are underway to investigate the issue of fiducial migration within soft tissue.

1.6.2 Clinical Experience with Extracranial Cases

Thus far, 34 patients with spinal lesions have been treated with the Cyberknife. In contrast, 12 pancreatic tumor patients underwent implantation of gold fiducial balls during a laparotomy for pancreatic carcinoma. These patients were treated with a highly conformal single fraction of 15 Gy using breathholding throughout the procedure. This treatment, which was administered as part of a dose escalation protocol, provided significant palliation from pretreatment symptoms.

2 CONCLUSION

Stereotactic radiosurgery has been evolving toward frameless technology that is both less invasive and more flexible. However, all other widely available radiosurgical systems continue to use stereotactic frames for localization and immobilization. Such frame-based radiosurgical systems can be adapted to fractionated treatment, but some compromise in precision is necessary. These devices are also not amenable to treatment outside the cranium, and typically require prolonged general anesthesia when used in children. The Cyberknife was developed in an attempt to overcome these restrictions, and although the initial clinical system has been limited by the hardware used for imaging and the software used in targeting, most of the original design objectives have been accomplished. The Cyberknife does not use skeletal fixation, its overall accuracy compares favorably with that achieved by conventional LINAC and Gamma Knife systems that rely on invasive stereotactic frames. In addition, treatment planning and delivery software has been shown to allow delivery of homogeneous conformal dose distribution to targets of irregular shape. Perhaps most importantly, this technology is finally making it possible to consider performing radiosurgery at almost any location within the body.

REFERENCES

1. Adler JR, Murphy MJ, Chang SD, Hancock SL. Image-guided robotic radiosurgery. Neurosurgery 44:1299–1307, 1999.
2. Lemieux L, Kitchen ND, Hughes SW, Thomas DG. Voxel-based localization in frame-based and frameless stereotaxy and its accuracy. Med Phys 21:1301–1310, 1994.
3. Murphy MJ, Cox RS. The accuracy of dose localization for an image-guided frameless radiosurgery system. Med Phys 23:2043–2049, 1996.
4. Winston KR, Lutz W. Linear accelerator as a neurosurgical tool for stereotactic radiosurgery. Neurosurgery 22:454–464, 1988.
5. Maciunas RJ, Galloway RL, Jr, Latimer JW. The application accuracy of stereotactic frames. Neurosurgery 35:682–694; discussion 694–685, 1994.
6. Schell MC, Bova FJ, Larson DA, Keavitt DD, Lutz WR, Podgorask EB, WU A. Stereotactic radiosurgery. AAPM Task Group 42 Report 45:6–8, 1995.
7. Schweikard A, Adler JR, Latombe JC. Motion planning in stereotaxic radiosurgery. Proc IEEE Int Conf Robotics Automation, pp 1990–1916, 1993.
8. Schweikard A, Tombropoulos RZ, Adler JR, Latombe JC. Treatment planning for a radiosurgical system with general kinematics. Proc IEEE Conf Robotics Automation, 1720–1727, 1994.
9. Chang SD, Adler JR, Murphy MJ. Stereotactic radiosurgery of spinal lesions. In: Maciunas RJ, ed. Advanced Techniques in Central Nervous System Metastasis. Park Ridge, Illinois: American Association of Neurologic Surgeons, 1998, pp 269–276.
10. Chang SD, Murphy M, Geis P, Martin DP, Hancock SL, Doty JR, Adler JR, Jr. Clinical experience with image-guided robotic radiosurgery (the Cyberknife)

in the treatment of brain and spinal cord tumors. Neurol Med Chir (Tokyo) 38:780–783, 1998.

11. Chang SD, Murphy MJ, Tombropoulos R, Adler JR. Robotic radiosurgery. In: Alexander E, Maciunas R, eds. Advanced Neurosurgical Navigation. New York: Thieme Medical and Scientific Publishers, 1998, pp 443–449.

12. Antonuk LE, Yorkston J, Huang W, Siewerdson JH, Boudry JM, El-Mohri Y, Marx MV. A real time, flat panel, amorphous silicon, digital x-ray imager. Radiographics 15:993–1000, 1995.

13. Weisfield RL, Street RA, Apte R, More A. An improved page size 127 mm pixel amorphous-silicon image sensor for x-ray diagnostic medical imaging applications. SPIE International Symposium on the Physics of Medical Imaging, February 1997.

14. Sandler HM, Bree RL, McLaughlin PW, Grosman HB, Lichter AS. Localization of the prostatic apex for radiation therapy using implanted markers. Int J Radiat Oncol Biol Phys 27:915–919, 1993.

15. Crook JM, Raymond Y, Salhani D, Yang B, Exche B. Prostate motion during standard radiotherapy as assessed by fiducial markers. Radiother Oncol 37:35–42, 1995.

22

Movement Disorders: Indications

Ahmed Alkhani and Andres M. Lozano
University of Toronto and Toronto Western Hospital,
Toronto, Ontario, Canada

1 INTRODUCTION

Neurosurgical interventions for movement disorders have increased in the last decade. Several disorders that are refractory to medical treatment are now being considered for surgery. Progress in understanding the underlying pathophysiology in these disorders and the anatomical and physiological relationships of basal ganglia components has helped identify potential targets for surgical interventions. In addition, advancement in neuroradiology, stereotactic localization, and intraoperative neurophysiological mapping has facilitated the localization of the targeted structures. This has resulted in improvement of surgical outcome and has made surgery a relatively safe and valuable option in the treatment of these disorders.

Currently, essential tremor (ET), Parkinson's disease (PD), and generalized dystonia (GD) are the three main movement disorders treated with stereotactic neurosurgical interventions. In this chapter, we will discuss indications for surgery, patient selection, rationale for surgery, and outcome for each of these movement disorders.

1.1   Essential Tremor

Essential tremor is a relatively common inherited disorder, with an estimated prevalence of 0.5 per 1000 persons older than the age of 40. Clinical symptoms usually start in early adulthood, with another peak of incidence in late ages. The illness is characterized by a 5 to 10 Hz tremor, which appears with maintenance of posture. Tremor amplitude may increase toward a target at the termination of movement (intention) [1]. The Essential Tremor Rating Scale is used to grade the severity of tremor: 0 = no tremor, 1 = slight, 2 = moderate amplitude, 3 = marked amplitude, 4 = severe amplitude [2]. Like most tremors, ET is worsened by emotion, fatigue, and exercise. It can be temporarily suppressed in the majority of patients by using oral ethanol. Beta blockers, such as propranolol, are usually helpful in controlling the tremor. Other drugs, including primidone and clonazepam, have also been effective [3]. Despite these medications, a small portion of ET patients continue to have severe tremor and significant motor disabilities. Patients with disabling tremor who have failed medical treatment are candidates for surgical intervention.

Neurons firing in synchrony with peripheral tremor are present in the ventral intermediate (Vim) thalamic nucleus. These so called "tremor cells" receive kinesthetic and cerebellar inputs and project primarily to the motor cortex. They can be identified intraoperatively through microelectrode recordings techniques. Intraoperative stimulation at sites with tremor cells will result in an immediate tremor arrest. Radiofrequency thalamotomy and thalamic deep brain stimulation (DBS) of the Vim nucleus are used in the treatment of ET.

Unilateral thalamotomy achieves 70% to 90% improvement in contralateral tremor as measured with the Tremor Rating Scale [4]. Reported complications of thalamotomy include paresthesia, dysequilibrium, and dysarthria. Thalamic DBS has been used in an attempt to avoid these permanent complications. Unilateral DBS is reported to improve contralateral tremor by 68% to 89%. Bilateral thalamic DBS has been advocated to help patients with bilateral and axial tremor. Deep brain stimulation has many of the side effects of lesioning, but these effects can usually be diminished or eliminated by decreasing stimulation intensity. However, adjusting stimulation parameters may reduce the effectiveness of DBS in controlling tremor [5,6].

1.2   Parkinson's Disease

Parkinson's disease is a neurodegenerative disorder characterized mainly by loss of dopaminergic pigmented neurons in the substantia nigra pars compacta (SNc). The incidence of PD is 3/1000 and may reach as high as 3% in individuals older than age 65 [7]. Early in the course of the disease, patients with PD usually have good control of their symptoms with medical treatment. However, with time and disease progression, PD patients receive fewer benefits in response to medication, and significant adverse effects can appear. Further dose increases may not produce better control of symptoms or may induce important side effects, including drug-induced dyskinesias. Many patients continue to have profound motor disabilities despite the best available pharmacotherapy. The unpredictable dramatic switching between "on" (good motor function) and "off" (akinetic, rigid, and tremor) states, experienced by a large number of patients later in the course of PD complicates the illness [8].

Stereotactic surgery for PD is not new. Stereotactic thalamotomy was used to treat tremor in the 1950s and 1960s. However, the introduction of L-dopa in the late 1960s and its striking benefits in PD symptoms resulted in almost total disappearance of surgery. In the early 1990s, the surgical option was re-explored. The promising results of radiofrequency lesioning in the posteroventral part of the internal segment of globus pallidus (GPi) (pallidotomy) in improving motor symptoms of PD and controlling drug-induced dyskinesias opened the door for developments in surgical treatment of PD [9–11].

1.2.1 Selection of Patients

Surgery is indicated for patients with PD who continue to have significant motor disabilities despite best medical management. All efforts should be exercised by a specialist in movement disorders to optimize the medical treatment by adjusting doses and frequencies of medications before considering surgical intervention. Patients with idiopathic PD who respond to L-dopa are good potential candidates for surgery. Patients with so called "Parkinson plus" syndromes, such as multiple systems atrophy or progressive supranuclear palsy, are often less responsive to L-dopa and are generally poor surgical candidates. Patients without significant disabling motor symptoms (grades 1 and 2) and those with end-stage (grade 5) PD are not the best candidates for surgery (Table 1) [12]. Cognitive and psychiatric disturbances, autonomic disturbances, and speech and swallowing difficulties are not uncommon in PD patients. These symptoms not only fail to improve, but may worsen after surgery. Younger patients derive more benefits from surgery, but advanced age is not a contraindication. Significant coexisting medical conditions, psychiatric disease, or focal abnormalities on brain images are relative contraindications.

1.2.2 Surgical Techniques

Magnetic resonance imaging (MRI) (the most commonly used image modality), computerized tomography (CT), or ventriculography can be used

TABLE 1   Hoehn and Yahr Staging of PD

Stage 0.0 = no signs of PD
Stage 1.0 = unilateral involvement only
Stage 1.5 = unilateral and axial involvement
Stage 2.0 = bilateral involvement without impairment of balance
Stage 2.5 = mild bilateral involvement with recovery on retropulsion
            (pull) test
Stage 3.0 = mild to moderate bilateral involvement, some postural
            instability; still able to walk and stand unassisted
Stage 5.0 = wheelchair bound or bedridden unless added

Abbreviation: PD, Parkinson's disease.

to localize surgical targets. Targets can be visualized directly on MRI or indirectly as a function of their relationship to the anterior and posterior commissures. A stereotactic frame is applied under local anesthesia before imaging is used to determine target coordinates. During the procedure, intraoperative mapping is used to verify the anatomical data obtained from images. Two forms of physiological mapping are available: macroelectrode stimulation and microelectrode recordings and stimulation. With macroelectrode stimulation, a 1- to 2-mm diameter electrode is used to deliver a current to the chosen target. Using voltage output of approximately 1 to 4 volts at 2 to 300 Hz current, both clinical benefits and adverse effects of stimulation are noted. Microelectrode recordings and stimulation permit the acquisition of direct measures of the activity of single neurons. Spontaneous and evoked single-unit activity is amplified and displayed on an oscilloscope or heard on a speaker. This information permits unambiguous definition of axonal and neuronal territories. These data are used to determine the boundaries of the targeted structure and to help in placing the lesion or electrode more accurately. Stimulation can be used to identify important structures close to the target. In targeting thalamic Vim nucleus, the thalamic somatosensory relay nucleus (ventral caudalis) can be localized. For GPi, the corticospinal and corticobulbar tract are identified, as well as the optic tract. For the subthalamic nucleus (STN), oculomotor nerve, corticospinal, and medial lemniscal sensory tracts can also be identified [13].

The two widely used techniques in functional neurosurgery currently are lesioning and chronic deep brain stimulation. In lesioning, a radiofrequency generator produces a lesion at a chosen target using the exposed electrode's tip (Fig. 1). The size of the lesion depends on the time of application (30 to 60 seconds), temperature at the electrode tip (45° to 90° C), and size of the electrode used (1 to 3 mm) [13,14]. In DBS, an electrode is

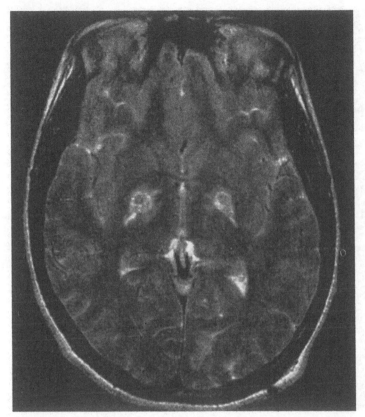

FIGURE 1   An axial cut T2 MRI scan for patient with DYT1 generalized dystonia treated with bilateral radiofrequency pallidotomy.

placed at the target and connected to a subcutaneous internal pulse generator fitted with a lithium battery (Figs. 2 and 3). Although radiofrequency lesioning induce immediate effects, which may last for years, DBS has the advantage being adjustable and reversible. This is particularly important in case of bilateral procedures. On the other hand, DBS is more expensive and carries the risk of infection or mechanical failure like any other implanted foreign body [15,16]. The widely used targets in the treatment of PD are the thalamic Vim nucleus, GPi, and STN.

Thalamic Vim.   Thalamotomy reduces or abolishes parkinsonian contralateral tremor in 80% to 90% of patients or, using a different measure, it improves tremor to grade 0 or 1 in about 75% of cases. Vim thalamotomy in PD is not effective for rigidity, bradykinesia, speech, or gait. Complica-

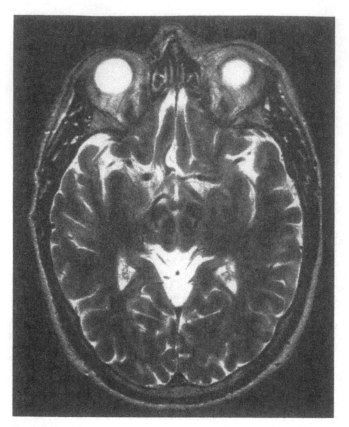

Figure 2 T2 axial magnetic resonance imaging (MRI) scan for a patient with advanced Parkinson's disease treated with bilateral subthalamic nuclei deep brain stimulation illustrating electrode positions.

tions of thalamotomy include paresthesias, ataxia, and aphasia. The incidence of these complications is significantly increased in bilateral thalamotomies. Because the benefits of thalamic procedures are restricted to tremor, currently thalamotomy/DBS are reserved only for PD patients who have tremor predominance [17].

Globus Pallidus (internal segment). According to current models, dopamine deficiency in PD causes hyperactivity of GPi and substantia nigra reticulata (SNr) (basal ganglia output) (Fig. 4) [18]. Using the Unified Parkinson's Disease Rating Scale (UPDRS) as an objective assessment for outcomes, pallidotomy produces improvement in contralateral bradykinesia, tremor, and rigidity during "off" state [10–12]. In a review analysis, pal-

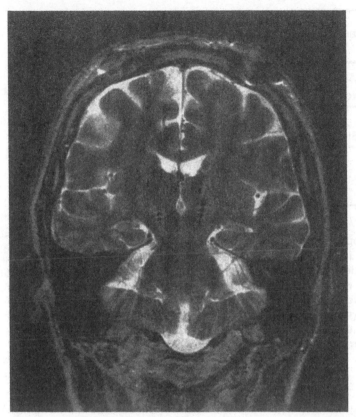

FIGURE 3 T2 coronal magnetic resonance imaging (MRI) scan for the same patient as Figure 2.

lidotomy results in a 45.3% improvement in the motor components of UPDRS during "off" state (range 0–108), 41.3% improvement in activity of daily living (ADL) as assessed by the Schwab and England Functional Scale for ADL, and 86.4% improvement in contralateral drug-induced dyskinesias scores during "on" state [19]. A recent study on long-term follow-up of pallidotomy illustrates sustained improvements for more than 5 years in "off" state symptoms and "on" state dyskinesias [20]. Cerebral hemorrhages, visual field defects, and contralateral motor weakness are the most significant morbidities, and these serious complications occur in 1% to 3% of patients. Postoperative morbidity occurs in 23.1% of cases. In 14% of cases, the morbidity is persistent [19]. These adverse effects appear to be more common with bilateral pallidotomies [21]. Deep brain stimulation

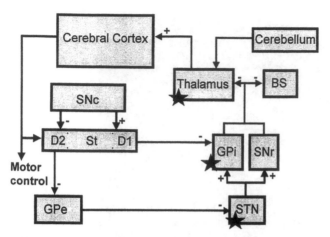

FIGURE 4 Proposed simplified functional model of the basal ganglia. This diagram illustrates only the main connections and surgical targets. D1 receptor denotes neurons expressing predominantly D1 dopamine receptors; D2 receptor denotes neurons with predominant D2 dopamine receptors; SNc and SNr, the pars compactica and pars reticulata of the substantia nigra, respectively; GPi and Gpe, the internal and external portions of the globus pallidus; and BS, the brainstem. Plus signs indicate excitation and minus signs inhibition. Stars indicate sites of surgical interventions.

in the GPi may accomplish similar clinical benefits and has the advantage that the stimulation-induced adverse events are reversible with stimulation parameter adjustment [15,16].

Subthalamic Nucleus. The STN is in a unique position to influence the activities of the entire output of the basal ganglia. The dopamine deficiency state in PD is thought to change the physiology of the striatum and external segment of the globus pallidus (GPe) to produce increased excitatory drive from the STN to the output nuclei of the basal ganglia (GPi and SNr). Bilateral STN stimulation improves both the axial and appendicular motor symptoms of PD [22]. Kumar et al. reported improvement in the total motor UPDRS score during "off" state by 53.8%, bradykinesia 55%, tremor 92.9%, rigidity 49.5%, postural instability 43.6%, gait 30%, and dyskinesias during "on" state by 41% after bilateral STN stimulation [23]. In addition, subthalamic nucleus stimulation improves the unpredictable fluctuation between "on" and "off" states in these patients and reduces the daily doses of anti-PD medications [23]. The long-term effect of STN stimulation is still to be determined.

1.3 Generalized Dystonia

Dystonia is a condition characterized by involuntary sustained muscle contractions that cause abnormal movements and posturing and often are associated with pain. It is classified as primary, idiopathic, or inherited; or
secondary due to underlying brain pathology, metabolic disease, or drugs. It
is also classified according to the affected body part as generalized, segmental, or hemidystonic. These conditions are often refractory to medical
treatment. Repeated local injections of botulinum toxin may help patients
with focal dystonias. However, its use is usually limited to small muscle
groups and can be complicated by development of antibodies to the toxin
with loss of efficacy. Thalamotomy has been used in the past, whereas more
recent reports described encouraging results in the use of pallidotomy and
pallidal stimulation in cases of primary generalized and segmental dystonias.
Globus pallidus interventions are thought to act through effects at down-
stream thalamic, cortical, and brainstem targets. In some reported cases,
clinical improvements may be delayed for days to weeks after surgery
[24,25]. The improvement can be especially striking in cases of hereditary
generalized dystonia like DYT1, an autosomal-dominant disease secondary
to trinucleotide GAG deletion in chromosome 9 [26]. Our knowledge of the
long-term use of these procedures for dystonias is still very limited.

2 CONCLUSIONS

Surgery is a useful method, and sometimes the only one, to treat patients
with various movement disorders. The advent of implantable DBS electrodes
has made this surgery much safer and probably has improved the control of
abnormal movements as well. For most patients at this time, DBS is preferable to lesioning. Coupled with the other advances in stereotactic technology, it may be tempting to view these procedures as "routine." However,
this is not so. The Vim nucleus is a relatively large and safe target that can
be localized with macrostimulation alone, but targeting the Gpi or the STN
is a more demanding task. For these cases, the most exquisite imaging possible is needed at a minimum, and the use of microelectrode recording is
ideal to ensure an adequate result. We would argue that microelectrode recording (MER) is also of value for surgery aimed at the Vim nucleus in
patients with tremor.

     At least as important as these technical considerations is the need for
careful patient selection. Before proceeding with any surgery for relief of a
movement disorder, patients should be seen by a neurologist with expertise
in this area, and standard measures for tremor or disability should be performed. Careful follow-up will allow the surgeon to assess his results and
to provide the best possible care.

REFERENCES

1. MF Brin, W Koller. Epidemiology and genetics of essential tremor. Mov Disord 1998;13(suppl 3):55–63.
2. S Fahn, E Tolosa, C Martin. Clinical rating scale for tremor. In: J Jankovic, E Tolosa, eds. Parkinson's disease and movement disorders. Munich: Urban and Schwarzenberg, 1988, pp 225–234.
3. PG Wasielewski, JM Burns, WC Koller. Pharmacological treatment of tremor. Mov Disord 1998;13(suppl 3):90–100.
4. JD Speelman, PR Schuurman, RMA de Bie, DA Bosch. Thalamic surgery and tremor. Mov Disord 1998;13 (suppl 3):103–016.
5. W Koller, R Pahwa, K Busenbark, J Hubble, S Wilkison, A Lang, P Tuite, E Sime, A Lozano, R Houser, T Malapira, D Smith, D Tarsy, E Miyawaki, T Norregaard, T Kormos, W Olanow. High-frequency unilateral thalamic stimulation in the treatment of essential and parkinsonian tremor. Ann Neurol 42(3): 292–299, 1997.
6. S Moghal, AH Rajput, C D'Arcy, R Rajput. Prevalence of movement disorders in elderly community residents. Neuroepidemiology 13:175–178, 1994.
7. PR Schuurman, A Bosch, PMM Bossuyt, GJ Bonsel, EJW van Someren, RMA de Bie, MP Merkus, JD Speelman. A comparison of continuous thalamic stimulation and thalamotomy for suppression of severe tremor. N Engl J Med 342: 461–468, 2000.
8. AE Lang, AM Lozano. Parkinson's disease: Second of two parts. N Engl J Med 339:1044–1053, 1998.
9. J Guridi, AM Lozano. A brief history of pallidotomy. Neurosurgery 41:1169–1180, 1997.
10. LV Laitinen, AT Bergenheim, MI Hariz. Leksell's posteroventral pallidotomy in the treatment of Parkinson's disease. J Neurosurg 76:53–61, 1992.
11. AE Lang, AM Lozano, E Montgomery, J Duff, R Tasker, W Hutchinson. Posteroventral medial pallidotomy in advanced Parkinson's disease. N Engl J Med 337:1036–1042, 1997.
12. JW Langston, H Widner, CG Goetz, D Brooks, S Fahn, T Freeman, R Watts. Core assessment program for intracerebral transplantations (CAPIT). Mov Disord 7:2–13, 1992.
13. A Lozano, W Hutchison, Z Kiss, R Tasker, K Davis, J Dostrovsky. Methods for microelectrode-guided posteroventral pallidotomy. J Neurosurg 84:194–202, 1996.
14. JL Vitek, RA Bakay, MR DeLong. Microelectrode-guided pallidotomy for medically intractable Parkinson's disease. Adv Neurol 74:183–198, 1997.
15. J Volkmann, V Sturm, P Weiss, J Kappler, J Voges, A Koulousakis, R Lehrke, H Hefter, HJ Freund. Bilateral high-frequency stimulation of the internal globus pallidus in advanced Parkinson's disease. Ann Neurol 44:953–961, 1998.
16. C Gross, A Rougier, D Guehl, T Boraud, J Julien, B Bioulac. High-frequency stimulation of the globus pallidus internalis in Parkinson's disease: A study of seven cases. J Neurosurg 87:491–498, 1997.

17. MN Linhares, R Tasker. Microelectrode-guided thalamotomy for Parkinson's disease. Neurosurgery 46(2):390–395, 2000.
18. MR DeLong. Primate models of movement disorders of basal ganglia origin. Trends Neurosci 13:281–285, 1990.
19. A Alkhani, AM Lozano. Pallidotomy for Parkinson's disease: A review of contemporary literature. J Neurosurg 94(1):43–49, 2001.
20. J Fine, J Duff, R Chen, B Chir, W Hutchison, AM Lozano, AE Lang. Long-term follow-up of unilateral pallidotomy in advanced Parkinson's disease. N Engl J Med 342(23):1708–1714, 2000.
21. G Vingerhoets, C van der Linden, E Lannoo, V Vandewalle, J Caemaert, M Wolters, D van den Abbeele. Cognitive outcome after unilateral pallidal stimulation in Parkinson's disease. J Neurol Neurosurg Psychiatry 66:297–304, 1999.
22. P Limousin, P Krack, P Pollack, A Benazzouz, C Ardouin, D Hoffmann, AL Benabid. Electrical stimulation of the subthalamic nucleus in advanced Parkinson's disease. N Engl J Med 339:1105–1111, 1998.
23. R Kumar, AM Lozano, YJ Kim, WD Hutchison, E Sime, E Halket, AE Lang. Double-blind evaluation of subthalamic nucleus deep brain stimulation in advanced Parkinson's disease. Neurology 51:850–855, 1998.
24. R Kumar, A Dagher, WD Hutchison, AE Lang, AM Lozano. Globus pallidus deep brain stimulation for generalized dystonia: Clinical and PET investigation. Neurology 53:871–874, 1999.
25. AM Lozano, R Kumar, RE Gross, N Giladi, WD Hutchison, JO Dostrovsky, AE Lang. Globus pallidus internus pallidotomy for generalized dystonia. Mov Disord 12:865–870, 1997.
26. WG Ondo, JM Desaloms, J Jankovic, RG Grossman. Pallidotomy for generalized dystonia. Mov Disord 13:693–698, 1998.

23

Technical Considerations in Movement Disorders Surgery

Philip Starr

University of California San Francisco,
San Francisco, California, U.S.A

1 INTRODUCTION

The major subcortical structures targeted for deep brain stimulation (DBS) or lesioning for the treatment of movement disorders include the nucleus ventralis intermedius (Vim) of the thalamus, the globus pallidus internal segment (GPi), and the subthalamic nucleus (STN). The major technical goal during surgery for movement disorders is to maximize both precision and safety. The methods for localization of the Vim, GPi, and STN are evolving and vary significantly between centers. Three types of methods may be used to determine target location before lesioning or chronic stimulator placement: image-guided stereotactic localization, microelectrode mapping, and intraoperative test stimulation through the lesioning or DBS electrode, often called "macrostimulation." The first of these is based on anatomy, whereas the latter two are based on physiology.

2 IMAGE-GUIDED LOCALIZATION

2.1 Targeting from the Commissures

Classically, image-guided localization has been based on identification of internal landmarks, usually the anterior and posterior commissures (AC and

PC), in reference to a coordinate system provided by a stereotactic frame rigidly fixed to the patient's head. The AC and PC may be visualized on ventriculography, computed tomography (CT), or magnetic resonance imaging (MRI). Anatomical targets within motor thalamus, GPi, and STN may all be localized indirectly by measuring fixed distances from these landmarks, based on the location of the targets with respect to the AC and PC.

Table 1 provides reasonable initial anatomical coordinates for each target, determined from standard brain atlases and clinical studies in which the anatomical target coordinates have been verified physiologically [1–4]. Lateral coordinates for Vim and Gpi are best expressed in terms of distance from the third ventricular wall rather then the midline. These anatomical coordinates must be considered only an approximate guideline, however, for the following reasons: (1) There is significant individual variability in the spatial position of these targets in AC-PC based coordinates [1,3]; (2) The optimal target point within each nucleus has not been determined with certainty, as very few studies correlate location of lesions or electrode leads with outcome [5,6]; (3) Optimal location within a given target may be different for lesioning versus chronic stimulation [7]; (4) The exact initial target position may also depend on the patient's symptomatology. In targeting for

TABLE 1 Approximate Anatomic Coordinates for Vim, GPi, and STN with Respect to the Commissures

Target nucleus	Coordinates in mm	Corresponds to:	References
Vim	Vertical = 0 Lateral = 11 from third ventricle wall AP = 6 anterior to PC	Anteroventral border of Vim, in the arm territory	[3,4]
Gpi	Vertical = −2 to −8 Lateral = 18 from third ventricular wall AP = 2 anterior to MCP	Inferior border of motor territory of Gpi, immediately superior to optic tract	[1,15,50, 89]
STN	Vertical = −4 to −6 Lateral = 12 AP = 2 to 3 posterior to MCP	Center of the STN	[4,72]

Abbreviations: *Vim*, Ventralis intermedius; *GPi*, Globus pallidus internal; *STN*, Subthalamic nucleus; *AP*, Anteroposterior; *MPC*, Midcommissural point.

thalamic surgery for tremor relief, for example, prominent leg rather than arm tremor might dictate a slightly more lateral approach in Vim [8].

2.2 Use of MR for Stereotactic Targeting

Magnetic resonance imaging-based stereotactic localization has the advantage of allowing direct visualization of at least some borders of the target nuclei, in addition to excellent visualization of the commissures. The borders of Gpi and STN, as well as the thalamocapsular border, are identifiable with appropriate pulse sequences. Thus, MRI-based stereotaxy provides the opportunity to adjust target coordinates according to individual variation in the positions of deep nuclei, resulting in improved accuracy over that which is achieved using indirect, AC-PC based coordinates [1,9]. Some MR pulse sequences useful for movement disorders surgery are listed in Table 2. In general, contiguous (zero interspace) slices are necessary to cover the target area. For two-dimensional-acquisition sequences, however, image resolution is enhanced by acquiring the images noncontiguously, as two interleaved sets. This avoids signal degradation that would otherwise occur when there is zero slice separation and images are acquired as a single set [10]. The field of view must be large enough to cover the fiducial markers; usually 26 cm is adequate. Typical matirx size is 256×256 or 256×512.

TABLE 2   Some MR Pulse Sequences Commonly Used for Movement Disorders Surgery

MR pulse sequence	Sample parameters	Comments
T-2 weighted fast spin echo	TR = 2500, TE = 110	Excellent for STN visualization, in the coronal plane
Inversion recovery-fast spin echo	TR = 3000, TE = 40, TI = 200	Excellent for GPi visualization, in the axial plane
Three-dimensional acquisition gradient echo	TR = 7, TE = 3.4, flip angle = 30°, bandwidth = 15 kHz	May be reformatted in any plane with minimal image degradation

Abbreviations: *MR*, Magnetic resonance; *STN*, Subthalamic nucleus; *GPi*, Globus pallidus internal.

Magnetic resonance imaging has the disadvantage, compared with CT and ventriculography, of several types of image distortion effects [11]. Image distortion may result in apparent positions of the target or fiducial markers on the image that are different from their actual positions in real space. Distortion effects can vary widely between different scanners, sequence protocols, and frame systems. Before using MRI as the sole modality for anatomical localization, the degree of distortion should be estimated by performing a phantom study [12]. Distortion effects may be partially corrected using computational algorithms [11], or CT-MR image fusion techniques [13,14]. Alternatively, some groups use a nonstereotactic MRI to plan "individualized" AC-PC based coordinates, then perform the actual stereotactic localization with ventriculography or with CT [4,15].

2.3 Frame Placement

Stereotactic procedures begin with fixation of the frame to the patient's head. "Scanner-dependent" frame systems, such as the Leksell (Atlanta, GA) series G frame or the Radionics (Burlington, MA) CRW-fn frame are frequently used for functional stereotaxy. These frames are designed to be fixed with the vertical axis parallel to the MR or CT gantry. Unless special surgical planning software is used to calculate the target coordinates, scanner-dependent stereotactic systems also require that images be obtained orthogonal to the frame axes.

It is important to place the frame with its axes orthogonal to standard anatomical planes of the brain. Frame misalignments are often described using the terms "pitch," "roll," and "yaw," following nautical terminology [16]. Good frame placement is facilitated by the use of the earplugs provided with most scanner-dependent systems. These align the frame with the external auditory canals. The use of the earplugs ensures that the mediolateral (X) axis of the frame is perpendicular to the midsagittal plane of the brain, thus avoiding any roll (lateral tilt) or yaw (rotation) of the frame with respect to the brain. To adjust the pitch, the anteroposterior axis of the frame may then be angled according to superfical landmarks so as to parallel the AC-PC line. A line between the inferior orbital rim and the external auditory canal is approximately parallel to the AC-PC [1], as is a line from the glabella to the inion [17]. The eyes and mouth should remain unencumbered by the frame, so as to allow visual field examination and airway access. Once the frame is aligned in all dimensions, the skull pins are advanced symmetrically. It is important to begin withdrawing the earplugs before the pins are fully tightened, to avoid severe pain in the external auditory canals. Intravenous sedation (such as 1–2 mg of Versed) is desirable when the earplugs are used.

Straight frame placement ensures that the preoperative images, as well as maps made from intraoperative physiological exploration, are interpretable in terms of familiar anatomy corresponding to standard brain atlases. In addition, the use of indirect targeting from the AC-PC line assumes that there is no pitch, yaw, or roll of the frame with respect to the brain; such deviations will reduce accuracy. When the frame is imperfectly aligned, computational algorithms [16] or surgical planning software [18] may be used to correct for this.

2.4 Surgical Planning Software

Surgical planning software is a useful, although not essential, adjunct to frame-based stereotactic targeting and is available from a variety of commercial sources including Elekta (Atlanta, GA), Radionics (Burlington, MA), and Sofamor-Danek (Memphis, TN) [18]. Such software usually provides a variety of functions. Among the most useful is multiplanar visualization of the probe trajectory based on a given arc and ring angle, which assists greatly in planning a trajectory that avoids large cortical vessels, sulci, or ventricles. Another helpful feature is semiautomated registration of the image set in stereotactic space as defined by the fiducial markers. This may improve targeting speed and reduce human error. Other functions are useful only in specific situations. Many software packages allow the user to reformat MR images along standard anatomical planes orthogonal to the AC-PC line and midsagittal plane. However, to preserve a high degree of resolution in the reformatted images, the original image set should be acquired volumetrically. This limits the choice of pulse sequences and is generally not necessary if the headframe is carefully placed orthogonal to standard anatomical planes. Computational fusion of nonstereotactically acquired images (usually MR) with stereotactic images (usually CT) is a useful function for operators whose MR units suffer from spatial distortion. Superposition of a "deformable" human brain atlas onto MR or CT images is a function used by many surgeons. However, accurately matching an individual brain to a standard atlas may not be possible, even if the atlas is "deformable." A reasonable alternative is to use MR pulse sequences, which provides maximal visualization of the target nucleus.

2.5 Limitations of Anatomical Targeting

A number of factors limit the accuracy of anatomical targeting that is based on historical data. These are summarized in Table 3. The accuracy of any stereotactic system, regardless of imaging modality, is limited by mechanical properties of the frame, and in CT- or MR-based stereotaxy by slice thick-

TABLE 3 Factors Limiting the Accuracy of Anatomical Targeting

Method	Factors limiting accuracy
Any method that uses historical images in conjunction with a frame-based coordinate system	1. Application accuracy of stereotactic system 2. Brain shifts that may occur after imaging
MR-based targeting	Image distortion
"Indirect" targeting by measuring fixed distances	1. Anatomic variability between individuals 2. Requires perfectly straight frame placement
"Direct" targeting by visualization of the target structure's boundaries	Imperfect visualization of the target structure
Any purely anatomical method	Anatomy ≠ physiology. A given physiological function may not always occur in the same anatomical structure

Abbreviation: *MR*, Magnetic resonance.

ness. The "application accuracy" of a stereotactic system is a term that describes the accuracy of the system as it is used clinically. The application accuracy of standard frame-based stereotactic systems, with 1-mm thick CT slices, has been measured to be approximately 1.5 mm at the 95% confidence limit [19]. The application accuracy of frameless systems is probably less than this [18,20], explaining the continued widespread use of frame-based systems for functional work, whereas tumor stereotaxis is now largely performed with frameless systems.

In practice, the theoretical maximum accuracy of a stereotactic system is rarely achieved, as many other factors in a given case can further decrease the accuracy of anatomical targeting (Table 3). Thus, image-guided stereotaxis alone is usually adequate for placing a stimulator or lesion probe within several millimeters of the target, but physiologic studies are important to adjust or confirm final placement.

The use of intraoperative MR, currently under investigation for tumor surgery [21], could improve stereotactic targeting for functional neurosurgery by providing a real time update of the actual probe position. Application of this technique to basal ganglia surgery, however, awaits improvements in the image quality for these units, as well as the development of MR-compatible, low-artifact instrumentation for guiding probes into place.

3 MICROELECTRODE RECORDING AND MICROSTIMULATION

3.1 Overview of Microelectrode Recording

Since its introduction by Albe-Fessard and Guiot [22] in the early 1960s, microelectrode recording (MER) has been performed in the human thalamus during surgery for parkinsonism and other movement disorders [23–33]. There is now a growing literature on microelectrode recording in the human GPi [34–41] and the human STN [42]. The most common technique is recording of single-unit, extracellular action potentials using high impedence (0.1-1.0 Mohm at 1000 Hz) tungsten or platinum-iridium microelectrodes [28,36,41,43].

The utility of microelectrode recording for target localization is based on several principles [28,36,41,43]. Transitions between gray and white matter may be identified, as extracellularly recorded action potentials in gray and white matter have distinguishable waveforms. Different basal ganglia nuclei have characteristic patterns of spontaneous discharge, which are relatively easy to identify. Some of these patterns are shown in Figure 1. Motor subterritories of a region can be distinguished from nonmotor regions by finding neurons whose discharge frequencies are modulated by movement. Localization within a motor region can be accomplished by mapping the receptive field of a movement-sensitive cell during motor examination of the patient, then comparing the cell's receptive field with the known somatotopic organization of the nucleus [36,41]. Microstimulation, or passing current through the microelectrode, can evoke motor and sensory phenomena and thus localize motor and sensory pathways. Finally, the spatial resolution of microelectrode techniques is high; structural boundaries may be identified with submillimetric precision [28,36,41,43].

"Semimicroelectrode" recording refers to the use of slightly larger-tipped, lower impedance electrodes that record from a small group of cells but are not fine enough to resolve individual action potentials. This technique may permit accurate identification of nuclear borders and movement-responsive cell regions [44], but does not allow detailed resolution of the discharge rate and pattern, which is especially useful for globus pallidus localization [36,41].

3.2 Hardware for Microelectrode Recording

Hardware for MER normally provides the following functions: amplification, filtering, visual display and audio monitoring of the microelectrode signal,

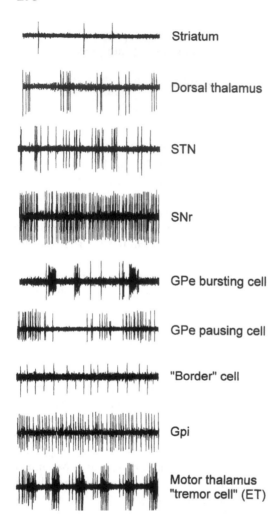

Striatum

Dorsal thalamus

STN

SNr

GPe bursting cell

GPe pausing cell

"Border" cell

Gpi

Motor thalamus
"tremor cell" (ET)

FIGURE 1 Microelectrode recordings from the thalamus and basal ganglia. Each trace represents a 1-second recording. Recordings are from patients with Parkinson's disease (upper 8 traces) or essential tremor (ET, lowest trace).

microstimulation, and impedance monitoring. Optional additional functions include data recording and storage, and on-line or off-line data analysis. Systems approved by the Food and Drug Administration (FDA) for microelectrode recording in the human are commercially available [45]. Alternatively, it is possible to put together one's own recording rack from individual components. This is less expensive than purchasing a commercial system, but is much more labor intensive [45].

In addition to good electronics, single-unit recordings require high quality microelectrodes and a low-noise environment. We mainly use platinum-coated tungsten microelectrodes, with 15 to 25 micron tip diameter and impedance 0.2 to 0.6 mΩ at 1 KHz [43]. Similar microelectrodes for extracellular single unit recording are commercially available from several sources, including Frederick Haer (Brunswick, Maine) and Microprobe, Inc. (Gaithersburg, Maryland). To reduce electrical noise at line frequency, it is important to place the headstage of the preamplifier close to the microelectrode itself, which usually involves mounting it on the stereotactic arc [43]. Alternatively, an actively shielded cable between electrode and amplifier may be used [43]. The best ground is usually the microelectrode guide tube or the stereotactic arc. Finally, it may be necessary to unplug electrical devices near the MER apparatus, such as an electrically powered operating room table or coagulation units.

3.3 Microelectrode Localization of GPi

On a frontal approach to the pallidum, the microelectrode usually encounters striatum, then the external globus pallidus (GPe), prior to GPi. The majority of striatal neurons have very low (0–10 Hz) spontaneous discharge rates (Fig. 1). Neuronal discharge patterns in GPe and GPi have characteristic discharge patterns that are specific to the disease state. Most published physiological data are for Parkinson's disease (PD) (Fig. 1) [34–41,43], but some data are available for dystonia and hemiballismus [46–48]. In PD, GPe neurons have spontaneous discharge rates of 30 to 60 Hz and typically discharge in "bursting" or "pausing" patterns. Globus pallidus internal neurons in PD are faster than GPe cells, with spontaneous discharge rates of 60 to 100 Hz. In dystonia and hemiballismus, GPi discharge rates may be much lower [46–48]. Cells with very regular discharge at 20 to 40 Hz, so-called "border" cells, are typically found in the white matter laminae surrounding GPe and GPi [49]. The optic tract (OT) can be identified by light-evoked fiber activity below the inferior margin of GPi [36,41].

Cells in GPi that are responsive to joint movements usually respond to movement of one or a small number of joints in a restricted region on the contralateral side of the body [36,37,41]. As the motor territory of GPi is somatotopically organized, with leg representations tending to be more dorsal and more medial than arm representations [41,50], the recorded distribution of neuronal receptive fields helps to determine the mediolateral coordinate of an electrode track. In patients with tremor, cells with discharges grouped at tremor frequency are often recorded [35,39]. Microstimulation can be used to localize both the corticospinal tract (CST) and the OT [36,41]. The CST in the internal capsule is identified by evoking muscle contractions (usually of the tongue, face, or hand) at low current thresholds, such as 10 microamperes at 300 Hz, 200 microsecond pulse width. The optic tract is identified when the patient reports visual phenomena (focal scintillating scotomata) at low current thresholds.

3.4 Microelectrode Localization of the Motor Thalamus

During thalamic surgery, MER is especially useful to identify cells that respond to active or passive movements and to identify sensory thalamus either by microstimulation or by recording cells with cutaneous receptive fields. Lenz et al detected 107 movement-related cells out of a total 1012 cells recorded along electrode trajectories that included both motor and sensory thalamus [30]. These cells usually respond to movements of one or a small number of contralateral joints [30,51]. They are further classified as passive or active cells according to whether their discharge frequencies are modulated by passive or active movements [30]. In the subhuman primate, active cells are more likely to be found in the pallidal receiving area (ventralis oralis anterior and posterior, or Voa and Vop, in the Hassler terminology), whereas passive cells are more likely to be found in the cerebellar receiving area (Vim) [52]. This may be true in human PD patients but has not been clearly confirmed [30].

As the microelectrode descends toward the thalamic target, the caudate nucleus may be encountered first. The next structure traversed, the dorsal thalamus, has relatively low spontaneous activity in the awake patient, but may show occasional bursts. Microelectrode entry into motor thalamus is often heralded by an increase in spontaneous activity, and can be confirmed by the identification of movement-responsive cells and/or cells discharging at tremor frequency. The posterior border of motor thalamus, formed by the lemniscal receiving area of sensory thalamus, contains neurons whose sensory receptive fields are extremely well localized [33]. This thin anterior rim of the sensory ventrocaudal nucleus (Vcae) contains cells responding to deep muscle pressure. The remainder of the ventrocaudal nucleus (Vcpe) responds to extremely light cutaneous stimuli [33]. Recording cutaneous sensory cells provides a precise, reproducible demarcation of the posterior edge of motor thalamus. The mediolateral position of a microelectrode track can be estimated by the somatotopic organization of motor and sensory cells, since face/jaw, arm and leg representations are organized along a medial to lateral axis. This is true of both cerebellar (Vim) and pallidal (Voa/Vop) receiving areas [30], as well as for the sensory nucleus Vc [33].

Microstimulation can identify the posterior and lateral borders of Vim. Laterally, low stimulation thresholds for evoked muscle contractions indicate that the electrode is at or has traversed the border between Vim and internal capsule. Posteriorly, low thresholds for evoked paresthesias indicate that the electrode has traversed the border between Vim and Vc [28].

3.5 Microelectrode Localization of STN

Single cell discharge characteristics in the human STN have been studied in the parkinsonian state [42], and are similar to those observed in the parkinsonian monkey [53]. A representative trace is shown in Figure 1. Since cell density in STN is extremely high, background noise is high and individual cells are hard to isolate [42,53]. Single neurons discharge at 20–50 Hz [42]. However, typical recordings are of multiple cells and therefore the apparent discharge frequency may be higher unless great care is taken to isolate individual cells. As the microelectrode passes through the inferior border of STN into SNr, the discharge pattern changes abruptly. Background noise diminishes greatly, single neurons again become easy to isolate, and the discharge rate is high (50–70) (Fig. 1) [42]. Microstimulation up to 100 microamperes may occasionally evoke corticobulbar responses, paresthesia, tremor arrest, or ocular deviation, but these effects are reported to be inconsistent [42].

3.6 Is MER Necessary?

The role of microelectrode recording during surgery for movement disorders, and particularly for pallidotomy, is actively debated. Some centers argue that it is essential [41,50,54], whereas others are adamant that it is not [55]. Rates of permanent morbidity have been similar, and relatively low, for both groups. Many reports that have documented clear benefits from pallidotomy, as measured by standard rating scales, come from centers that use microelectrode recording [56–61]. In some recent well-documented series, however, pallidotomy without microelectrode recording yielded similar short-term results (up to 1 year) as centers that perform pallidotomy with microelectrode recording [14,15,62,63]. In one of these series, longer term follow-up produced a diminution in benefit [64], to a greater extent than the long-term studies performed by the MER groups [58]. Thus, when used for pallidotomy, MER may permit more complete lesioning of the motor territory of the target, which may be associated with more durable benefit.

4 IMPEDANCE MONITORING AND STIMULATION THROUGH A MACROELECTRODE

Additional intraoperative physiologic confirmation of the brain target may be obtained using the lesioning probe or deep brain stimulator. These "macroelectrodes" are typically about 1 mm in diameter and thus much too large to record cellular activity, but they can be used for impedance monitoring or electrical stimulation. Because the macroelectrode has a low impedance, the impedance of the surrounding brain tissue contributes significantly to current flow in response to applied voltage. Gray and white matter have different impedances, so it is possible to detect transitions between gray and white matter if the impedance to a test pulse is measured as the macroelectrode descends.

Electrical stimulation through the lesion probe or DBS lead, or "macrostimulation," affects a larger volume of tissue than microstimulation, as the probe tip and the current flow are several orders of magnitude larger. Macrostimulation provides the final intraoperative check on target localization just before lesioning or permanent stimulator placement, and has been used during surgery for movement disorders for many years [65,66]. As with microstimulation, macrostimulation can evoke visual, motor, and cutaneous sensory responses by effects on structures that border the target. In GPi, proximity of the probe to inferior and posteromedial borders is indicated by the current thresholds for activating optic tract and corticobulbar/corticospinal tracts, respectively [41]. In motor thalamus, proximity to posterior and lateral borders is indicated by activation of sensor thalamus and corticobulbar tract, respectively. In STN, proximity to posteromedial and lateral borders may be indicated by activation of lemniscal fibers and corticobulbar tract, respectively [4,67]. During STN surgery, macrostimulation may also evoke oculomotor effects [67] or mood changes [68], although the exact structures or pathways responsible for these effects are not yet clear.

For patients with tremor, intraoperative tremor suppression provides another indication of adequacy of probe placement. This has long been known for thalamic surgery [65,69–71], but appears to be true for surgery of GPi and STN as well [72]. In STN, intraoperative suppression of rigidity has also been used as a guide to placement of chronic STN stimulators [4,73].

Caution is advised, however, when using acute stimulation to predict the effects of lesioning or chronic stimulation. Symptoms other than tremor may not respond immediately to acute intraoperative test stimulation. During GPi pallidotomy, for example, bradykinesia often fails to improve with acute test stimulation through the lesion probe, but this does not predict a poor long-term effect of lesioning for bradykinesia [41]. After implantation of a DBS lead into GPi, symptomatic benefit may require time (from hours up to several weeks) to appear [74], again illustrating the point that failure to improve with brief test stimulation does not necessarily imply an incorrect lead placement. Pallidotomy and chronic pallidal stimulation for dystonia are also associated with long delays (weeks or months) between surgery and symptomatic benefit [75,76]. With the exception of tremor control, therefore, we use intraoperative macrostimulation mainly to confirm appropriate voltages for adverse effects, rather than to assess for clinical benefit.

In any of the surgical targets discussed here, motor symptoms may be partially or completely suppressed by simple placement of the macroelectrode, even before stimulation or lesioning. This "microlesion effect," when observed, provides evidence that the probe is within or has passed through the motor territory of the target nucleus. Unless a permanent lesion is subsequently made deliberately, this effect is generally temporary. For DBS procedures, failure to observe a microlesion effect does not necessarily predict a poor outcome from chronic stimulation.

5 METHODS OF LESIONING

The most common technique for creation of a permanent lesion is that of radiofrequency (RF) thermocoagulation, developed in the 1940s and 1950s [77,78]. Alternating current at radiofrequency (approximately 500,000 Hz) is passed through a monopolar electrode at the lesioning site, to a large surface area dispersive electrode taped to the patient's skin. In the immediate region of the active electrode, the rapidly oscillating electrical field produces movement of electrolytes that is sufficient to cause significant frictional heating [77]. The temperature at the lesion center is monitored with a thermistor on the active electrode tip. In the brain, temperatures over 45° C produce permanent tissue destruction. Acutely, RF lesioning produces a central zone of coagulation necrosis surrounded by edema [79]. With a commercially available RF electrode of active tip dimensions 1.1 × 3 mm (Radionics, Burlington, MA), the diameter of the coagulum, in laboratory tests, varies nearly linearly from 1 to 4 mm for temperatures from 60° to 80° C applied for 60 seconds [41,77]. Thus, once the target site is selected based on anatomical targeting and physiological confirmation, the size of the lesion can be planned according to the predicted spread of the zone of coagulation at different times and temperatures. The lesion may also be "shaped" to the target structure by making multiple lesions, either along a single lesioning track or multiple adjacent tracks [36,41].

Other techniques for lesion generation are being explored. Lesioning of the thalamus and GPi by stereotactic radiosurgery has been reported [55,80–82]. With this technique, the lesion is generated by radiation necrosis. There is a latent period between treatment and clinical effect. Only image-based anatomical targeting is used to guide lesion location, without physiological verification. Chemical lesioning of GPi, by infusion of excitotoxins, has been successful in a primate model of parkinsonism [83]. This technique has the theoretical advantage of being axon-sparing, thus potentially avoiding damage to white matter structures surrounding the target. Historically, however, the size of the lesion using chemical infusion techniques has been difficult to control [84,85].

6 SPECIAL TECHNICAL CONSIDERATIONS FOR DBS

6.1 DBS Hardware

The most commonly used brain electrodes for DBS are the Medtronic (Minneapolis MN) model 3387 and model 3389 quadripolar leads. The leads have four platinum-iridium contacts, 1.5 mm in length, separated by 3 mm center to center (model 3387) or 2 mm center to center (model 3389). The lead is connected to a battery-operated, programmable implanted pulse generator (IPG), which is placed subcutaneously in the infraclavicular area. The pulse generator may be single channel for use with one DBS lead (Itrel II, Medtronic) or dual-channel for use with bilateral DBS leads (Kinetra, Medtronic). Any one or any combination of the four lead contacts may be used for monopolar stimulation (with the pulse generator as the cathode), and any two contacts or groups of contacts may be used together for bipolar stimulation. The pulse width, stimulation amplitude, and stimulation frequency (up to 185 Hz), as well as the choice of active contacts and stimulation mode (bipolar or monopolar) are all adjustable by the physician using an external programming unit. The patient may turn the stimulator on or off at any time using an external magnet. Stimulation parameters may vary but typically range as follows: Pulse width = 60–210 μs, amplitude = 1–4 V, and frequency 130–185 Hz.

6.2 Operative Techniques for DBS

Once the lead is in place, it must be anchored to the skull. The Medtronic lead implant kit provides a burr hole cap with a groove for lead anchoring, designed to fit in a 14-mm burr hole. The first-generation burr hole cap can be difficult to use as it tends to alter the vertical position of the lead, often necessitating intraoperative fluoroscopy to track and correct changes in the lead position. Other anchoring techniques have been reported. Some surgeons anchor the lead in the burr hole with methylmethacrylate or hydroxyapatite bone source while the proximal end is still fixed in position on the stereotactic arc or micropositioner [4]. After removal of the stylet and micropositioner, the lead may also be fixed to the skull with a miniplate [86].

After the lead is anchored, it may be temporarily externalized for several days of in-hospital testing, or it may be immediately internalized and attached to a lead extender and pulse generator. The lead extender attaches to the DBS lead under the scalp, and is tunneled to an infraclavicular incision to attach to the IPG. A pocket is dissected bluntly over the pectoralis fascia to hold the IPG. The connector on the lead extender should be positioned over the skull and fixed into place with a suture or a groove drilled in the bone. We place it behind the ear, superolateral to the mastoid. If the connector is placed in the soft tissues of the neck, constant motion between the lead and the connector may cause lead fracture, and tension on the lead could easily cause failure of the anchoring system, resulting in lead migration.

6.3   MR imaging of DBS Components

The manufacturer of the Medtronic DBS system cautions against MRI of their device outside of a limited range of imaging parameters and field strengths. Nevertheless, MR imaging of DBS lead is important for postoperative documentation of exact lead location, as well as for preoperative stereotactic localization in cases where a second lead is implanted in a patient who already has one pre-existing lead. Detailed testing of the Medtronic DBS components (model 3387 lead and ITREL 2 pulse generator) for heating, movement, or large induced currents within an MR coil suggests that MR imaging of these components is safe [87]. Many groups perform MR imaging of these components, and no adverse events have been reported as of late 1999 [87,88]. The strong magnetic field of the MR can turn the IPG on or off, so the IPG should be set to zero volts before MR so that the patient does not experience transient discomfort that may be associated with alternation of the device between on and off states.

With any MR pulse sequences, the lead produces a metal artifact that is larger than the actual lead size and may be irregular in shape. The use of a fast spin echo MR technique may result in a smaller artifact in comparison with inversion recover-fast spin echo or gradient echo techniques.

REFERENCES

1. Starr PA, Vitek JL, DeLong ML, Bakay RAE. MRI-based stereotactic targeting of the globus pallidus and subthalamic nucleus. Neurosurgery 44:303–314, 1999.
2. Maeda T. Lateral coordinates of nucleus ventralis intermedius target for tremor alleviation. Stereotact Funct Neurosurg 52:191–199, 1989.
3. Kelly PJ, Derome P, Guiot G. Thalamic spatial variability and the surgical results of lesions placed with neurophysiologic control. Surg Neurol 9:307–315, 1978.
4. Benabid AL, Benazzouz A, Gao D, Hoffman D, Limousin P, Koudsie A, Krack P, Pollak P. Chronic electrical stimulation of the ventralis intermedius nucleus

of the thalamus and of other nuclei as a treatment for Parkinson's disease. Techniques Neurosurg 5:5–30, 1999.

5. Vitek JL, Bakay RAE, DeLong MR. Microelectrode guided GPi pallidotomy for medically intractable Parkinson's disease. Adv Neurol 74:183–198, 1997.
6. Gross RE, Lombardi WJ, Lang AE, Duff J, Hutchison WD, Saint-Cyr JA, Tasker RR, Lozano AM. Relationship of lesion location to clinical outcome following microelectrode-guided pallidotomy for Parkinson's disease. Brain 122:405–416, 1999.
7. Bejjani B, Damier P, Arnulf I, Bonnet AM, Vidailhet M, Dormont D, Pidoux B, Cornu P, Marsault C, Agid Y. Pallidal stimulation for Parkinson's disease: Two targets? Neurology 49:1564–1569, 1997.
8. Keller TM, Tcheng TK, Burkhard PR, Richard H, Tamas LB. Stereotactically guided thalamotomy for treatment of parkinsonian tremor isolated to the lower extremity. J Neurosurg 89:314–316, 1998.
9. Roberts DW, Darcey TM, Mamourian A, Lee MJ. Direct stereotactic targeting of the globus pallidus: An MRI-based anatomic variability study. Stereotact Funct Neurosurg 65:1–5, 1995.
10. Vlaardingerbroek M, den Boer J. Magnetic resonance imaging. Berlin: Springer-Verlag, 1996, pp 107–113.
11. Sumanaweera TS, Adler JR, Napel S, Glover GH. Characterization of spatial distortion in magnetic resonance imaging and its implications for stereotactic surgery. Neurosurgery 35:696–704, 1994.
12. Walton L, Hampshire A, Forster DMC, Kemeny A. A phantom study to assess the accuracy of stereotactic localization, using T1-weighted magnetic resonance imaging with the Leksell stereotactic system. Neurosurgery 38:170–178, 1996.
13. Alexander EA, Kooy HM, Herk M, Schwartz M, Barnes PD, Tarbell N, Mulkern RV, Holupka EJ, Loeffler JS. Magnetic resonance image-directed stereotactic neurosurgery: Use of image fusion with computerized tomography to enhance spatial accuracy. J Neurosurg 83:271–276, 1995.
14. Scott R, Gregory R, Hines N, Carroll C, Hyman N, Papanasstasiou V, Leather C, Rowe J, Silburn P, Aziz T. Neuropsychological, neurological and functional outcome following pallidotomy for Parkinson's disease: A consecutive series of eight simultaneous bilateral and twelve unilateral procedures. Brain 121: 659–675, 1998.
15. Giller CA, Dewey RB, Ginsburg MI, Mendelsohn DB, Berk AM. Stereotactic pallidotomy and thalamotomy using individual variations of anatomic landmarks for localization. Neurosurgery 42:56–62, 1998.
16. Krauss JK, King DE, Grossman RG. Alignment correction algorithm for transformation of anterior commissure/posterior commissure based coordinates into frame coordinates in image-guided functional neurosurgery. Neurosurgery 42: 806–811, 1998.
17. Tamas LB, Tcheng TK. Selective thalamotomy for tremor: A new look at an old procedure. Techniques Neurosurg 5:65–72, 1999.
18. Germano I, Heilbrun MP. Interactive computer-assisted image-guided technology as an adjuvant to neurosurgery for movement disorders. In: Germano IM

(ed). Neurosurgical Treatment of Movement Disorders. Park Ridge, IL: American Association of Neurological Surgeons, 1998, pp 219–226.

19. Maciunas RJ, Galloway RL, Latimer JW. The application accuracy of stereotactic frames. Neurosurgery 35:682–695, 1994.
20. Kaus M, Steinmeier R, Sporer T, Ganslandt O, Fahlbusch R. Technical accuracy of a neuronavigation system measured with a high-precision mechanical micromanipulator. Neurosurgery 41:1431–1437, 1997.
21. Black PM, Alexander E, Martin C, Moriarty T, Nabavi A, Wong TZ, Schwartz RB, Jolesz F. Craniotomy for tumor treatment in an intraoperative magnetic resonance imaging unit. Neurosurgery 45:423–433, 1999.
22. Albe-Fessard D, Arfel G, Guiot G, Hardy J, Vourc'h G, Hertzog E, Aleonard P, Derome P. Dérivation d'activités spontanées et évoquées dans les structures cérébrales profondes de l'homme. Rev Neurol 106:89–105, 1962.
23. Bertrand G, Jasper H, Wong A, Mathews G. Microelectrode recording during stereotactic surgery. Clin Neurosurg 16:328–356, 1966.
24. Ohye C, Narabayashi H. Physiological study of presumed ventralis intermedius neurons in the human thalamus. J Neurosurg 50:290–297, 1979.
25. Ohye C, Saito Y, Fukamachi A, Narabayashi H. An analysis of the spontaneous rhythmic and non-rhythmic burst discharges in the human thalamus. J Neurol Sci 22:245–259, 1974.
26. Fukamachi A, Ohye C, Narabayashi J. Delineation of the thalamic nuclei with a microelectrode in stereotaxic surgery for parkinsonism and cerebral palsy. J Neurosurg 39:214–225, 1973.
27. Gaze RM, Gillingham FJ, Kalyanaraman S, Porter RW, Donaldson AA, Donaldson IML. Microelectrode recordings from the human thalamus. Brain 87: 691–706, 1966.
28. Lenz FA, Dostrovsky JO, Kwan HC, Tasker RR, Yamashiro K, Murphy JT. Methods for microstimulation and recording of single neurons and evoked potentials in the human central nervous system. J Neurosurg 68:630–634, 1988.
29. Lenz FA, Tasker RR, Kwan HC, Schnider S, Kwong R, Murayama Y, Dostrovsky JO, Murphy JT. Single unit analysis of the human ventral thalamic nuclear group: Correlation of thalamic "tremor cells" with the 3–6 Hz component of parkinsonian tremor. J Neurosci 8:754–764, 1988.
30. Lenz FA, Kwan HC, Dostrovsky JO, Tasker RR, Murphy JT, Lenz YE. Single unit analysis of the human ventral thalamic nuclear group. Activity correlated with movement. Brain 113:1795–1821, 1990.
31. Lenz FA, Kwan HC, Martin RL, Tasker RR, Dostrovsky JO, Lenz YE. Single unit analysis of the human ventral thalamic nuclear group. Tremor related activity in functionally identified cells. Brain 117:531–543, 1994.
32. Lenz FA, Normand SK, Kwan HC, Andrews D, Rowland LH, Jones MW, Seike M, Lin YC, Tasker RR, Dostrovsky JO, Lenz YE. Statistical prediction of the optimal site for thalamotomy in parkinsonian tremor. Mov Disord 10:318–328, 1995.
33. Lenz FA, Dostrovsky JO, Tasker RR, Yamashiro K, Kwan HC, Murphy JT. Single unit analysis of the human ventral thalamic nuclear group: Somatosensory responses. J Neurophysiol 59:299–316, 1988.

34. Hutchison WD, Lozano AM, Davis KD, Saint-Cyr JA, Lang AE, Dostrovsky JO. Differential neuronal activity in segments of globus pallidus in Parkinson's disease patients. Neuroreport 5:1533–1537, 1994.
35. Hutchison WD, Lozano AM, Tasker RR, Lang AE, Dostrovsky JO. Identification and characterization of neurons with tremor-frequency activity in human globus pallidus. Exp Brain Res 113:557–563, 1997.
36. Lozano A, Hutchison W, Kiss Z, Tasker R, Davis K, Dostrovsky J. Methods for microelectrode-guided posteroventral pallidotomy. J Neurosurg 84:194–202, 1996.
37. Stereo D, Beric A, Dogali M, Fazzini E, Alfaro G, Devinsky O. Neurophysiological properties of pallidal neurons in Parkinson's disease. Ann Neurol 35: 586–591, 1994.
38. Taha JM, Favre J, Baumann TK, Burchiel KJ. Characteristics and somatotopic organization of kinesthetic cells in the globus pallidus of patients with Parkinson's disease. J Neurosurg 85:1005–1012, 1996.
39. Taha JM, Favre J, Baumann TK, Burchiel KJ. Tremor control after pallidotomy in patients with Parkinson's disease: Correlation with microrecording findings. J Neurosurg 86:642–647, 1997.
40. Hutchison WD, Levy R, Dostrovsky JO, Lozano AM, Land AE. Effects of apomorphine on globus pallidus neurons in Parkinsonian patients. Ann Neurol 42:767–775, 1997.
41. Vitek JL, Bakay RAE, Hashimoto T, Kaneoke Y, Mewes K, Zhang J, Rye D, Starr P, Baron M, Turner R, DeLong MR. Microelectrode-guided pallidotomy: Technical approach and application for medically intractable Parkinson's disease. J Neurosurg 88:1027–1043, 1998.
42. Hutchison WD. Neurophysiological identification of the subthalamic nucleus in surgery for Parkinson's disease. Ann Neurol 44:622–628, 1998.
43. Hutchison WD. Microelectrode techniques and findings of globus pallidus. In: Krauss JK, Grossman RG, Jankovic J, (eds). Pallidal surgery for the treatment of parkinson's disease and movement disorders. Philadelphia: Lippincott-Raven, 1998, pp 135–152.
44. Yokoyama T, Sugiyama K, Nishizawa S, Yokota N, Ohta S, Uemura K. Subthalamic nucleus stimulation for gait disturbance in Parkinson's disease. Neurosurgery 45:41–50, 1999.
45. Starr PA. The Axon Guideline System 3000. Neurosurgery 44:1354–1356, 1999.
46. Vitek JL, Chockkan V, Zhang JY, Kaneoke Y, Evatt M, DeLong MR, Triche S, Mewes K, Hashimoto T, Bakay RAE. Neuronal activity in the basal ganglia in patients with generalized dystonia and hemiballismus. Ann Neurol 46:22–35, 1999.
47. Lenz FA, Suarez JI, Metman LV, Reich SG, Karp BI, Hallett M, Rowland LH, Dougherty PM. Pallidal activity during dystonia: Somatosensory reorganisation and changes with severity. J Neurol Neurosurg Psychiatry 65:767–770, 1998.
48. Suarez JI, Metman LV, Reich SG, Dougherty PM, Hallett M, Lenz FA. Pallidotomy for hemiballismus: Efficacy and characteristics of neuronal activity. Ann Neurol 42:807–811, 1997.

49. DeLong MR. Activity of pallidal neurons during movement. J Neurophysiol 34:414–427, 1971.
50. Guridi J, Gorospe A, Ramos E, Linazasoro G, Rodriguez MC, Obeso JA. Stereotactic targeting of the globus pallidus internus in Parkinson's disease: Imaging versus electrophysiological mapping. Neurosurgery 45:278–289, 1999.
51. Raeva SN. Localization in human thalamus of units triggered during "verbal commands," voluntary movements and tremor. Electroencephalogr Clin Neurophys 63:160–173, 1986.
52. Vitek JL, Ashe J, DeLong MR, Alexander G. Physiologic properties and somatotopic organization of the primate motor thalamus. J Neurophysiol 71:1498–1513, 1994.
53. Bergman H, Wichmann T, Karmon B, DeLong MR. The primate subthalamic nucleus. II. Neuronal activity in the MPTP model of parkinsonism. J Neurophysiol 72:507–520, 1994.
54. Alterman R, Sterio D, Beric A, Kelly PJ. Microelectrode recording during posteroventral pallidotomy: Impact on target selection and complications. Neurosurgery 44:315–323, 1999.
55. Young RF, Vermeulen SS, Grimm P, Posewitz A. Electrophysiological target localization is not required for the treatment of functional disorders. Stereotact Funct Neurosurg 66(suppl 1):309–319, 1997.
56. Baron MS, Vitek JL, Bakay RAE, Green J, Kaneoke Y, Hashimoto T, Turner RS, Woodard JL, Cole SA, McDonald WM, DeLong MR. Treatment of advanced Parkinson's disease by posterior GPi pallidotomy: 1-year results of a pilot study. Ann Neurol 40:355–366, 1996.
57. Dogali M, Fazzini E, Kolodny E, Eidelberg D, Sterio D, Devinsky O, Beric A. Stereotactic ventral pallidotomy for Parkinson's disease. Neurology 45:753–761, 1995.
58. Fazzini E, Dogali M, Stereo D, Eidelberg D, Beric A. Stereotactic pallidotomy for Parkinson's disease: A long-term follow-up of unilateral pallidotomy. Neurology 48:1273–1277, 1997.
59. Krauss JK, Desaloms JM, Lai EC, King DE, Jankovic J, Grossman RG. Microelectrode-guided posteroventral pallidotomy for treatment of Parkinson's disease: Postoperative magnetic resonance imaging analysis. J Neurosurg 87:358–367, 1997.
60. Lang AE, Lozano A, Montgomery E, Duff J, Tasker R, Hutchinson W. Posteroventral medical pallidotomy in advanced Parkinson's disease. New Engl J Med 337:1036–1042, 1997.
61. Uitti RJ, Wharen RE, Turk MF, Lucas JA, Finton MJ, Graff-Radford NR, Boylan KB, Georss SJ, Kall BA, Adler CH, Caviness JN, Atkinson EJ. Unilateral pallidotomy for Parkinson's disease: Comparison of outcome in younger versus older patients. Neurology 49:1072–1077, 1997.
62. Kishore A, Turnbull IM, Snow BJ, de la Fuente-Fernandez R, Schulzer M, Mak E, Yardley S, Calne DB. Efficacy, stability and predictors of outcome of pallidotomy for Parkinson's disease. Six-month follow-up with additional 1-year observations. Brain 120:729–737, 1997.

63. deBie RMA, deHaan RJ, Nijssen PCG, Wijnand A, Rutgers F, Beute GN, Bosch DA, Haaxma R, Schmand B, Schuurman PR, Staal MJ, Speelman JD. Unilateral pallidotomy in Parkinson's disease: A randomised, single-blind, multicentre trial. Lancet 354:1665–1669, 1999.
64. Samii A, Turnbull IM, Kishore A, Schulzer M, Mak E, Yardley S, Calne DB. Reassessment of unilateral pallidotomy in Parkinson's disease: A 2-year follow-up study. Brain 122:417–425, 1999.
65. Hassler R, Riechert T, Munginger F, Umbach W, Ganglberger JA. Physiological observations in stereotaxic operations in extrapyramidal motor disturbances. Brain 83:337–350, 1960.
66. Ohye C, Kubota K, Hongo T, Nagao T, Narabayashi H. Ventrolateral and subventrolateral thalamic stimulation. Arch Neurol 11:427–434, 1964.
67. Rezai AR, Hutchison W, Lozano AM. Chronic subthalamic nucleus stimulation for Parkinson's disease. In: Rengachary SS, Wilkins RH, (eds). Neurosurgical Operative Atlas. Park Ridge, IL: American Association of Neurological Surgeons, 1999, pp 195–207.
68. Bejjani B, Damier P, Arnulf I, Thivard L, Bonnet A, Dormont D, Cornu P, Pidoux B, Samson Y, Agid Y. Transient acute depression induced by high-frequency deep brain stimulation. N Engl J Med 340:1476–1500, 1999.
69. Benabid AL, Pollak P, Gao D, Hoffmann D, Limousin P, Gay E, Payen I, Benazzouz A. Chronic electrical stimulation of the ventralis intermedius nucleus of the thalamus as a treatment of movement disorders. J Neurosurg 84:203–214, 1996.
70. Hirai T, Miyazaki M, Nakajima H, Shibazaki T, Ohye C. The correlation between tremor characteristics and the predicted volume of effective lesions in stereotaxic nucleus ventralis intermedius thalamotomy. Brain 106:1001–1018, 1983.
71. Tasker RR, Organ LW, Hawrylyshyn P. Investigation of the surgical target for alleviation of involuntary movement disorders. Appl Neurophysiol 45:261–274, 1982.
72. Rodriguez MC, Guridi OJ, Alvarez L, Mewes K, Macias R, Vitek J, DeLong MR, Obeso JA. The subthalamic nucleus and tremor in Parkinson's disease. Mov Disord 13:111–118, 1998.
73. Limousin P, Krack P, Pollak P, Benazzouz A, Ardouin C, Hoffman D, Benabid AL. Electrical stimulation of the subthalamic nucleus in advanced Parkinson's disease. N Engl J Med 339:1105–1111, 1998.
74. Gross C, Rougier A, Guehl D, Boraud T, Julien J, Bioulac B. High-frequency stimulation of the globus pallidus internalis in Parkinson's disease: A study of seven cases. J Neurosurg 87:491–498, 1997.
75. Lozano AM, Kumar R, Gross RE, Giladi N, Hutchison WD, Dostrovsky JO, Lang AE. Globus pallidus internus pallidotomy for generalized dystonia. Mov Disord 12:865–870, 1997.
76. Krauss JK, Pohle T, Weber S, Ozdoba C, Burgunder J. Bilateral stimulation of the globus pallidus internus for treatment of cervical dystonia. Lancet 354:837–838, 1999.

77. Cosman ER. Radiofrequency lesions. In Gildenberg PL, Tasker RR, (eds). Text-book of Stereotactic and Functional Neurosurgery. New York: McGraw-Hill, 1997, pp 973–986.
78. Sweet WH, Mark VH. Unipolar anodal electrolyte lesions in the brain of man and cat: Report of five human cases with electically produced bulbar or mesencephalic tractotomies. Arch Neurol Psychiatry 70:224–234, 1953.
79. Dieckmann G, Gabriel E, Hassler R. Size, form and structural peculiarities of experimental brain lesions obtained by thermocontrolled radiofrequency. Confin Neurol 26:134–142, 1965.
80. Rand RW, Jacques DB, Melbye RW, Copcutt BG, Fisher MR, Levenick MN. Gamma knife thalamotomy and pallidotomy in patients with movement disorders: Preliminary results. Stereotact Funct Neurosurg 61:65–92, 1993.
81. Freidman JH, Epstein M, Sanes JN, Lieberman P, Cullen K, Lindquist C, Daamen M. Gamma knife pallidotomy in advanced Parkinson's disease. Ann Neurol 39:535–538, 1996.
82. Duma CM, Jacques DB, Kopyov OV, Mark RJ, Copcutt B, Farokhi HK. Gamma knife radiosurgery for thalamotomy in parkinsonian tremor: A five year experience. J Neurosurg 88:1044–1049, 1998.
83. Lieberman DM, Corthesy ME, Cummins A, Oldfield EA. Reversal of experimental parkinsonism by using selective chemical ablation of the medial globus pallidus. J Neurosurg 90:928–934, 1999.
84. Gildenberg PL. Studies in stereoencephalotomy VIII. Comparison of the variability of subcortical lesions produced by various procedures. Confin Neurol 17:299–309, 1957.
85. White RJ, MacCarty CS, Bahn RC. Neuropatholic review of brain lesions and inherent dangers in chemopallidectomy. A M. A. Arch Neurol 2:12–18, 1960.
86. Favre J, Taha JM, Steel T, Burchiel KJ. Anchoring of deep brain stimulation electrodes using a microplate. Technical note. J Neurosurg 85:1181–1183, 1996.
87. Tronnier VM, Staubert A, Hahnel S, Sarem-Aslani AS. Magnetic resonance imaging with implanted neurostimulators: An in vitro and in vivo study. Neurosurgery 44:118–126, 1999.
88. Rezai AR, Lozano AM, Crawley AP, Joy MLG, Davis KD, Kwan CL, Dostrovsky JO, Tasker RR, Mikulis DJ. Thalamic stimulation and functional magnetic resonance imaging: Localization of cortical and subcortical activation with implanted electrodes. J Neurosurg 90:583–590, 1999.

24

Intractable Tremor: Ablation Versus Stimulation

Emad N. Eskandar and G. Rees Cosgrove

Massachusetts General Hospital and Harvard Medical School, Boston, Massachusetts, U.S.A.

1 INTRODUCTION

Tremor is defined as an involuntary rhythmical movement and is often categorized in three positions: hands in repose (*rest*), hands held up with arms outstretched (*postural*), and during movement (*intention*). The amplitude, frequency, and severity of the tremor may vary from patient to patient but can cause severe functional disability.

Essential tremor (ET) is one of the most common movement disorders and is characterized by disabling intentional tremor not secondary to Parkinson's disease (PD) or other underlying neurological conditions. It is an idiopathic disorder characterized by a 4 to 12 Hz tremor of the extremities that is most prominent during purposeful movement. About half of the cases are familial and transmitted in an autosomal-dominant mode with variable penetrance [21]. This disorder has been termed "benign essential tremor," because tremor is the only major symptom, but it can produce significant disability including inability to feed or drink, control hand movements, or even talk on a telephone. The onset is insidious and can occur at any age but has a bimodal age distribution with peak incidence in the second and sixth decades. The disease has a variable progression and most often affects the upper extremities. Recent studies have supported the finding that both thalamotomy and thalamic stimulation can be quite effective in controlling medically refractory essential tremor [3–5,9,13,14,17,19,25,27,38].

Essential tremor must be differentiated from a parkinsonian tremor, which is generally present at rest with a frequency of 3 to 5 Hz and is suppressed by movement. It can, however, be both postural and intentional and is often resistant to dopamine replacement therapy. Parkinson's disease patients with unilateral disease or marked asymmetry in their symptoms and in whom tremor is the predominant cause of disability may also benefit from thalamotomy or thalamic stimulation [3–5,8,14–17,19,20,22,24,26,27,29, 41]. However, the effects of thalamotomy or thalamic stimulation on the other cardinal symptoms of PD are much less predictable and may, in some cases, cause worsening of symptoms. Therefore, PD patients with predominant dyskinesias, bradykinesia, or rigidity should be considered for other treatment modalities, such as pallidotomy, pallidal stimulation, or subthalamic stimulation. In addition, as PD is a progressive disease, it is reasonable to expect that even patients with tremor-predominant PD will eventually develop the more disabling symptoms of akinesia and rigidity.

Tremors secondary to other underlying neurological conditions must also be differentiated from ET. These include disabling intention tremor caused by damage of the cerebellum or cerebellar tracts from cerebrovascular accidents, trauma, or multiple sclerosis [2,6,10,14,18,23]. These conditions often imply more diffuse CNS pathology and therefore the outcome of thalamic surgery is less predictable and complication rates may be higher.

2   ANATOMY AND PATHOPHYSIOLOGY

The role of the ventrolateral thalamus in movement disorders and the optimal location for therapeutic lesions have long been the subject of debate. Part of the difficulty lies in the fact that numerous anatomical classification schemes are in use. The most widely used schemes are the Anglo-American terminology and Hassler terminology. In the Anglo-American terminology, the ventrolateral nuclei are divided from anterior to posterior into the ventralis anterior (VA), ventralis lateralis (VL), and ventralis posterior (VP), whereas in the Hassler terminology the same nuclei are divided into lateral polaris (LPO), ventralis oralis anterior (Voa), ventralis oralis posterior (Vop), ventralis intermedius (Vim) and ventralis caudalis (VC) (Fig. 1). The Hassler nomenclature will be used in this discussion as it appears to correlate with the relevant anatomy and physiology.

The main pallidal output pathways terminate in the ventrolateral thalamus, particularly the Voa nucleus, which in turn projects back to the premotor cortex. In contrast, the Vop and Vim nuclei receive multiple inputs,

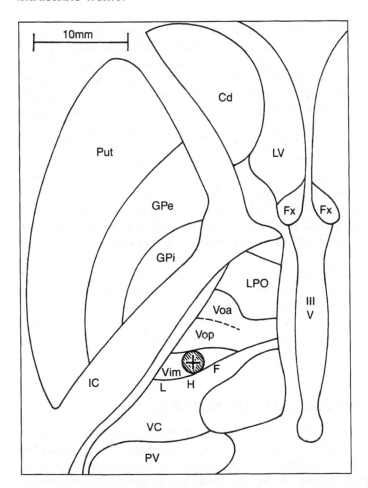

FIGURE 1 Axial section through the thalamus at 1.5 mm above the AC-PC plane. Abbreviations are as follows: Gpe—globus pallidus externa; Gpi—globus pallidus interna; IC—internal capsule; VC—ventralis caudalis; Vim—ventralis intermedius; Voa—ventralis oralis anterior; Vop—ventralis oralis posterior. L, H, and F refer to the somatotopic representation of the leg, hand, and face in the VC and Vim nuclei.

including afferents from the contralateral cerebellum through the brachium conjunctivum. The Vop and Vim nuclei then project to the motor and premotor cortices. The VC nucleus is the primary thalamic relay for the medial lemniscal and spinothalamic tracts, and projects to the somatosensory cortex. Microelectrode recordings in the area of Vim reveal neurons that respond to kinesthetic stimulation, that is, movement of the joints and squeezing of muscle bellies, whereas neurons in VC respond to tactile stimulation [8,38]. Furthermore, neurophysiological recordings have also revealed cells that fire synchronously with the observed tremor (tremor cells), further implicating the Vim in the pathology of tremor [38]. Whether the presence of these cells indicates that the genesis of tremor lies within Vim, or that Vim is simply part of a larger loop mediating tremor is not clear. In either case, there is a considerable amount of clinical evidence that Vim lesions are effective in alleviating tremor. Lesions placed more anteriorly, in the Vop nucleus, or large lesions including both Vim and Vop lead to improvement in tremor and rigidity, although bradykinesia is often unaffected or sometimes worsened by such lesions [18,34,39,43]. These findings support the contention that thalamotomy is best reserved for patients with Parkinson's disease in whom tremor is the predominant complaint or in patients with intractable essential tremor.

In patients with ET, the goal of thalamotomy is to permanently abolish tremor by placing a small lesion in the Vim nucleus of the thalamus. In thalamic stimulation, the goal is to place the probe 2 to 3 mm anterior to the junction of Vim and VC so that the stimulating current inactivates a portion of Vim while avoiding stimulation of the VC nucleus or the internal capsule.

3 INDICATIONS FOR THALAMIC SURGERY

The indications for thalamotomy or thalamic stimulation are similar. Patients should have tremor that is refractory to medical therapy and represents the predominant form of disability. The best candidates for thalamic surgery are patients with incapacitating benign essential tremor and those with tremor-predominant PD that is unilateral or asymmetric. Patients with PD who have other motor signs should be considered for surgery aimed at other targets, such as the globus pallidus internus (Gpi) or the subthalamic nucleus (STN). Thalamic surgery may also be useful in patients with tremor secondary to multiple sclerosis or trauma, although the results are less predictable because of the associated injury to other brain structures inherent in these afflictions.

Patients being considered for thalamic surgery should be evaluated by an experienced movement disorders team to ensure that they are good candidates for surgery and that all appropriate medical therapies have been tried. Medical therapy for patients with ET should include adequate trials of propanolol, mysoline, and clonazepam, whereas therapy for patients with PD should include Sinemet, dopamine agonists, and anticholinergics. An essential element of this evaluation is to determine the major cause of the patient's disability so that realistic goals and expectations can be agreed on before surgery.

It is important to confirm the clinical diagnosis of benign essential tremor or idiopathic PD, as a variety of neurodegenerative diseases can present with tremor in their early stages. Patients with these other neuro-degenerative diseases appear to have a much poorer prognosis after thala-motomy. Evidence of dementia or other cognitive decline, speech disorders, serious systemic disease, and advanced age are also considered contraindi-cations to surgery. As a final point, bilateral thalamotomies are generally associated with a prohibitively high complication rate and should not be undertaken.

4 OPERATIVE TECHNIQUE—THALAMOTOMY AND THALAMIC STIMULATION

4.1 Anaesthetic Considerations

Patients are kept NPO on the evening before surgery and are generally ad-vised to withhold their antiparkinsonian and antitremor medication on the morning of surgery to ensure that the tremor will be evident throughout the surgery. Surgery is performed under local anesthesia and requires the full cooperation of the patient; therefore, the intraoperative use of sedating agents should be avoided.

4.2 Stereotactic Imaging

A magnetic resonance imaging (MRI) compatible stereotactic frame is af-fixed to the cranial vault after infiltration of the pin insertion sites with local anaesthetic. Stereotactic sagittal T1-weighted MR images are obtained first to identify the anterior commissure (AC) and the posterior commissure (PC) and measure the AC-PC length. Text T1-weighted axial images are obtained through the basal ganglia and thalamus parallel to the AC-PC plane. Addi-tional images in the coronal plane with fast spin echo inversion (FSE IR) recovery sequences to accentuate the gray-white matter borders of the thal-amus and internal capsule can be used, depending on the experience of the center. Alternatively, three-dimensional volumetric acquisition series can be acquired that allow thinner sections and reconstruction in any plane, but these series generally require 10 to 12 minutes and are thus subject to move-ment artifacts.

A variety of MR sequences can be used for targeting, but it is imper-ative that each center verify the spatial accuracy of their stereotactic frame in their scanner with phantoms. At our center, we prefer to complement the MRI targeting with computed tomographic (CT) images parallel to the in-

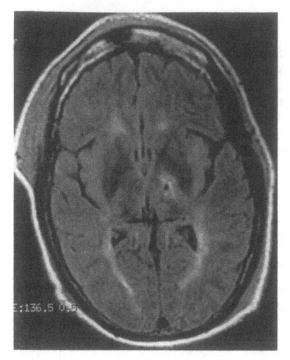

FIGURE 2 Thalamotomy. Axial T2-weighted magnetic resonance images after thalamotomy.

tercommissural line and through the area of interest. Computed tomographic images, although geometrically accurate, do not provide the intrinsic anatomical detail that MR images provide and should not be used alone for targeting purposes. The target coordinates from both the MRI and CT images are then compared for accuracy. Some centers have continued to use the classic method of ventriculography to localize the target; however, recent studies have shown that surgery guided by CT/MRI alone is just as effective and may have a lower complication rate [8,11].

4.3 Target Selection

A variety of stereotactic atlases provide detailed anatomical representations of thalamic and basal ganglia anatomy. There is some controversy regarding optimal target location in the thalamus, but the following parameters are generally agreed on. The initial target is located at a point about 5 mm posterior to the mid AC-PC plane, 13.5 to 15 mm lateral to the midline, and 0 to 1 mm above the level of the intercommissural plane. When the third ventricle is dilated, it is wise to add 1 to 2 mm to the lateral dimension. Alternatively, one can measure 11 mm lateral to the wall of the third ventricle. The spatial resolution of modern MRI scanners continues to improve, but the detailed nuclear anatomy of the thalamus is still impossible to discern. Therefore, intraoperative physiological confirmation of the lesion location through stimulation or a combination of stimulation and microelectrode recording remains essential.

4.4 Surgical Technique

With the patient in a comfortable position, the scalp is infiltrated with local anaesthetic and a parasagittal incision is made for a burr hole placed 2.5 cm from the midline at the level of the coronal suture. The dura and pia is coagulated, avoiding any cortical veins to allow for atraumatic introduction of the electrode. At this point, the stereotactic arc is brought into position and the electrode guide tube is lowered into the burr hole directly over the pial incision. The burr hole is filled with fibrin glue or the skin is temporarily closed around the guide tube with nylon sutures to prevent excessive loss of cerebrospinal fluid (CSF) and brain settling.

4.5 Microelectrode Recording

Microelectrode recordings in the ventrolateral thalamus reflect the connectivity of the various nuclei as reviewed by Tasker [34]. Recordings in the Vop nucleus frequently reveal voluntary cells that are less noisy than those in Vim or VC. These cells change their firing rate in advance or at the beginning of their related movements [28]. Some cells may increase their firing shortly before the movement, whereas others may show a decreased rate or become rhythmic at the onset or completion of a movement. Recordings in Vim reveal moderately noisy high voltage neurons that respond to contralateral passive joint movement, squeezing of muscle bellies, or pressure on deep structures such as tendons. In patients with tremor, kinesthetic cells fire rhythmically at tremor frequency. Recordings in VC reveal very noisy spontaneous activity and many high voltage cells. These cells generally respond to superficial light touch such as light brushing of the skin or a puff of air. These cells respond faithfully without fatigue. The largest volume of VC is occupied by tactile cells representing the face and manual digits. The floor of the thalamus can be identified by the sudden loss of spontaneous neuronal activity as the microelectrode leaves the gray matter of the thalamus and enters the white matter of the zona incerta. A careful analysis of the neuronal activity of these various cell types can confirm that the appropriate target in Vim thalamus is selected.

4.6   Macrostimulation

Macrostimulation using an electrode with a 2-mm exposed tip can also be used to delineate the optimal lesion location. Stimulation is performed with square wave pulses at 0.5 to 2.0 volts at a frequency of 2 Hz to obtain motor thresholds and at 50 to 75 Hz to assess for amelioration of symptoms or sensory responses.

The typical thalamotomy target (Vim) is directly anterior to the appropriate somatotopic area in VC and just medial to the internal capsule. Occasionally, the mere introduction of the electrode reduces the tremor, indicating that the electrode is in good position. More often, because of individual variation, targeting error, and the small size of Vim, the electrode may be in a suboptimal position and require adjustment. If the electrode is placed too anteriorly in the Vop nucleus, low frequency stimulation may induce movement in the contralateral limbs. This movement is focal at threshold, beginning at one joint and involving greater parts of the contralateral limbs as stimulation intensity is increased [34]. Because VC is the relay nucleus for superficial tactile sensation, high frequency stimulation can induce parasthesias at much lower thresholds than that of the Vim nucleus. Therefore, low threshold (0.25 to 0.5 volts) parasthesias of the fingertips or mouth indicate that the electrode is too posterior and needs to be moved anteriorly.

In addition to the anterior-posterior differences between the thalamic nuclei, there is also a clear medial-to-lateral somatotopy within both Vim and VC. Neurons in VC representing the face are found more medial; those representing the lower limbs more lateral near the internal capsule; and those representing the upper extremity and hand intermediate (Fig. 3). The definition of this somatotopic distribution is important as the lesion or the stimulating electrode in Vim should be placed directly anterior to the appropriate site in the VC nucleus [7,15]. Thus lesions for tremor involving the upper extremity should be placed more medial than lesions for tremor involving the lower extremities.

If the electrode is in good position, low frequency (2 Hz) stimulation within Vim usually drives the tremor, whereas high frequency (75 Hz) stimulation suppresses it. Suppression of tremor with 0.5 to 2.0 volts is the goal and indicates accurate targeting. In addition, high frequency stimulation should be used to ensure that there is no evidence of neurological impairment such as motor, speech, or cognitive difficulties.

4.7   Lesion Generation

Once the target has been confirmed, a test lesion is made at 46° to 48° C for 60 seconds. During this time, the patient is tested neurologically for

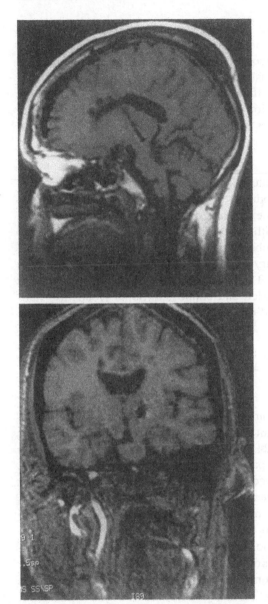

FIGURE 3 Thalamic stimulator. Sagittal (**top**) and coronal (**bottom**) magnetic resonance images demonstrating a stimulator in the Vim nucleus of the thalamus.

contralateral motor dexterity and sensation along with verbal skills. If there is improvement in tremor and no neurological deficits, then a permanent lesion is made at 75° C for 60 seconds. During the lesioning, the neurological status of the patient is continuously monitored and lesioning is halted if any impairment or change is noted. If complete abolition of the tremor has not been accomplished, then the lesion may be enlarged as guided by the intra-operative physiological responses and recordings.

4.8   Stimulator Placement

Once the optimal target coordinates have been obtained, the deep brain stim-ulating (DBS) electrode is introduced to the appropriate depth. By tempo-rarily connecting the lead to an external stimulator, the inhibitory effect on tremor can be assessed along with the presence of any side effects. If tremor suppression is obtained, the probe is secured in place using the burr hole cap or bone cement. The primary incision is closed and the patient is then placed under general anesthesia. The infraclavicular pocket for the stimulator is made and the leads are tunneled and connected. Some groups use fluo-roscopic guidance to ensure that the electrode has not migrated during the procedure.

5   RESULTS

5.1   Thalamotomy

The general finding that thalamotomy is an effective treatment for tremor in patients with tremor-predominant Parkinson's disease has been known for some time (Table 1) [8,14–16,24,26,30,36,39]. In a study of the long-term effects of thalamotomy on 60 patients, Kelly and Gillingham found that contralateral tremor was abolished in 90% of patients undergoing unilateral thalamotomy at the first postoperative evaluation [16]. Subsequent evalua-tions revealed that the effect diminished somewhat over time so that at 4 years, 86% of patients remained tremor free, whereas at 10 years, 57% of surviving patients remained tremor free. Rigidity was also improved by thal-amotomy in 88% of patients initially and in 55% of patients at 10 years. There was no effect of thalamotomy on bradykinesia or other manifestations of Parkinson's disease, such as mental deterioration or gait disturbance. More recent series reflect a similar distribution. Jankovic et al reported a series of 42 patients who underwent thalamotomy for intractable tremor [14]. Of these patients, 72% had complete abolition of tremor, whereas an addi-tional 14% had significant improvement in tremor. There was a small but statistically insignificant effect on rigidity and no effect on bradykinesia. In another series reported by Fox et al, 34 of 36 (94%) PD patients had com-

TABLE 1   Summary of Thalamotomy and Thalamic Stimulation Studies

Study	PD patients number	Good outcome	ET patients number	Good outcome
Thalamotomy				
Fox et al, 1991	36	86%		
Goldman et al, 1992			8	100%
Jankovic et al, 1995	42	86%	6	83%
Kelly et al, 1987	12	100%		
Kelly et al, 1980	60	90%		
Linhares et al, 2000	40	75%		
Lund et al, 1996	53	94%		
Nagaseki et al, 1986	27	96%	16	94%
Wester et al, 1990	33	79%		
Thalamic stimulation				
Benabid et al, 1996	80	86%	20	69%
Blond et al, 1992	10	80%	4	75%
Huble et al, 1996			10	90%
Koller et al, 1997	29	71%	29	90%
Limousin et al, 1999	73	85%	37	89%
Ondo et al, 1998	19	82%	14	83%

Abbreviations: *PD*, Parkinson's disease; *ET,* essential tremor.

plete abolition of contralateral tremor, whereas 29 of 34 (85%) remained tremor free at 1 year [8].

Similar results are obtained in patients with intractable essential tremor, with 80% to 100% of patients having marked or moderate improvement (Table 1) [9,14,25]. In a series of eight patients with ET treated with thalamotomy reported by Goldman et al, tremor was absent or markedly reduced in all patients at a mean follow-up of 17 months [9]. Jankovic et al treated six ET patients with thalamotomy. Overall, 5 of 6 or 83% of patients had moderate to marked improvement in their tremor at a mean follow-up of 59 months [14]. Patients with intractable cerebellar intention tremor respond at somewhat lower rates, with 60% to 80% of patients having significant improvement in tremor [10,14,23].

5.2 Thalamic Stimulation

Long-term studies of thalamic stimulation reveal results largely comparable to thalamotomy. Patients with tremor-predominant PD have sustained response rates of 80% to 95%, whereas patients with ET have response rates of 70% to 85% [3–5,13,17,19,27,29,38]. There have been two recent large series looking at thalamic stimulation for the treatment of intractable tremor. In a multicenter American trial reported by Koller et al, 29 patients with ET and 24 patients with parkinsonian tremor were treated with high-frequency unilateral thalamic stimulation [17]. Moderate to marked improvement occurred in 90% of ET patients and 71% of PD patients. The effects were largely maintained at 1 year. The results of a multicenter European trial were similar. In this study, a total of 74 patients with parkinsonian tremor and 37 patients with ET were treated with thalamic stimulation [19]. Overall, there was a moderate to marked improvement in 85% of treated sides in patients with PD and in 89% of patients with ET. There are few studies directly comparing thalamotomy and thalamic stimulation in the modern era. The best recent study was a prospective randomized trial of 68 patients from an experienced group in the Netherlands [29]. A total of 68 patients with either PD (n = 45), ET (n = 13), or MS (n = 10) were randomized to receive either thalamotomy or thalamic stimulation. The primary outcome measure was functional improvement as measured by the Frenchay's Activity Index. Secondary outcome measures included the severity of residual tremor, adverse effects of intervention, and patient self-assessment of functional outcome. All measures were obtained at 6 months after surgery. As expected, tremor was either completely abolished or greatly suppressed in 27 of 34 (79%) thalamotomy patients and in 30 of 33 (91%) thalamic stimulation patients. However, the improvement in functional status was significantly greater in the thalamic stimulation group than in the thalamotomy group. More than twice as many patients undergoing deep brain stimulation reported that their functional status had improved, as compared to those undergoing thalamotomy. One patient died postoperatively from an intracranial hemorrhage after thalamic stimulation (a risk inherent to both techniques), but the overall neurological complication rate was better for the stimulator group (6/34, or 18%) than the thalamotomy group (16/34, or 47%).

This well-designed study confirms the prevailing clinical impression that thalamic stimulation appears equally effective in controlling tremor as thalamotomy and may be associated with fewer side effects. However, this study also demonstrated that tremor control is not necessarily equivalent to functional improvement. The greater functional improvement in the thalamic stimulation group as compared to the thalamotomy group may be attributable to reduced side effects, to the fact that the amount of current can be titrated in the stimulation group to maximize benefit while avoiding side effects, or to a different mechanism of action of stimulation. The limitations of this study include the fact that assessments were not blinded. Furthermore, the duration of the study is short, and more long-term studies will be needed before definitive conclusions can be reached regarding the duration of benefit.

5.3 Complications of Thalamic Surgery

Thalamotomy shares the same general risks associated with other stereotactic procedures, namely hemorrhage and infection, that occur in about 2% to 5% of patients. The mortality rate is between 0.5% and 1%. Other specific complications of thalamotomy are the result of inaccurate lesion placement or overly large lesions. Lesions placed too laterally may result in contralateral weakness caused by injury of the posterior limb of the internal capsule. Many patients, about 25%, have transient contralateral facial weakness presumably secondary to edema involving the internal capsule [8]. The percentage of patients suffering from transient contralateral arm weakness ranges from 3% to 30%, and 1% to 15% of patients go on to suffer mild but persistent contralateral weakness [8,14,20]. Another major source of morbidity relates to difficulties with speech. About 30% of patients have transient dysarthria or dysphasia, whereas about 10% go on to have persistent deficits [8,14]. Lesions placed too posterior may cause contralateral hemisensory deficits caused by injury of the VC nucleus. Correspondingly, there may be numbness or parasthesias of the mouth or fingers in 1% to 5% of patients [7,35]. Transient confusion occurs in about 10% to 20% of patients, and mild cognitive and memory deficits may persist in about 1% to 5% of patients [14,35]. Older patients and patients with pre-existing cognitive deficits or evidence of tissue loss on CT scan appear to be at a higher risk for impaired postoperative cognition [7]. Left thalamic lesions are associated with an increased risk for deficits in learning, verbal memory, and dysarthria, whereas right thalamic lesions are associated with impaired visuospatial memory and nonverbal performance abilities [40]. Bilateral thalamotomies are associated with deficits in memory and cognition in up to 60% of patients along with increased risk of hypophonia (decreased speech volume), dysarthria, dysphasia, and abulia [7].

The risk of intracerebral hemorrhage for thalamic stimulation is similar to that for thalamotomy—between 2% and 5% [29]. In addition, specific risks are associated with implanting hardware that are familiar to neurosurgeons, such as infection, migration, and hardware malfunction. In a multicenter American study of 53 patients, the complications included two perioperative hemorrhages that resolved without sequelae, one perioperative seizure, two wound infections, one stimulator malfunction, and one instance of hardware erosion [17]. In a multicenter European trial of 111 patients treated with thalamic stimulation, complications related to the surgery included three subdural hematomas, one thalamic hematoma (that resolved without sequelae), two infections, and one patient with transient cognitive deficits [19]. Few studies directly compare the two techniques; however, as mentioned above, the recent study by Schurman et al suggests that there may be fewer neurological complications with thalamic stimulation [29].

6 DISCUSSION

The decision to use thalamotomy or thalamic stimulation is not clearcut. The advantages of thalamotomy are that it is an established technique with which there is considerable experience. The surgery is relatively more straightforward and is of shorter duration than thalamic DBS. Once the surgery is complete, there are no further concerns about hardware infection, migration, or malfunction. Furthermore, once the lesion is made, there are no adjustments to be made to the stimulator. This can be an important consideration for patients who live in remote areas or, for example, international patients for whom frequent visits for adjustments are not practical. However, thalamotomy creates an irreversible lesion and has the potential to cause permanent neurological deficits. If the lesion is too large or is not placed properly, there is no recourse. Of course, in experienced hands and with careful attention to detail, the neurological risk should be small. Thalamotomy also has a major disadvantage in that it cannot be safely performed bilaterally because of the increased risk of severe neurological complications such as hypophonia, dysarthria, and cognitive deficits.

Thalamic stimulation has been available for a relatively short period; however, it is rapidly becoming an established technique. In an increasing number of studies, thalamic stimulation appears to be at least as effective as thalamotomy for the alleviation of tremor. One major advantage is that stimulators can be placed bilaterally with less risk of neurological complications. Because the stimulators are adjustable, it should, in theory, be possible to titrate the magnitude of stimulation to achieve the maximal possible benefit while avoiding side effects. As no lesion is made, the technique is easily reversible, thereby leaving the door open for new restorative therapies that may become available in the near future. In the only recent study prospectively comparing the two techniques, patients undergoing thalamic stimulation had similar tremor control, a better functional outcome, and fewer neurological complications when compared with patients undergoing thalamotomy. Nevertheless, thalamic stimulation has a number of disadvantages. The surgery is more complex and requires general anesthesia for the internalization of the pulse generator. Patients with implanted stimulators require a good deal more follow-up for adjustments, battery replacement, repair of malfunctions, and so on. As with all implanted hardware, the stimulator is subject to infection, migration, and malfunction. Finally, the equipment used for thalamic stimulation is expensive and pulse generators typically need to be replaced every 3 to 5 years.

Both thalamotomy and thalamic stimulation can impart useful functional improvement in selected patients with intractable essential tremor or tremor-predominant PD. Based on the available evidence, we recommend stimulation as the first option because it appears to provide good relief of tremor with potentially fewer side effects and does not create an irreversible lesion. However, thalamotomy remains an effective and proven technique that can be used when patients decide against a stimulator or when other considerations mitigate against placement of a stimulator.

Given the rapid advances in functional neurosurgery, it is likely that the treatment strategies for patients with intractable tremor will gradually evolve over time. The optimal management of these patients will continue to require a combined approach, with medical therapy providing the first line of treatment and thalamic surgery providing an option for selected patients who can no longer be adequately managed with medications alone.

REFERENCES

1. Alterman RL, Kall BA, Cohen H, Kelly PJ. Stereotactic ventrolateral thalamotomy: Is ventriculography necessary? Neurosurgery 37(4):717–721, 1995.
2. Arsalo A, Hanninen A, Laitinen L. Functional neurosurgery in the treatment of multiple sclerosis. Ann Clin Res 5:74–79, 1973.
3. Benabid AL, Pollak P, Gervason C, Hoffman D, Gao DM, Hommel M, Perret JE, de Rougemont J. Long-term suppression of tremor by chronic stimulation of the ventral intermediate thalamic nucleus. Lancet 337(16):403–406, 1991.
4. Benabid AL, Pollak P, Gao D, Hoffman D, Limousin P, Gay E, Payen I, Benazzouz A. Chronic electrical stimulation of the ventralis intermedius nucleus of the thalamus as a treatment of movement disorders. J Neurosurg 84:203–214, 1996.
5. Blond S, Caparros-Lefebvre D, Parker F, Assaker R, Petit H, Guieu JD, Christiaens JL. Control of tremor and involuntary movement disorders by chronic stereotactic stimulation of ventral intermediate thalamic nucleus. J Neurosurg 77:62–68, 1992.
6. Bullard DE, Nashold BS. Stereotaxic thalamotomy for treatment of posttraumatic movement disorders. J Neurosurg 61:316–321, 1984.
7. Burchiel KJ. Thalamotomy for movement disorders. Neurosurg Clin N Am 6(1):55–71, 1995.
8. Fox MW, Ahlskog E, Kelly PJ. Stereotactic ventrolateralis thalamotomy for medically refractory tremor in post-levodopa era Parkinson's disease patients. J Neurosurg 75:723–730, 1991.
9. Goldman MS, Ahlskog E, Kelly P. The symptomatic and functional outcome of stereotactic thalamotomy for medically intractable essential tremor. J Neurosurg 76:924–928, 1992.

10. Goldman MS, Kelly PJ. Symptomatic and functional outcome of stereotactic ventralis lateralis thalamotomy for intention tremor. J Neurosurg 77:223–229, 1992.

11. Hariz MI, Bergenhiem AT. Clinical evaluation of CT guided versus ventriculography guided thalamotomy for movement disorders. Acta Neurochir 123: 147, 1993.

12. Hassler R, Riechert T. Indikationen und Lokalisations methode der gezielten Hirnoperationen. Nervenarzt 25:441, 1954.

13. Huble JP, Busenberg KL, Wilkinson S, Penn RD, Lyons K, Koller WC. Deep brain stimulation for essential tremor. Neurology 46:1150–1153, 1996.

14. Jankovic J, Cardoso F, Grossman R, Hamilton WJ. Outcome after stereotactic thalamotomy for parkinsonian, essential, and other types of tremor. Neurosurgery 37:680–687, 1995.

15. Kelly PJ, Ahlskog JE, Goerss SJ, Daube JR, Duffy JR, Kalls BA. Computer-assisted stereotactic ventralis lateralis thalamotomy with microelectrode recording control in patients with Parkinson's disease. Mayo Clin Proc 62:655–664, 1987.

16. Kelly PJ, Gillingham FJ. The long-term results of stereotaxic surgery and l-dopa therapy in patients with Parkinson's disease. J Neurosurg 53:332–337, 1980.

17. Koller W, Pahwa R, Busenbark K, Hubble J, Wilkinson S, Lang A, Tuite P, Sime E, Lazano A, Hauser R, Malapira T, Smith D, Tarsy D, Miyawaki E, Norregaard T, Kormos T, Olanow CW. High frequency unilateral thalamic stimulation in the treatment of essential and parkinsonian tremor. Ann Neurol 42:292–299, 1997.

18. Krayenbuhl H, Ysargil MG. Relief of intention tremor due to multiple sclerosis by stereotaxic thalamotomy. Confin Neurol 22:368–374, 1962.

19. Limousin P, Speelman JD, Gielen F, Janssens M. Multicentre European study of thalamic stimulation in parkinsonian and essential tremor. J Neurol Neurosurg Psych 66:289–296, 1999.

20. Linhares MN, Tasker RR. Microelectrode-guided thalamotomy for Parkinson's disease. Neurosurgery 46(2):390–398, 2000.

21. Lou JS, Jankovic J. Essential tremor. Clinical correlates in 350 patients. Neurology 41:234–238, 1991.

22. Lund-Johansen M, Hugdahl K, Wester K. Cognitive function in patients with Parkinson's disease undergoing stereotaxic thalamotomy. J Neurol Neurosurg Psychiatry 60:564–571, 1996.

23. Marks PV. Stereotactic surgery for post-traumatic cerebellar syndrome: An analysis of seven cases. Stereotact Funct Neurosurg 60:157–167, 1993.

24. Matsumoto K, Shichijo F, Fukami T. Long-term follow-up review of cases of Parkinson's disease after unilateral or bilateral thalamotomy. J Neurosurg 60: 1033–1044, 1984.

25. Nagaseki Y, Shibazaki T, Hirai T, Kawashima Y, Hirato M, Wada H, Miyazaki M, Ohye C. Long-term follow-up results of selective VIM-thalamotomy. J Neurosurg 65:296–302, 1986.

26. Narabayashi H, Maeda T, Yokochi F. Long-term follow-up study of nucleus ventralis intermedius and ventrolateralis thalamotomy using a microelectrode technique in parkinsonism. Appl Neurophysiol 50:330–337, 1987.

27. Ondo W, Jankovic J, Schwartz K, Almaguer M, Simpson RK. Unilateral thalamic deep brain stimulation for refractory essential tremor and Parkinson's disease tremor. Neurology 51:1063–1069, 1998.

28. Raeva S. Localization in human thalamus of units triggered during verbal commands, voluntary movements, and tremor. Electroenceph Clin Neurophysiol 63:160–173, 1986.

29. Schuurman PR, Bosch DA, Bossuyt PMM, Bonsel GJ, van Someren EJ, de Bie RM, Merkus MP, Speelman JD. A comparison of continuous thalamic stimulation and thalamotomy for suppression of severe tremor. N Engl J Med 342(7):461–468, 2000.

30. Selby G. Stereotactic surgery for the relief of Parkinson's disease. Part 2. An analysis of results in a series of 303 patients. J Neurol Sci 5:343–375, 1967.

31. Shinoda Y, Futami T, Kakei S. Input-output organization of the ventrolateral thalamus. Stereotact Funct Neurosurg 60:17–31, 1993.

32. Starr PA, Vitek JL, Bakay RA. Deep brain stimulation for movement disorders. Neurosurg Clin N Am 9(2):381–402, 1998.

33. Tasker RR, Dostrovsky JO, Dolan EJ. Computerized tomography is just as accurate as ventriculography for functional stereotactic thalamotomy. Stereotact Funct Neurosurg 57:157–166, 1991.

34. Tasker RR, Kiss ZH. The role of the thalamus in functional neurosurgery. Neurosurg Clin N Am 6(1):73–104, 1995.

35. Tasker RR, Siqueira J, Hawrylyshyn P, Organ L. What happened to VIM thalamotomy for Parkinson's disease? Appl Neurophysiol 46:68–83, 1983.

36. Tasker RR. Deep brain stimulation is preferable to thalamotomy for tremor suppression. Surg Neurol 49:145–154, 1998.

37. Tomlinson FH, Jack CR, Kelly PK. Sequential magnetic resonance imaging following stereotactic radiofrequency ventralis lateralis thalamotomy. J Neurosurg 74:579–584, 1991.

38. Troster AI, Fields JA, Pahwa R, Wilkinson SB, Strait-Troster KA, Lyons K, Kieltyka J, Koller WC. Neuropsychological and quality of life outcome after thalamic stimulation for essential tremor. Neurology 53:1774–1780, 1999.

39. Van Buren JM, Li CL, Shapiro DY, Henderson WG, Sadowsky DA. A qualitative and quantitative evaluation of Parkinsonians three to six years following thalamotomy. Confin Neurol 35:202–235, 1973.

40. Vilkki J, Laitinen LV. Effects of pulvinotomy and ventrolateral thalamotomy on some cognitive functions. Neuropsychologia 14:67–78, 1976.

41. Wester K, Huglie-Hanssen E. Stereotaxic thalamotomy—experiences from the levodopa era. J Neurol Neurosurg Psychiatry 53:427–430, 1990.

25

Parkinsonism: Ablation Versus Stimulation

Bryan Rankin Payne
Louisiana State University, New Orleans, Louisiana, U.S.A.

Roy A. E. Bakay
Rush Medical College, Rush-Presbyterian-St. Luke's
Medical Center, Chicago, Illinois, U.S.A.

1 INTRODUCTION

The surgical treatment of Parkinson's disease (PD) has a storied history. The end of the first chapter was in the 1960s and coincided with the introduction of L-dopa, the first effective medical therapy for PD. The limitations of pharmacotherapy with L-dopa for this disorder were known within several years of its introduction, but the reintroduction of surgical treatment lagged. Thalamic nucleus ventralis intermedius (Vim) lesioning for tremor continued at a much reduced rate during the 1970s and 1980s, but pallidotomy was rarely performed and, except for reference in neurosurgery textbooks, all but disappeared. It was not until 1992 that Laitinen and colleagues published the results of posteroventral pallidotomy for PD in drug-resistant patients [1]. Initially described by Svennilson based on the work of Leksell [2], the posteroventral pallidotomy relieved all the cardinal signs of PD (tremor, rigidity, bradykinesia) and was found to be very effective in the alleviation of drug-induced dyskinesias [1,3]. After this report there was a resurgence of interest in the procedure, and many centers around the world began performing pallidotomies to treat drug-resistant PD.

The genesis of deep brain stimulation (DBS) in the treatment of PD was the observation during preablative electrophysiological testing during thalamotomies when stimulation at greater than 100 Hz led to tremor arrest [3–5]. This observation and the recognition that bilateral thalamotomies were associated with significant morbidity led several centers to try chronic stimulation of the Vim in an attempt to minimize morbidity associated with bilateral procedures [6–8]. The clinical success in alleviating tremor with this approach was equivalent to lesioning and the incidence of dysarthria was reduced. The natural progression of events led to chronic deep brain stimulation of other targets historically lesioned for the control of other symptoms of PD. Siegfried and Lippitz reported their results of chronic DBS of the pallidum and demonstrated efficacy with this approach [9]. Since then, many centers have reported their findings with chronic DBS of the pallidum [10–12].

Advances in understanding the pathophysiology of PD suggested that the subthalamic nucleus (STN) might also be a potential target for ablation in the treatment of PD. The STN has excitatory connections with both output nuclei of the basal ganglia [globus pallidus internal (GPi) and substantia nigra reticularis (SNr)] and is overactive in PD [13,14]. Based on these findings, Benabid and colleagues explored DBS of the STN for PD [15]. The dramatic success of STN DBS suggested this target as a possible site for ablation. The results of several small series of unilateral and bilateral subthalamotomies show that reduction of the cardinal symptoms of PD can be achieved with this procedure [16,17].

Presented here is a brief description of the benefits and drawbacks of the various ablative and DBS targets currently available. It should be noted that many of these procedures, particularly DBS, are relatively new, and long-term results and scientifically stringent studies are not available for review. However, general guidelines can be stated with the caveat that new information is becoming available at an astounding pace.

2   MECHANISM OF ACTION

The manner in which ablative lesions affect the pathophysiology of PD is relatively straightforward. Abnormal activity of various nuclei within the sensorimotor pathway of the basal ganglia-thalamocortical circuits is ameliorated by lesioning, thus removing the abnormal signal from the circuit. This does not restore normal transmission from the surgical site but does release the efferent target nucleus from the abnormal signal.

The simplest way to conceive of DBS is as a physiological but not anatomical lesion. This may be clinically accurate, but there is evidence that other factors are associated with its mechanism of action. Depending on the stimulation parameters of the electrode, distance from the electrode, and baseline firing patterns, neurons may be inhibited or activated [18,19]. Similarly, axons may be inhibited or activated, depending on their distance from the electrode and their orientation to it [19]. Regardless, the clinical effects of lesioning and chronic stimulation, as well as patterns of cortical stimulation, are similar [20,21].

3 ABLATIVE LESIONS

3.1 Thalamotomy

Thalamotomy is one of the oldest procedures used in the treatment of PD. Ablation of the Vim, ventralis oralis posterior nuclei (Voa) of the thalamus, or both is associated with excellent tremor control of the contralateral limbs. Reports have shown that several large series of patients exhibited excellent and long-lasting tremor relief in the order of 73% to 93% of patients [3,22–28]. Most authors also found some beneficial effect on rigidity. Akinesia and bradykinesia are not affected, although drug-induced dyskinesias may benefit if the anterior motor thalamus (Voa, Vop) is included.

A major drawback to thalamotomy, even in patients with PD dominated by tremor, is the relatively high incidence of adverse effects in the range of 9% to 23% of patients. This is particularly true after bilateral procedures. Bilateral thalamotomies are associated with irreversible speech disturbances, dysarthria, dysphagia, or balance problems in more than 25% of patients. Even unilateral procedures are associated with significant permanent morbidity, including paresthesias (11%), gait disturbance (6%), dysarthria (3%), and hand ataxia (14%) [27]. Because of the high incidence of significant complications associated with bilateral procedures, this approach is seldom recommended. However, because of the ability to change stimulation parameters with DBS and effectively avoid permanent complications, this modality is preferable in cases requiring bilateral surgery. Thalamic DBS stimulation has been demonstrated to have an equal efficiency and a decreased rate of complications [27,28], but a role will remain for unilateral thalamotomy in situations of individual choice, economical exclusion, or limited access to medical expertise for follow-up and maintenance (Table 1).

3.2 Pallidotomy

The reintroduction of the posteroventral pallidotomy for Parkinson's disease was a major step in establishing surgical intervention as an accepted treat-

TABLE 1   Differences in Treatment Modalities

	Ablation	Dbs
Tissue destruction	Yes	Minimal and therefore reversible
Effect	Irreversible and permanent but can be enlarged by a repeat procedure	Stimulator parameters are adjustable to maximize beneficial effects and minimize adverse effects. Effects also reversible by turning off stimulator.
Safety	Procedural safety similar until lesioning, where the risks increase. Rare infection (<1%).	Adjustability and reversibility add to safety. Infection rate higher (~4%) and usually requires removal of device.
Postoperative maintenance	Minimal	Frequent parameter adjustability better changes, and repair of mechanical failures results in heavy postoperative maintenance and requires special expertise.
Bilateral procedures	Second side carries much higher risks, especially for speech.	Bilateral treatment relatively safe because of adjustability.

ment. All the cardinal symptoms of the disease are improved and drug-induced dyskinesias are effectively eliminated [1,3,29–34]. A randomized trial of unilateral pallidotomy demonstrated statistically significant improvement in all the cardinal symptoms of PD as well as drug-induced dyskinesias compared to best medical management at 6 months [29]. Refinement of lesion location and maximization of lesion size with the use of microelectrode recording have allowed benefits to be maintained. The 2-year results of pallidotomy demonstrate long-term benefit in studies using microelectrode recording [29,30] and in one without microelectrode recording [31].

The relative benefit of pallidotomy over thalamotomy in PD is significant. Because PD is a progressive disease, the treatment of tremor with thalamotomy, even if it is the predominant symptom, may be short sighted.

The systematic improvement after unilateral pallidotomy results in a significant improvement in the quality of life in patients with advanced PD [34]. Unilateral pallidotomy, especially on the nondominant side, has the advantage over DBS of being effective without requiring further intervention (DBS parameter programming, battery replacement, etc.) on the part of physicians or effort by the patient and his family. One study with short-term follow-up on a small number of patients failed to demonstrate a difference in safety or efficacy between unilateral pallidotomy and unilateral GPi DBS [35]. Further studies are needed.

Bilateral pallidotomies are performed with less risk than bilateral thalamotomies but are still associated with greater risk than a unilateral procedure. The additional benefit of a second, contralateral pallidotomy is usually less than the initial procedure if the two procedures are staged [32] and the incidence of complications is higher. Possibly the reason less benefit is often seen after a second procedure is because of persisting ipsilateral benefits from the initial procedure. Also, the more severely affected side is usually treated first. However, we have noted an improvement in axial symptoms after a second, contralateral procedure (usually DBS for the second procedure) that was significant. Some authors feel that bilateral pallidotomies can be performed without increased risk of speech and swallowing difficulties [1,33], but this is not the experience of most investigators [36]. Whether there is a significant risk of cognitive or psychological changes after bilateral pallidotomy is difficult to determine. In a large series of bilateral pallidotomies, there were no clinical changes of this type [33], but it was noted as a complication in two of four patients treated in another series [37]. Lesion location may play a role in determining cognitive changes after pallidotomy. Some evidence suggests that lesions outside the sensorimotor pallidum may be associated with these changes [38]. A DBS for the second side after a unilateral pallidotomy is probably a better choice than a second pallidotomy.

3.3 Subthalamotomy

Subthalamotomy has theoretical advantage over other ablative lesions, but these are mitigated by two factors. The advantages are that it would affect both output nuclei of the basal ganglia (GPi and SNr). The disadvantages are the risk of ablating the adjacent corticospinal and corticobulbar tracts, and the risk of iatragenic hemiballismus, dyskinesias, or chorea. There are limited reports of using the STN as an ablative target, and although symptomatic improvement was reported, there were also incidences of induced movement disorders [16,39]. However, positive outcomes after subthalamotomy with a low incidence of adverse events have been reported [17,40].

Another factor working against development of the STN as an ablative target has been the emergence of STN stimulation for the treatment of PD.

Because stimulation parameter changes allow for minimization of risk, little effort has been expended in developing the target for ablation. However, there are advantages to ablative lesions, including the decreased risk of infection (no foreign bodies), lower cost, less follow-up (no programming), and no need for battery replacements. The ability to reverse adverse clinical effects is a powerful incentive to use stimulation; however, further clinical study is required before subthalamotomy can be rejected as an alternative.

4 DEEP BRAIN STIMULATION

4.1 Thalamus

For historical reasons, the Vim of the thalamus was the first DBS target attempted in the treatment of PD [6]. Vim stimulation provides excellent and stable contralateral palliation of tremor in more than 80% of patients, with minimal risks [3,6,7,8,41,42]. In a randomized trial of thalamotomy and Vim DBS, the efficiency was equivalent and the safety better with DBS. There is little other clinical benefit in Vim DBS in PD. Stimulation of the Vim is, in general, preferable to ablation, but the target itself has little advantage over the GPi and STN in the treatment of PD symptoms. Similar to thalamotomy, most benefit is seen in tremor, with little change in other cardinal PD signs. Globus pallidus interna and STN DBS both are effective against tremor and STN stimulation may be equally effective as thalamic stimulators. Motor fluctuations and dyskinesias develop over time in nearly all PD patients, and thalamic stimulation is of little value in their treatment. Rigidity and dyskinesias may benefit from a thalamic stimulator if the Vop is included in the stimulation field (similar to thalamotomy), but this improvement is less than that of other stimulation targets [27]. At present, the Vim of the thalamus is an attractive target for DBS in patients with essential tremor, but it should be used sparingly in patients with PD because of the limited number of symptoms effectively treated.

4.2 Globus Pallidus

Since first described in 1994 [43], several centers have reported results using chronic GPi stimulation for PD [3,11,12,44,45]. The application of DBS in the pallidum was a natural step after the success of chronic stimulation of the Vim in reproducing the benefits of thalamotomy. Similar to lesions and stimulation of the thalamus, DBS of the GPi produces clinical improvement comparable to lesioning of the nucleus. The GPi lies just above the optic tract and adjacent to the internal capsule. Because no lesion is created with DBS, the risk of injury to these structures is minimized. In addition, changes in stimulation parameters allow for fine-tuning of the stimulator to maximize benefit and permit changes during progression of the disease. There is also evidence that bilateral stimulation is less likely than ablative lesions to affect speech, swallowing, and cognitive functions, and may in some instances improve or reverse them [37,46]. A significant drawback to chronic stimulation is the limited ability to affect more than a portion of the posterior GPi. This may be why there is variable improvement in gait after GPi DBS [47]. The effective stimulation field is generally symmetrical and could affect adjacent structures (internal capsule) before maximum clinical benefit is often reached. The relative benefits and drawbacks of various treatment modalities must always be considered and one only forms pallidotomy over GPi DBS [48]. It is clear that the effectiveness of unilateral pallidotomy diminishes with time [49], but it is not established that the same is true of DBS.

4.3 Subthalamic Nucleus

The efficacy of using the STN as a target for chronic stimulation in the symptomatic improvement of PD has been shown [3,15,50–52]. Because the STN exerts control over both input nuclei (GPi and SNr) of the thalamus in PD, it might be expected to be a superior target for stimulation than the GPi if the development of involuntary movements could be prevented. This has been shown to be possible; however, superiority over GPi stimulation in general or for specific symptomatic indications remains to be demonstrated. Similar to chronic stimulation elsewhere, the benefits are primarily contralateral and like GPi stimulation, benefit all the cardinal symptoms of PD. There is evidence that STN stimulation has only marginal or unpredictable effect on the alleviation of drug-induced dyskinesias [52], but our experience has been more positive.

Only short series directly comparing the effectiveness of GPi to STN stimulation in the symptomatic control of PD are available [53]. Both Veterans Administration and National Institutes of Health-funded studies are underway, with the objective of determining if there are significant differences in the effectiveness of GPi and STN stimulation. At this time, it can only be said that both targets are effective.

5 RELATIVE COST OF ABLATION VERSUS STIMULATION

Many of the costs associated with the creation of an ablative lesion and placement of a deep brain stimulator are similar (Table 2). These include preoperative imaging, operating room time for burr hole creation and target identification and hospital stay. The time difference between that needed for

TABLE 2 Costs of Ablation Versus Deep Brain Stimulation

Initial	Both	Cost ($)	Ablation	Cost ($)	Deep brain stimulation*	Cost ($)
Capital investment	Imaging station for preoperative planning stereotactic frame Z-drive and x-y stage Data collection station (microelectrode recording)	Costs vary widely depending on supplier(s)	Lesion generator $35,000–15,000	Costs vary widely depending on supplier		
Per procedure	Preoperative imaging OR time for intracranial procedure Postoperative imaging Hospital stay	Variable			Lead	$1895
					Extension	$495
					Generator	$7245
					OR time for generator placement	Variable
					OR time for generator replacement	Variable
					Generator	$7245
					Lead	ICP
					programming	#95970

*Costs for Medtronic's Activa® system.
Abbreviation: OR, Operating room.

creation of an ablative lesion and that for placement of a stimulator is probably negligible. Costs unique to an ablative lesion are the acquisition of the radiofrequency lesion generator and associated electrodes. For a DBS, there are the additional costs of the DBS lead, extension, and generator for each patient. Additionally, there is a need for a second procedure under general anesthesia to place the generator. After both procedures, there is routine medical follow-up, but DBS requires a variable number of visits to program the stimulator to maximize effectiveness. Deep brain stimulation also requires replacement of the pulse generator when the battery runs down, and the lead may need to be replaced occasionally. Additional costs are associated with deep brain stimulation relative to ablative lesions, but the reversibility, flexibility, and lower risk of adverse effects currently make it a more attractive procedure in general and especially when bilateral procedures are required.

REFERENCES

1. Laitinen LV, Bergenheim AT, Hariz MI. Leksell's posteroventral pallidotomy in the treatment of Parkinson's disease. J Neurosurg 76:53–61, 1992.
2. Svennilson E, Torvik A, Lowe R, Leksell L. Treatment of parkinsonism by stereotactic thermolesions in the pallidal region. A clinical evaluation of 81 cases. Acta Psychiat Neurol Scand 35:358–377, 1960.
3. Starr PA, Vitek JL, Bakay RAE. Ablative surgery and deep brain stimulation for Parkinson's disease. Neurosurgery 43:989–1015, 1998.
4. Ohye C, Kubota K, Hooper HE, et al. Ventrolateral and subventrolateral thalamic stimulation Arch Neurol 11:427–434, 1964.
5. Hassler R, Reichert T, Mundinger F, et al. Physiological observations in stereotaxic operations in extrapyramidal motor disturbances. Brain 83:337–350, 1960.
6. Benabid AL, Pollak P, Gervason C, Hoffmann D, Gao DM, Hommel M, Perret JE, de Rougemont J. Long-term suppression of tremor by chronic stimulation of the ventral intermediate thalamic nucleus. Lancet 337:403–406, 1991.
7. Blond S, Caparros-Lefebvre D, Parker F, Assaker R, Petit H, Guieu JD, Christiaens JL. Control of tremor and involuntary movement disorders by chronic stereotactic stimulation of the ventral intermediate thalamic nucleus. J. Neurosurg 77:62–68, 1992.
8. Tasker RR. Deep brain stimulation is preferable to thalamotomy for tremor suppression. Surg Neurol 49:145–154, 1998.
9. Siegfried J, Lippitz B. Chronic electrical stimulation of the VL-VPL complex and of the pallidum in the treatment of movement disorders: Personal experience since 1982. Stereotact Funct Neurosurg 62:71–75, 1994.
10. Kumar R, Lozano AM, Montgomery E, Lang AE. Pallidotomy and deep brain stimulation of the pallidum and subthalamic nucleus in advanced Parkinson's disease. Mov Disord 13(suppl 1):73–82, 1998.

11. Pahwa R, Wilkinson S, Smith D, Lyons K, Miyawaki E, Koller WC. High-frequency stimulation of the globus pallidus for the treatment of Parkinson's disease. Neurology 49(1):249–253, 1997.

12. Gross C, Rougier A, Guehl D, Boraud T, Julien J, Bioulac B. High-frequency stimulation of the globus pallidus internalis in Parkinson's disease: A study of seven cases. J Neurosurg 87(4):491–498, 1997.

13. DeLong MR, Crutcher MD, Georgopoulos AP. Primate globus pallidus and subthalamic nucleus: Functional organization. J Neurophysiol 53(2):530–543, 1985.

14. DeLong MR. Primate models of movement disorders of basal ganglia origin. Trends Neurosci 13:281–285, 1990.

15. Limousin P, Pollak P. Benazzouz A, Hoffmann D, Le Bas JF, Broussolle E, Perret JE, Benabid AL. Effect on parkinsonian signs and symptoms of bilateral subthalamic nucleus stimulation. Lancet 345:91–95, 1995.

16. Obeso JA, Alvarez CM, Marcins RJ. Lesions of the subthalamic nucleus (STN) in Parkinson's disease (PD). Neurology 48(A136), 1997.

17. Gill SS, Heywood P. Bilateral dorsolateral subthalamotomy for advanced Parkinson's disease. Lancet 350:1224, 1997.

18. Schlag J, Villablanca J. A quantitative study of temporal and spatial response patterns in a thalamic cell population electrically stimulated. Brain Res 8:255–270, 1968.

19. Ranck JB. Which elements are excited in electrical stimulation of mammalian central nervous system: A review. Brain Res 98:417–440, 1975.

20. Caparros-Lefebvre D, Ruchoux MM, Blond S, Petit H, Percheron G. Long-term thalamic stimulation in Parkinson's disease: Postmortem anatomoclinical study. Neurology 44:1856–1860, 1994.

21. Davis K, Taub E, Houle S, Lang AE, Dostrovsky JO, Tasker RR, Lozano AM. Globus pallidus stimulation activates the cortical motor system during alleviation of parkinsonian symptoms. Nat Med 3(6):671–674, 1997.

22. Kelly PJ, Gillingham FJ. The long-term results of stereotaxic surgery and L-dopa therapy in patients with Parkinson's disease: A 10 year follow-up study. J Neurosurg 53:332–337, 1980.

23. Nagaseki Y, Shibazaki T, Hirai T. Long-term follow-up results of selective VIM-thalamotomy. J Neurosurg 65:296–302, 1986.

24. Jankovic J, Cardoso F, Grossman R. Outcome after stereotaxic thalamotomy for parkinsonian, essential, and other types of tremor. Neurosurgery 37:680–687, 1995.

25. Matsumoto K, Schichijo F, Fukami T. Long-term follow-up review of cases of Parkinson's disease after unilateral or bilateral thalamotomy. J Neurosurg 60:1033–1044, 1984.

26. Narabayashi H, Maeda T, Yokochi F. Long-term follow up study of nucleus ventralis intermedius and ventrolateralis thalamotomy using a microelectrode technique in parkinsonism. Appl Neurophysiol 50:330–337, 1987.

27. Schuurman PR, Bosch DA, Bossuyt PMM, Bonsel GJ, Van Someren, EJW, de Bie, RMA, Merkus MP, Speelman JD. A comparison of continuous thalamic

stimulation and thalamotomy for suppression of severe tremor. N Engl J Med 342(7):461–468, 2000.

28. Tasker RR, Munz M, Junn FS Kiss ZH, Davis K, Dostrovsky JO, Lozano AM. Deep brain stimulation and thalamotomy for tremor compared. Acta Neurochir 68:49–53, 1997.

29. Vitek JL, Bakay RAE, Freeman A, et al. Randomized clinical trial of GPi pallidotomy versus best medical therapy for Parkinson's disease. Ann Neurol 2000. Submitted for publication.

30. Lang AE, Lozano AM, Montgomery E, et al. Posteroventral medial pallidotomy in advanced Parkinson's disease [see comments]. N Engl J Med 337(15):1036–1042, 1997.

31. Samii A, Turnbull IM, Kishore A, et al. Reassessment of unilateral pallidotomy in Parkinson's disease. A 2-year follow-up study [see comments]. Brain 122(Pt 3):417–425, 1999.

32. Alterman RL, Kelly PJ. Pallidotomy technique and results: The New York University experience. Neurosurg Clin N Am 9(2):337–343, 1998.

33. Iacono RP, Shima F, Lonser RR, et al. The results, indications, and physiology of posteroventral pallidotomy for patients with Parkinson's disease [see comments]. Neurosurgery 36(6):1118–1125; discussion 1125–1127, 1995.

34. Martinez-Martin P, Valldeoriola F, Molinuevo JL, Nobbe FA, Rumia J, Tolosa E. Pallidotomy and quality of life in patients with Parkinson's disease: An early study. Mov Disord 15(1):65–70.

35. Merello M, Nouzeilles, MI, Kuzis Gabriela, et al. Unilateral radiofrequency lesion versus electrostimulation of posteroventral pallidum: A prospective randomized comparison. Mov Disord 14(1):50–56, 1999.

36. Favre J, Taha JM, Nguyen TT, et al. Pallidotomy: A survey of current practice in North America. Neurosurgery 39(4):883–890; discussion 890–892, 1996.

37. Ghika J, Ghika-Schmid F, Fankhauser H, et al. Bilateral contemporaneous posteroventral pallidotomy for the treatment of Parkinson's disease: Neuropsychological and neurological side effects. Report of four cases and review of the literature. J Neurosurg 91(2):313–321, 1999.

38. Lombardi WJ, Gross RE, Trepanier LL, et al. Relationship of lesion location to cognitive outcome following microelectrode-guided pallidotomy for Parkinson's disease: Support for the existence of cognitive circuits in the human pallidum. Brain 123(Pt 4):746–758, 2000.

39. Guridi J, Obeso JA. The role of the subthalamic nucleus in the origin of hemiballism and parkinsonism: New surgical perspectives. In: Obeso JA, DeLong MR, Ohye C, Marsden CD, eds. The basal ganglia and new surgical perspectives for Parkinson's disease. Advances in Neurology, Vol. 74. Philadelphia: Lippincott-Raven, 1997, pp 235–247.

40. Gill S, Heywood P. Bilateral subthalamic nucleotomy can be accomplished safely. Mov Disord 13(2):201, 1998.

41. Koller W, Pahwa R, Busenbark K, et al. High-frequency unilateral thalamic stimulation in the treatment of essential and parkinsonian tremor. Ann Neurol 42:292–299, 1997.

42. Limousin P, Speelman JD, Gielen F, et al. Multicenter European study of thalamic stimulation in parkinsonism and essential tremor. J Neurol Neurosurg Psychiatry 66:289–296, 1999.
43. Siegfried J, Lippitz B. Bilateral chronic electrostimulation of ventroposterolateral pallidum: A new therapeutic approach for alleviating all parkinsonian symptoms. Neurosurgery 35(6):1126–1130, 1994.
44. Kumar R, Lozano AM, Duff J. Comparison of the effects of microelectrode-guided posteroventral medial pallidotomy and globus pallidus internus deep brain stimulation. Neurology 48(suppl):A430, 1997.
45. Linden C, Caemaert J, Vandewalle V. Chronic unilateral stimulation of the internal globus pallidus in advanced Parkinson's disease: A 3 month follow-up in 9 patients. Neurology 48(suppl):A430, 1997.
46. Fields JA, Troster AI, Wilkinson SB, et al. Cognitive outcome following staged bilateral pallidal stimulation for the treatment of Parkinson's disease. Clin Neurol Neurosurg 101:182–188, 1999.
47. Nieuwboer A, De Weerdt W, Dom R, Nuttin, B, Peeraer L, Pattyn A. Walking ability after implantation of a pallidal stimulator: Analysis of plantar force distribution in patients with Parkinson's disease. Parkinsonism Related Disord 4:189–199, 1998.
48. Tronnier VM, Fogel W, Kronenbuerger W, Steinvorth S. Pallidal stimulation: An alternative to pallidotomy? J Neurosurg 87:700–705, 1997.
49. Fine J, Duff J, Chen R, Chir B, et al. Long-term follow-up of unilateral pallidotomy in advanced Parkinson's disease. N Engl J Med 342:1708–1714, 2000.
50. Limousin P, Krack P, Pollack P, et al. Electrical stimulation of the subthalamic nucleus in advanced Parkinson's disease. N Engl J Med 339:1105–1111, 1998.
51. Kumar R, Lozano AM, Kim YJ, et al. Double-blind evaluation of subthalamic nucleus stimulation. Mov Disord 13:907–914, 1998.
52. Krack P, Pollack P, Limousin P, et al. From off-period dystonia to peak dose chorea: The clinical spectrum of varying subthalamic nucleus activity. Brain 122:1133–1146, 1999.
53. Burchiel KJ, Anderson VC, Favre J, Hammerstad JP. Comparison of pallidal and subthalamic nucleus deep brain stimulation for advanced Parkinson's disease: Results of a randomized, blinded pilot study. Neurosurgery 45:1375–1382, 1999.

26

Surgery for Other Movement Disorders

Zvi Israel
Hadassah University Hospital, Jerusalem, Israel

Kim Burchiel
Oregon Health and Science University, Portland, Oregon, U.S.A.

1 INTRODUCTION

The main hyperkinetic movement disorders, dystonia, hemiballism, and chorea are all characterized by reduced basal ganglia output to the thalamus, leading to disinhibition of thalamocortical pathways and, thus, involuntary movements.

2 PATHOPHYSIOLOGY

Using the most accepted model of parallel direct and indirect basal-ganglia thalamocortical motor circuitry popularized by DeLong [1], a pathophysiological basis for movement disorders has been proposed. Essentially, the Globus pallidus interna (GPi) is innervated by both *direct* inhibitory input from the putamen and *indirect* inhibitory/excitatory pathways from the putamen through the globus pallidus externa (GPe) and subthalamic nucleus (STN). Putaminal activity is regulated by input from the substantia nigra pars compacta (SNc) and by excitatory input from the thalamic centromedian nucleus (CM).

The model for hyperkinetic disorders proposes that abnormally reduced GPi output results in disinhibition of thalamocortical neurons. The precise pathophysiological differences between the various hyperkinetic disorders may be secondary to differences in balance between the direct and the indirect striato-pallidal pathways. Thus, for example, hemiballismus results from lesions of the subthalamic nucleus. In terms of the model, this would leave the inhibitory direct pathway unopposed, thus reducing GPi output.

Dystonia is the most investigated but least understood of the hyperkinetic movement disorders. Supportive evidence for reduced GPi output in dystonia comes from microelectrorecordings performed during pallidotomy. Neuronal activity within the pallidal (Vop) and cerebellar (Vim) receiving areas of the motor thalamus is also altered in dystonia. The degree to which the changes in pallidal activity contribute to the changes in thalamic activity may be different for the various etiologies of dystonia.

This description is necessarily somewhat simplified and recent observations, primarily from microelectrorecordings in primate models have challenged some of the concepts of this model (see the reference by Vitek for a review of this evidence). Nevertheless, it does seem likely that in ballismus and chorea, reduced STN input is the main factor determining reduced GPi output, whereas in dystonia this results from a hyperactive putaminal input.

3 DYSTONIA

Dystonia is characterized by slow, involuntary, sustained, or intermittent muscle contraction in agonist-antagonist and adjacent or distal muscle groups, frequently causing twisting, repetitive spasmodic movements or abnormal postures [2,3].

3.1 Classification

Dystonia may be classified according to etiology as primary or secondary, according to its age of onset and according to its pattern of distribution [4–6] (Table 1) and is often described in terms of all three. Thus dystonia may represent a *disease entity*, for example, idiopathic hereditary dystonia or a *symptom* of another neurological disease. A number of hereditary patterns of idiopathic (or primary torsion) dystonia have been described, although an identical sporadic form occurs too. Several of the genes involved in various forms of primary dystonia have been identified. Early-onset dystonia (DYT1), for example, is associated with a gene at 9q 32-34 [7,8].

Dystonia as a symptom is secondary to a central nervous system (CNS) insult such as trauma, toxin exposure, cerebrovascular accident (CVA), tumor, infection, or certain drugs. Neurodegenerative diseases such as Parkinson's disease, Huntington's chorea, and Wilson's disease may also include dystonia as a symptom. Both primary and secondary forms of dystonia may present in generalized or focal forms.

TABLE 1   Classification of Dystonias

Etiology	Primary	Hereditary
		Sporadic
	Symptomatic	Associated with hereditary neurological syndromes
	Secondary to	Birth injury
		Postnatal head trauma
		Encephalitis
		Stroke
	Associated with	Parkinsonism
Age at onset	Childhood	0–12 years
	Adolescent	13–20 years
	Adult	>20 years
Distribution	Focal	Spasmodic torticollis
		Writer's cramp
		Blepharospasm
		Oral facial dyskinesias
	Segmental	Dystonia musculorum deformans
	Multifocal	Lesch-Nyhan syndrome
	Generalized	Drugs (phenothiazines, levodopa, butyrophenones)
	Hemidystonia	

3.2 Clinical Features

The characteristic features of dystonia include:

1. excessive co-contraction of antagonist muscles during voluntary movement
2. overflow of contraction to remote muscles not normally used in that voluntary movement
3. spontaneous spasms of co-contraction

Dystonic movements are typically involuntary, slow, sustained, contorting, and "wrapping," although superimposed rapid jerks and tremors may also occur. Abnormal, disabling posturing occurs involving proximal, appendicular, and axial muscles. Different subtypes of dystonia may give rise to variable clinical patterns. Thus, the distribution, task-relatedness, and other neurological conditions may all contribute to the specific clinical picture in an individual patient.

Primary dystonia mostly occurs in childhood. This typically begins as a focal problem and progresses somatotopographically. Younger onset seems associated with a more aggressive and prolonged course [9]. Secondary dystonias of neurosurgical interest are listed in Table 2. Focal dystonias are distinct and limited problems. They are not usually associated with a positive family history, are of adult onset, and are managed quite differently. For example, hemifacial spasm is best treated by microvascular decompression of the facial nerve.

3.3 Treatment

3.3.1 Medical Management

Various drugs have been used to palliate dystonia. These include trihexyphenidyl, benztropine, clonazepam, baclofen, carbamazepine, levodopa, bromocriptine, and amantadine. Certain subtypes of dystonia are remarkably responsive to trihexyphenidyl (artane) or L-dopa. However, for the most part, drug effects are unreliable, and anticholinergic side effects certainly can become problematic at the high drug doses needed for improvement.

Torticollis can, in experienced hands, be treated with injections of botulinum toxin into the affected muscles. This interferes with neuromuscular transmission, weakens the injected muscle, and relieves the focal dystonia. This can be effective for up to 3 to 4 months, when injections need to be repeated. Ultimately antibodies can develop to the toxin, which becomes ineffective.

3.3.2 Stereotactic Surgery

Compared with Parkinson's disease and tremor, dystonia is a relatively infrequent condition and few neurosurgeons have accumulated significantly sized series. Furthermore, comparison and meta-analysis of results are restricted because of the choice of different sites for lesions, differing techniques, variable methods of assessing outcomes, and often-inadequate follow-up.

TABLE 2 Etiology of Secondary Dystonias of Neurosurgical Interest

Birth injury
Postnatal head injury
Encephalitis
Meningitis
Stroke
Others

3.3.2.1 Indications. Surgery is not useful for every dystonic patient and indeed, in some, surgery is not indicated at all. Careful adherence to selection criteria will prevent unrealistic hopes in the unsuitable candidate and will likely improve overall outcome of surgical candidates. Tasker's experience has led him to suggest that surgery is most successful for dystonia of *distal* limb musculature where the main disability is the dystonia itself rather than any accompanying neurological deficits [9]. Progressive disease, cognitive impairment, and pseudobulbar effects are considered to be contraindications. When ablative surgery is contemplated, speech and gait difficulties are also relative contraindications.

3.3.2.2 Procedures. Stereotactic surgery for dystonia has until recently consisted mostly of ablative lesions in either the thalamus or pallidum. More recently, as experience with deep brain stimulation (DBS) for other movement disorders has increased and the technique has been shown to be safe, occasional reports using DBS for dystonia have also been appearing in the literature [10–20].

3.3.2.3 Technique for Thalamotomy and Pallidotomy. In contemporary practice, the target is chosen using frame-based stereotactic localization. Magnetic resonance (MR) has largely replaced computed tomography (CT) and ventriculography, although the latter is still in use in at least one major European institution. Images are imported to a computer workstation. Functional software is used to help select an optimal initial target. Targets established from a human stereotactic atlas can be registered in the program based on distances from the AC-PC (anterior commissure, posterior commissure) planes. These software programs also help correct for small frame rotations (coronal roll, axial yaw, and sagittal pitch) and to some extent for variable ventricular anatomy.

Microelectrorecording and stimulation are used to "map out" the target area and assist in deciding on the ideal final target for lesioning or DBS lead placement. Mapping techniques may use simultaneous microstimulation electromyogram (EMG), and passive limb movements to define a thalamic or pallidal homunculus and visual evoked potentials to localize the optic tract. Finally, thermal lesions are made while continually assessing the patient's neurological status. If deep brain stimulation has been chosen, the electrode is introduced and its position verified with fluoroscopy.

3.3.2.4 Thalamotomy and Pallidotomy: Results. The published literature on the use of thalamotomy and pallidotomy in the treatment of dystonia has been the subject of several excellent reviews [9,21]. Various nuclei of the motor thalamus have been targeted, either alone or in conjunction with other thalamic or extrathalamic nuclei for the treatment of dystonia. As mentioned previously, this diversity of approach makes analysis extremely difficult. Furthermore, many patients were operated bilaterally, and this clearly influenced the complication rate. Tasker's own series, published in 1988 [22], described the results of Vim or Vop thalamotomy in 49 patients with primary and secondary dystonia. Both phasic and tonic movements of upper and lower limbs were markedly improved by 40% to 69%. Significant improvement of 20% to 30% was noted for facial, neck, and trunk movements. Speech, locomotion, and dexterity were also improved, but in a minority of patients. The main complication observed was dysarthria, primarily in those patients operated bilaterally. However, approximately one-third of his patients regressed over a period of up to 6 years postoperatively. This may have occurred in patients whose disease was progressing preoperatively.

The major factors that determined the change of target from the thalamus to the pallidum for dystonia were the improved understanding of the functional organization of the basal ganglia-thalamocortical circuitry and the success of pallidotomy in the treatment of L-dopa-induced dyskinesias ("off" dystonia) in parkinsonian patients. Although pallidotomy has, since the 1950s, been known to be effective for dystonia [23], analysis of the results of early series is difficult, again because of a diverse choice of target, differing lesioning techniques, small numbers of patients treated, and variable follow-up. Since 1996, there has been renewed interest in pallidotomy for dystonia [24–36]. However, the largest contemporary clinical series consists of only eight patients [28], and thus, the relatively small numbers again confound categorical conclusions concerning efficacy. In most patients, the posterolateral (sensorimotor) part of the GPi has been targeted. Improvement is evident immediately intraoperatively. All patients, including those with primary or secondary dystonia, have been reported to benefit substantially from pallidotomy. Motor functioning and activities of daily living improve, whereas dystonic symptoms and disability decline. Contralateral, distal dystonias seem to improve most. Axial dystonias appear more resistant and probably benefit more from bilateral pallidotomy.

The trend toward deep brain stimulation and away from neuroablative lesions has occurred at the same time as the trend from thalamotomy to pallidotomy for the treatment of dystonia. It is, therefore, likely that there will never be a large enough series of dystonia patients treated with pallidotomy to allow accurate analysis of pallidotomy for dystonia.

3.3.2.5 Deep Brain Stimulation. Working with thalamic DBS for the management of parkinsonism and tremor, the early pioneers of DBS often noticed symptomatic improvement of any accompanying dystonia. Sellal et al implanted a DBS system in the contralateral ventroposterolateral thalamus of a patient with postraumatic hemidystonia. The patient experienced improved posture and movement until the system was removed 8 months later because of poor wound healing [10].

More recently, reports of pallidal stimulation for dystonia have been appearing in the literature [11–18], but experience is very limited. In contrast to pallidotomy for dystonia, often no immediate intraoperative benefit is reported, but rather, a slowly progressive clinical improvement may be seen over a period of several weeks. Furthermore, upon turning off the DBS, dystonia returns some hours later, but upon reactivation, can take days to resolve.

Tronnier et al reported on three patients with generalized dystonia, (two primary and one secondary) after bilateral pallidal stimulation and follow-up times of between 6 and 18 months. All three patients experienced significant relief in both axial and limb dystonia [19]. Loher et al have published a case of one patient with secondary hemidystonia. This patient had previously undergone thalamotomy with good tremor control but only transient improvement of the hemidystonia. They implanted a contralateral GPi DBS system. Reduced dystonic movements, posturing, and dystonia-associated pain were associated with functional gain in a follow-up period of 4 years [20]. One other report also describes the utility of GPi DBS in managing intractable dystonia-associated pain.

4 CHOREA

Chorea describes brief, abrupt, irregular, unpredictable, involuntary muscle contractions that are nonrhythmic, unpatterned, and have variable timing. Commonly involved are the distal parts of the extremities and the orofacial muscles. Chorea may appear as a symptom of Huntington's disease or other neurodegenerative disorders or may be secondary to other system diseases (Table 3).

Early experience with a modest number of patients showed both pallidotomy and thalamotomy to improve contralateral chorea [9]. More recently, Vim-Vop thalamotomy has been reported to alleviate choreiform movements [37]. Pallidotomy has been described in the contemporary literature as relieving contralateral chorea in a patient with Huntington's however, the exact site of the lesion is unclear and may have included parts of both the GPi and GPe [38]. One case of chorea treated with bilateral posteroventral pallidotomy was reported to remarkably improve; however, follow-up time was short (only 7 months) [39]. Only two groups have so far reported experience with DBS for chorea. Thalamic Vim stimulation improved contralateral symptoms in two children with modest follow-up of 4 and 18 months [40]. Choreoathetoid head movements were improved by DBS of the pallidal GPi [41]. Thus, whereas both the thalamic vim and the

TABLE 3   Etiology of Chorea

Neurodegenerative Diseases	Huntington's disease
	Wilson's disease
	Ataxia telangiectasia
Infection	Sydenham's chorea
Autoimmune	Systematic lupus erythematosus
Drugs	Levodopa
	Anticholinergics
	Antipsychotics
Metabolic Disorders	Hyperthyroidism
	Oral contraceptive pill
	Pregnancy
Vascular lesions	
Idiopathic	

pallidal GPi seem to be effective targets for both ablation and deep brain stimulation in the control of contralateral chorea, experience is sparse.

5   HEMIBALLISM

Hemiballism consists of forceful, wide-amplitude flinging movements, usually only of one side of the body. Proximal musculature and associated axial musculature are affected. Many patients also demonstrate additional distal choreiform movements. Ballism is unique in that it is the only abnormal involuntary movement disorder produced by a single, small lesion in a specific brain nucleus, the subthalamic nucleus. Thus, a primate model for ballism could be studied. This elegantly demonstrated that the abnormal activity sustaining the ballism was channeled through the medial GPi and the Vim as lesions of both these nuclei could abolish the dyskinesia [42]. Globus pallidus interna pallidotomy [43], Vim thalamotomy [44,45], and chronic thalamic DBS [46] are all effective at controlling hemiballism in humans. However, the best target is unknown, as the paucity of cases has not allowed these techniques to be subjected to comparison by way of a modern randomized trial.

6   CONCLUSIONS

Stereotactic surgery can undoubtedly significantly palliate some of the dystonia syndromes and dystonia-associated symptoms. Vim thalamotomy is effective for distal dystonic movements, but symptoms may recur over time. More recently, lesioning or stimulating the sensorimotor area of the GPi has been shown to possibly be more effective; however, adequate follow-up has yet to be documented. The surgical treatment of dystonia is a discipline that is still evolving. Dystonia surgery should be subjected to analysis by way of a modern, well-designed, randomized (and probably multicenter) trial to determine the best site and best mode of therapy.

Surgeons considering operating for the relief of chorea or hemiballism may choose a target for lesioning or stimulator placement based on reviewing the literature and their own experience. However, they should be aware that published experience for surgery on these patients is limited, and the small targets often recommended (in the pallidum or STN) may be best localized with the help of microelectrode recording. This is especially so in these patients, whose movements often mandate the use of general anesthesia and in whom macrostimulation will be of limited intraoperative benefit.

REFERENCES

1. Wichmann T, DeLong MR. Models of basal ganglia function and pathophysiology of movement disorders. Surgical Treatment of Movement Disorders. Neurosurg Clin N Am 9:223–236, 1998.
2. Marsden CD, Fahn S. Surgical approaches to the dyskinesias: Afterword. In: Marsden CD, Fahn S, eds. Neurology 2: Movement Disorders. London: Butterworth Scientific, 1982, pp 345.
3. Ad hoc Committee Meeting Proceedings, Dystonia Medical Research Foundation, 1984.
4. Marsden CD. Investigation of dystonia. In: Fahn S, Marsden CD, Calne DB, eds. Advances in Neurology 50: Dystonia 2. New York: Raven Press, 1988, pp 35–44.
5. Fahn S. Concept and classification of dystonia. In: Fahn S, Marsden CD, Calne DB, eds. Advances in Neurology 50: Dystonia 2. New York: Raven Press, 1988, pp 1–8.
6. Tasker RR, Doorly T, Yamashiro K. Thalamotomy in generalized dystonia. In: Fahn S, Marsden CD, Calne DB, eds. Advances in Neurology 50: Dystonia 2. New York: Raven Press, 1988, pp 615–631.
7. Ozelius L, Kramer PL, Moskowitz CB, Kwiatkowski DJ, Brin MF, Bressman SB, Schuback DE, Falk CT, Risch N, deLeon D. Human gene for torsion dystonia located on chromosome 9q32-34. Neuron 2:1427–1434, 1989.
8. The genetics of dystonia. http://www.dystonia-foundation.org/genetic.html. July 1998.
9. Tasker RR. Surgical treatment of the dystonias: In: Gildengerg P, and Tasker RR, eds. Textbook of Stereotactic and Functional Neurosurgery. McGraw Hill, 1997, pp 1015–1032.
10. Sellal F, Hirsch E, Barth P, Blond S, Marescaux C. A case of symptomatic hemidystonia improved by ventroposterolateral thalamic electrostimulation. Mov Disord 8:515–518, 1993.

11. Funk T, Vesper J, Wagner F, et. al. Deep brain stimulation of the globus pallidus internus for generalized dystonia. Poster #1355, AANS, San Francisco, 2000.
12. Krauss JK, Pohle T, Weber S, Ozdoba C, Burgunder JM. Bilateral stimulation of globus pallidus internus for treatment of cervical dystonia. Lancet 354:837–838, 1999.
13. Kumar R, Dagher A, Hutchison WD, Lang AE, Lozano AM. Globus pallidus deep brain stimulation for generalized dystonia: Clinical and PET investigation. Neurology 53:871–874, 1999.
14. Coubes P, Echenne B, Roubertie A, Vayssiere N, Tuffery S, Humbertclaude V, Cambonie G, Clanstres M, Frerebeau P. Treatment of early onset generalized dystonia by chronic bilateral stimulation of the internal globus pallidus. Neurochirurgie 45:139–144, 1999.
15. Brin MF, Germano I, Danisi FO, et. al. Deep brain stimulation of pallidum in intractable dystonia. Mov Disord 13:274, 1998.
16. Brin MF, Deep brain stimulation for dystonia and other movement disorders. American Academy of Neurology, April 1999.
17. Benabid AL, Pollack P, Limousin P et. al. Chronic stimulation of the ventro-lateral thalamic nucleus in dystonia. Focus on Dystonia, 26, 1994
18. Caputo E, Krack P, Tamma F, et. al. Dystonic tremor treated by unilateral pallidal deep brain stimulation after secondary failure of thalamic stimulation. Mov Disord 13:135, 1998.
19. Tronnier VM, Fogel W. Pallidal stimulation for generalized dystonia: Report of three cases. J Neurosurg 92:453–456, 2000.
20. Loher TJ, Hasdemir MG, Burgunder JM, Krauss JK. Long-term follow-up study of chronic globus pallidus internus stimulation for posttraumatic hemi-dystonia. J. Neurosurg 92:457–460, 2000.
21. Vitek JL. Surgery for dystonia. In: Bakay R, ed. Surgical Treatment of Movement Disorders. Neurosurgery Clinics of North America 9(2):345–366, 1998. WB Saunders.
22. Tasker RR, Doorly T, Yamashiro K. Thalamotomy in generalized dystonia. Adv Neurol 50:615–631, 1988.
23. Cooper IS. 20-year follow up study of the neurosurgical treatment of dystonia musculorum deformans. Adv Neurol 14:423–452, 1976.
24. Iacono RP, Kuniyoshi SM, Lonser RR, Morenski JD, Bailey L. Simultaneous bilateral pallidoansotomy for idiopathic dystonia musculorum deformans. Pediatr Neurol 14:145–148, 1996.
25. Vitek JL, Bakay RA. The role of pallidotomy in Parkinson's disease and dystonia. Curr Opin Neurol 10:332–339, 1997.
26. Weetman J, Anderson IM, Gregory RP, Gill SS. Bilateral posteroventral pallidotomy for severe antipsychotic induced tardive dyskinesia and dystonia. J Neurol Neurosurg Psych 63:554–556, 1997.
27. Lozano AM, Kumar R, Gross RE, Giladi N, Hutchison WD, Dostrovsky JO, Lang AE. Globus pallidus internus pallidotomy for generalized dystonia. Mov Disord 12:865–870, 1997.
28. Ondo WG, Desaloms JM, Jankovic J, Grossman RG. Pallidotomy for generalized dystonia. Mov Disord 13:693–698, 1998.

29. Vitek JL, Zhang J, Evatt M, Mewes K, Delong MR, Hashimoto T, Triche S, Bakay RA. GPi pallidotomy for dystonia: Clinical outcome and neuronal activity. Adv Neurol 78:211–219, 1998.

30. Bhatia KP, Marsden CD, Thomas DG. Posteroventral pallidotomy can ameliorate attacks of paroxysmal dystonia induced by exercise. J Neurol Neurosurg Psychiatry 65:604–605, 1998.

31. Lin JJ, Lin SZ, Lin GY, Chang DC, Lee CC. Application of bilateral sequential pallidotomy to treat a patient with generalized dystonia. Eur Neurol 40:108–110, 1998.

32. Lenz FA, Suarez JI, Metman LV, Reich SG. Karp BI, Hallett M, Rowland LH, Dougherty PM. Pallidal activity during dystonia: Somatosensory reorganization and changes with severity. J Neurol Neurosurg Psychiatry 65:767–770, 1998.

33. Justesen CR, Penn RD, Kroin JS, Egel RT. Stereotactic pallidotomy in a child with Hallervorden-Spatz disease. J Neurosurg 90:551–554, 1999.

34. Lin JJ, Lin GY, Shih C, Lin SZ, Chang DC, Lee CC. Benefit of bilateral pallidotomy in the treatment of generalized dystonia. Case Report. J Neurosurg 90:974–976, 1999.

35. Vitek JL, Chockkan V, Zhang JY, Kaneoke Y, Evatt M, DeLong MR, Triche S, Mewes K, Hashimoto T, Bakay RA. Neuronal activity in the basal ganglia in patients with generalized dystonia and hemiballismus. Ann Neurol 46:22–35, 1999.

36. Lai T, Lai JM, Grossman RG. Functional recovery after bilateral pallidotomy for the treatment of early onset primary generalized dystonia. Arch Phys Med Rehabil 80:1340–1342, 1999.

37. Kawashima Y, Takahashi A, Hirato M, Ohye C. Stereotactic Vim-Vo-thalamotomy for choreatic movement disorder. Acta Neurochir Suppl 52:103–106, 1991.

38. Laitenan LV, Hariz MI. Movement disorders. In: Youmans JR, ed. Neurological Surgery. Philadelphia: WB Saunders, 1996, pp 3575–3609.

39. Fujimoto Y, Isozaki Y, Yokochi F, Yamakawa K, Takahashi H, Hirai S. A case of chorea-acanthocytosis successfully treated with posteroventral pallidotomy. Rinsho Shinkeigaku 37:891–894, 1997.

40. Thompson TP, Kondziolka D, Albright AL. Thalamic stimulation for choreiform movement disorders in children. Report of two cases. J Neurosurg 92:718–721, 2000.

41. Kraus JK, Loher TJ, Pohle T et. al. Chronic GPi stimulation for treatment of cervical dystonia and choreoathetotic head movements. Open paper #777, CNS, San Antonio, September 2000.

42. Crossman AR, Brotchie JM. Primate models for the study of basal ganglia physiology and dysfunction. In: Krauss JK, Grossman RG, Jankovic J, eds. Pallidal surgery for the treatment of Parkinson's Disease and Movement Disorders. Philadelphia: Lippincott-Raven, 1998.

43. Suarez JI, Metman LV, Reich SG, Dougherty PM, Hallett M, Lenz, FA. Pallidotomy for hemiballismus: Efficacy and characteristics of neuronal activity. Ann Neurol 42:807–811, 1997.

44. Cardoso F, Jankovic J, Grossman RG, Hamilton WJ. Outcome after stereotactic thalamotomy for dystonia and hemiballismus. Neurosurgery 36:501–507, 1995.
45. Levesque MF, Markham C, Nakasato M. MR-guided ventral intermediate thalamotomy for post-traumatic hemiballismus. Stereotac Funct Neurosurg 58:88, 1992.
46. Siegfried J, Lippitz B. Chronic electrical stimulation of the VL-VPL complex and of the pallidum in the treatment of movement disorders: Personal experience since 1982. Stereotac Funct Neurosurg 62:71–75, 1994.

27

Functional Neurosurgery Using the Radionics Stereoplan System

James M. Schumacher

Center for Movement Disorders, University of Miami,
Miami, Florida, U.S.A. and McLean Hospital,
Harvard Medical School, Boston, Massachusetts, U.S.A.

1 INTRODUCTION

Since the early 1990s, there has been a renewal of interest in functional neurosurgical techniques in Parkinson's disease and other movement disorders. A better understanding of the neuroanatomical and neurophysiological basis of these disorders has fueled this renewal. Compared to the use of X-rays and ventriculograms, the advent of computed tomographic (CT)-guided stereotaxy was a godsend. With increasing need for accurate placement of instruments in smaller nuclei, magnetic resonance imaging (MRI)-guided techniques were used. The major disadvantage of using MRI alone was evident in its inherent magnetic image distortion (Walton, 1996). Magnetic resonance imaging provides a better target image, but when used alone it can lead to misplacement of an electrode or needle.

The Radionics workstation incorporates CT/MRI image fusion, Stereoplan target planning, anatomical atlas, and the NeuroMap micro/semimicroelectrode recording system. This system provides the surgeon with a safe, accurate, easy-to-operate system for functional techniques such as lesioning, biopsy, drug delivery, or placement of deep brain stimulators. Using early versions of Image Fusion and Stereoplan, the Oxford Movement Disorder Group demonstrated the system's accuracy to 1 mm (Aziz, 1998). Today, with later versions of the software and the use of the NeuroMap microelectrode recording systems, the software has become more user friendly and the frontiers of precision have been pushed a step further.

2 IMAGE FUSION

In our clinical program at Neurological Associates Center for Movement Disorders, all functional neurosurgical procedures are based on image fusion using CT and MRI. The patient starts the day with an MRI using the Siemens 1.5 Tesla MP Range (3-mm axial cuts) program that provided good visualization of nuclear groups in the basal ganglia and brainstem (Fig. 1). The patient is placed under local anesthesia and the Radionics CT frame and localizer are placed with the use of temporary ear bars. The frame is placed with rough approximation to the AC-PC line from external auditory meatus to the inferior orbital rim. A noncontrast CT scan is then done (GE scanner, 3-mm cuts). The MRI and CT data are stored on optical disc and transferred to the Radionics workstation. Unlike previous software versions that fused the MRI image to the CT bone density, the newer 2.0 version rapidly fuses the two images pixel to pixel. Previous versions of Image Fusion required that the MRI and CT images be nearly coplanar. The 2.0 fuses the images rapidly, even if the scan images are not matched.

3 TARGET PLANNING

In the operating room, data from Image Fusion are transferred to Radionics Stereoplan program and the CT fiducials are rapidly localized. The axial fused MRI image is then brought to the screen and target planning begins. For reference during target planning, the AC-PC line is used to fuse the images with anatomical brain slices from the Schaltenbrand brain atlas (Schaltenbrand, 1977). Targets in the basal ganglia are calculated roughly using Guiot's diagram (Guiot, 1968) and as modified by Benabid (Benabid, 1998). These targets are further refined directly on the MRI axial, coronal, and sagital images in the Stereoplan program. Once anterior-posterior, lateral, and vertical coordinates are determined, the ring and slide numbers are entered into the system to provide the safest trajectory to the target, avoiding sulci, fissures, and the ventricular system (Fig. 2). This technique is especially useful when working with a patient with some degree of atrophy and large ventricles and sulci. Once the surgeon is satisfied with the target and

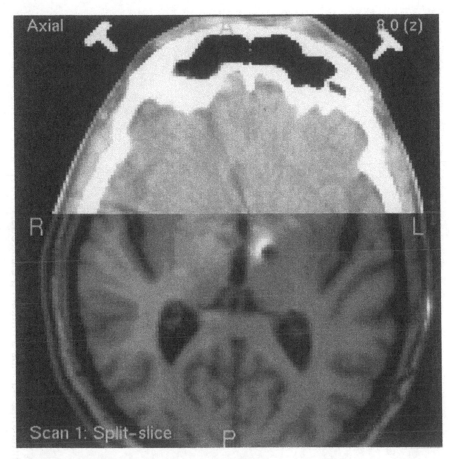

FIGURE 1 Split images of magnetic resonance imaging and computed tomography in Image Fusion. Good overlap of anatomical structures is seen between the two studies. Patient has had a previous left subthalamic nucleus stimulator.

trajectory, the coordinates are transferred to the Radionics Cossman, Roberts, Wells (CRW) stereotactic frame.

4 NEUROPHYSIOLOGICAL LOCALIZATION

Before placement of chronic stimulating electrodes or lesioning a target, neurophysiological localization is performed. At our center, we have shared in the development of the Radionics NeuroMap neurophysiology station.

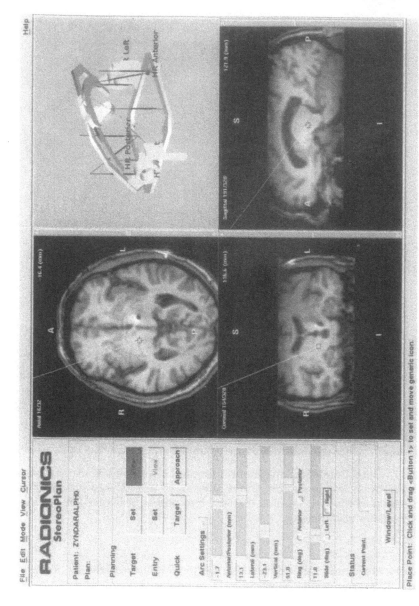

FIGURE 2   Fused magnetic resonance image on the Stereoplan workstation showing trajectory for placement of subthalamic nucleus stimulating electrode.

This unit is a compact computer using a Windows NT workstation. The workstation contains a series of amplifiers and filters that allow monitoring and refinement of up to eight channels of electrophysiological data from the patient. Data are displayed in real time and can be printed or archived for later analysis. For a typical patient undergoing a basal ganglia procedure, we use one channel only for semimicroelectrode recording and mapping of the region of interest. A second channel can be used for simultaneous electromyographic (EMG) data in a patient with tremor or dystonia. The electrode is mounted on the Radionics microdrive and connected to a pre-amp mounted on the CRW frame. Recording from the brain is typically started 12 mm above the target. Either microelectrodes or semimicroelectrodes can be used in this system.

For intraoperative recording, we are currently investigating the use of semimicroelectrodes. The 40-micron tip tungsten semimicroelectrode, (1 megaOhm $\pm$ 10% at 1 kHz) provides robust signals that accurately declare the margins of the target nuclei. For example, characteristic firing patterns of thalamic, subthalamic, pallidal, or nigral neurons can be identified and recorded (Fig. 3). In some procedures, such as thalamic mapping, kinesthetic response of neuronal activity can also be observed.

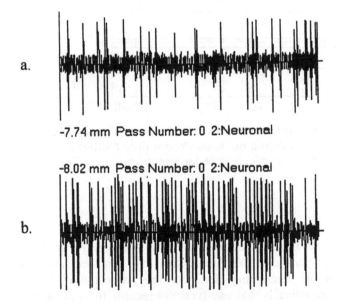

a.

-7.74 mm Pass Number: 0 2:Neuronal

-8.02 mm Pass Number: 0 2:Neuronal

b.

FIGURE 3 **a.** Semimicroelectrode recording from the subthalamic nucleus showing "pauser cells." **b.** Semimicroelectrode recording from the substantia nigra reticulata (SNr) showing fast activity.

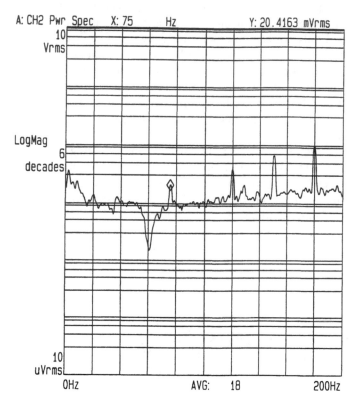

Avg   Type: RMS   Number: 20
[FFT]   Update Rt: 1   Overlap: 0 %
Date: 21.04.00 Time: 09:25:00

A: CH2 Pwr Spec   X: 75   Hz   Y: 20.4163 mVrms
10
Vrms

LogMag
6
decades

10
uVrms
OHz   AVG: 18   200Hz

FIGURE 4 Real-time fast Fourier transformation spectral analysis of neuronal activity in the subthalamic nucleus. Predominant activity is noted at 4 Hz and 75 Hz with harmonics in the far spectrum.

This technique has the advantage of allowing more precise mapping of the target's nuclear perimeter. With these data, one can then tailor the placement of the chronic stimulating electrode. The greatest limitation of semimicroelectrode recording is that one typically records from more than one neuron at a time. Semimicroelectrode recording provides a strong and reliable neuronal signal but makes determination of cell firing frequency difficult. To quantify frequencies of neuronal groups, we are currently in-

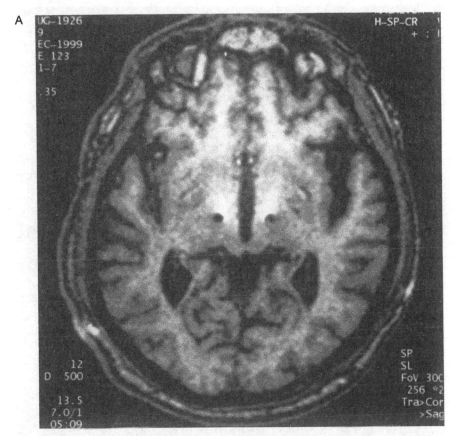

A

FIGURE 5   **A.** Patient with bilateral subthalamic nucleus stimulators (axial image).

vestigating the use of real-time fast Fourier transformation (FFT) analysis of semimicroelectrode signals (Fig. 4).

Once the nucleus of interest is mapped, the Medtronic Activa stimulating electrode can be placed and tested in the awake patient. The Radionics radiofrequency generator is used if a lesion such as a pallidotomy or thalamotomy is planned.

Macrostimulation, impedance calculations, and physical responses are evaluated before placement of a permanent lesion. To evaluate the placement of electrodes or lesions, all patients undergo postoperative magnetic resonance imaging (MRI) (Fig. 5).

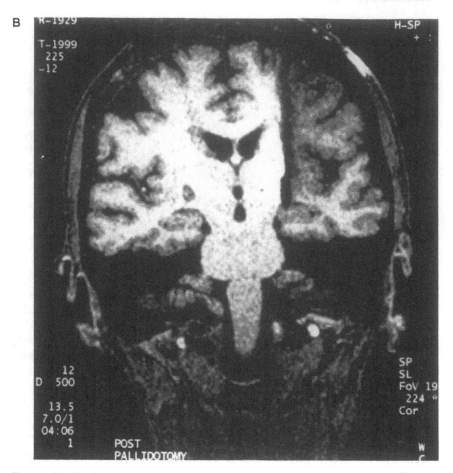

FIGURE 5   B. Patient with a Gpi stimulator and a pallidotomy (coronal image).

5   DISCUSSION

Safety is the most important part of any neurosurgical procedure. Functional stereotactic techniques demand a high level of forethought, caution, and preparation. A well-planned, successful procedure can modify the function of the brain to the patient's advantage. The surgeon should always work toward making the procedure as precise and noninvasive to the patient as is possible.

Second only to patient selection, the most critical part of stereotactic surgery is initial acquisition of targets and accurate placement of electrodes.

Technical advances in the field, such as image fusion, neuronavigation, and neurophysiological analysis provide better clinical outcome. It is our opinion that no stereotactic functional procedure should be based on MRI alone. The inherent distortion in the MR image can lead the surgeon astray. As a fisherman trying to snare a fish in the stream knows the prey is not exactly where it appears to be. To be successful, the thoughtful neurosurgeon must learn how to deal with distortion. Fusion of MRI on a CT image corrects this distortion and allows precise targeting.

Further confirmation of target is obtained through micro- or semimicroelectrode recording. The use of microelectrode recording is often debated, but we feel it adds another degree of accuracy and allows mapping the perimeters of the nucleus. Better placement of the chronic electrode is obtained by this technique. In our center, we are finding that semimicroelectrodes are dependable and provide adequate confirmation of target. Further advances with this technique, such as fast Fourier analysis, are promising and should provide more information about the nucleus of interest.

One shortcoming of the Radionics system is the fusion of the patient's anatomy with the Scaltenbrand atlas. Because every patient's anatomy is different, the atlas provides only a rough approximation and should never be used to plan target coordinates. Using the patient's own brain anatomy provided by MRI/CT fusion is reliable and accurate.

Some clear advantages of this workstation are accuracy, dependability, and expediency. Image Fusion and Stereoplan allow "first pass" target acquisition instead of multiple passes in an attempt to make up for MRI distortion.

Single-cell recording is important for research investigations to define functionality and cell firing frequency, but is a technical challenge because of the nature of the tiny electrode tip. Semimicroelectrodes are easy to use and give the surgeon a better map of the target nuclear boundaries. In addition, the developing Fourier analysis technique may help define the signature of the target nucleus and its predominant cell-firing frequencies.

As a tribute to the Radionics system, no patient in our center has thus far required repositioning of an electrode or lesion. Future directions with this system include real-time tracking of the probe along the workstation trajectory with simultaneous NeuroMap data displayed on the workstation screen

REFERENCES

1. Walton L, Hampshire A, Forster, Kemeny A. A phantom study to assess the accuracy of stereotactic localization, using T1-weighted magnetic resonance imaging with the Leksell stereotactic system. Neurosurgery 38:170–176, 1996.

2. Papanastassio V, Rowe J, Scott R, Silburn P, Davies L, Aziz T. Use of the Radionics Image Fusion and Stereoplan programs for target localization in functional neurosurgery. J Clin Neurosci 5:28–32.
3. Schaltenbrand G, Wahren W. Atlas for Stereotaxy of the Human Brain 2nd ed. Stuttgart: Georg Thieme Publishers, 1977.
4. Guiot G, Arfel G, Derome P. La chirurgie stereotaxique des tremblements de repos et d'attitude. Gaz Med France 75:4029–4056, 1968.
5. Benabid A, Benazzouz A, Hoffmann D, Limousin P, Krack P, Pollak P. Long-term electrical inhibition of deep brain targets in movement disorders. Mov Disord 13:119–125, 1998.

28

Computer-Assisted Image-Guided Stereotaxis in Movement Disorder Surgery

Paul A. House
University of Utah Health Sciences Center,
Salt Lake City, Utah, U.S.A.

Robert E. Gross
Emory University School of Medicine, Atlanta, Georgia, U.S.A.

1 INTRODUCTION

The field of functional neurosurgery has developed hand in hand with that of stereotaxis. Although Meyer first performed ablation of basal ganglia structures for control of tremor in 1942 as an open procedure, the safety of these procedures was significantly improved by the development of the stereotactic apparatus [1]. A number of stereotactic frames (and atlases) have been developed, most notably by Spiegel and Wycis [2], Talairach [3], Leksell [4], and Brown, Roberts, and Wells [5]. Successful placement of percutaneous lesions and implants relies on the precise subcortical localization each of these devices affords.

A number of technological advances have further improved the accuracy and safety of stereotactic procedures. First have been the improvements in imaging techniques, evolving from ventriculography to three-dimensional (3D) computed tomography (CT) and magnetic resonance imaging (MRI).

At the same time, the development of faster microprocessors has enabled a symbiosis of advanced imaging techniques, computational technology, and stereotaxis, leading to the advent of computer-assisted image-guided stereotaxis. This chapter will address the application of this technology to functional procedures for movement disorders.

2 ADVANTAGES OF COMPUTER-ASSISTED IMAGE GUIDANCE

Computer-assisted image guidance provides significant advantages for functional movement disorder procedures (Table 1). These advantages improve the accuracy of target localization by various methods (including anatomical formulaic, and atlas-registration techniques), and significantly decrease the number of steps and time required for target site calculation. The benefits of computer assistance at various stages of the procedures are best exemplified by a step-by-step analysis of the use of these techniques during a typical procedure for movement disorders, the implantation of a subthalamic nucleus (STN) deep brain stimulator for Parkinson's disease.

3 STEREOTACTIC PROCEDURES FOR MOVEMENT DISORDER SURGERY

3.1 Frame Application and Fiducial Localization

Under laboratory conditions, "frameless" computer-assisted image guidance is capable of submillimeter targeting accuracy [6], but rigid frame fixation

TABLE 1 Advantages of Using Computer-Assisted Image Guidance in Functional Neurosurgery

---

Rapid fiducial localization
Referencial localization of every point in a three-dimensional volume
Rapid correction of tilt, twist and rotation of head and frame within the scanner
Rapid correction of tilt, twist and rotation of frame in relation to the ICL
Rapid formulaic targeting based on distance from the ICL
Ability to merge multiple data sets (such as different MRI sequences, fMRI, PET)
Ability to superimpose (and morph) computer-based stereotactic atlas for target selection
Ability to superimpose post-operative imaging on operative planning to check accuracy

---

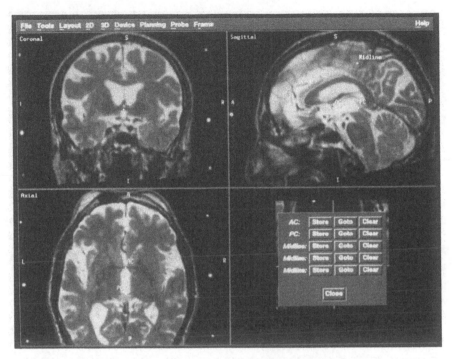

FIGURE 1 Screen from image-guided navigational workstation (Stealth, Medtronic Sofamor Danek, Broomfield, CO) showing the reformation of the volumetric data set parallel or orthogonal to the intercommissural line (AC-PC) and the vertical midline. AC, anterior commissure, PC, posterior commissure.

continues to be used for most functional intracranial neurosurgical procedures to provide the highest accuracy possible. Many stereotactic frame systems are currently in production. However, this discussion will focus on the Leksell G frame (Elekta Instruments, Atlanta, Georgia) used in conjunction with the StealthStation (Medtronic Sofamor Danek, Broomfield, Colorado), one of several commercially available computer-assisted image-guidance systems.

Frame-based stereotactic procedures first involve affixing the frame with four skull pins under local anesthetic. The frame base is fitted with a temporary fiducial-containing cage, the localizer. Imaging with CT, MRI (one or more sequences), magnetic resonance angiography (MRA), or venography (MRV) is then undertaken with the frame resting rigidly on a holder. More than one dataset can be merged before fiducial localization to

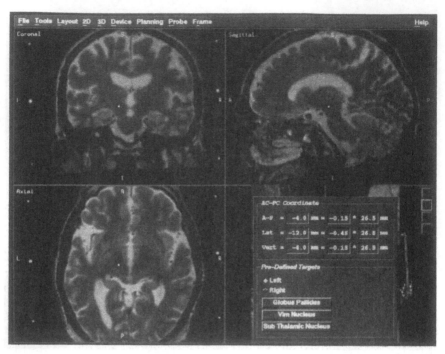

FIGURE 2 Screen from image-guided navigational workstation showing the positioning of a formulaically-calculated target for a pallidal procedure using the workstation software.

allow estimation and consideration of potential image distortions (as with MR), or to allow consideration of different types of information (parenchyma, vasculature, etc.) Computer workstations allow effortless shifting between datasets.

Previous techniques that did not use computer assistance required that the base ring be coplanar with the plane of the scanner gantry to maintain the geometry upon which target-centered stereotactic devices rely. This is not the case with computer-assisted techniques. The fiducials in any axial plane (not necessarily the one in which the target lies) are imported into the software using a cursor. Thereafter, the fiducials in each adjacent slice of the scan are automatically detected, generating a complete volumetric representation of the fiducial localizer. This registration allows the software to know the precise geometry of the localizer within the scanner, thereby eliminating the need to adjust the fiducial localizer position during scanning and leading to considerable economy of time.

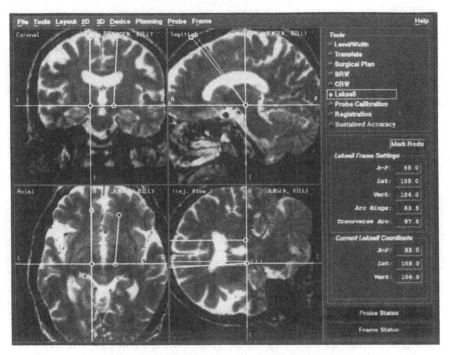

FIGURE 3 Screen from image-guided navigational workstation showing the use of trajectory views to view the course of an implanted electrode following trajectory planning. Only in the "trajectory view" is the entire course of the electrode "in plane."

3.2 Target Localization

After fiducial localization, the potential stereotactic target is calculated. In many instances, the target is calculated in relation to the intercommissural line (ICL) using standard formulas as pioneered by Talairach [7]. Previously, calculations required that the base ring lie parallel to the ICL to prevent geometric errors in projecting distances perpendicular to the ICL (or the use of complicated geometric calculations). This was accomplished by careful placement of the frame on the patient's head in relation to external landmarks or repositioning of the frame after a sagittal scout. Computer-assisted image guidance obviates this step by allowing reformation of the 3D imaging volume in a plane parallel to the ICL (Fig. 1). Once the anterior commissure and posterior commissure are marked, the image set is automatically corrected for tilt and rotation. The midline is manually identified at three points, and the software then automatically corrects for twist errors.

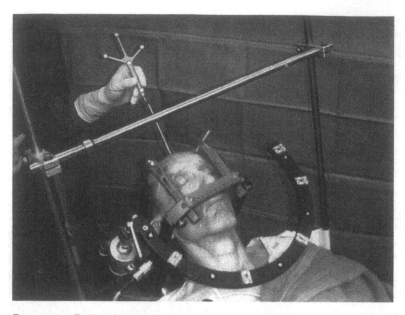

FIGURE 4 Following registration of the Leksell™ base ring to the arc of the Stealth™ frameless stereotactic system, using Framelink® software, the coordinates in frame-space of any point on the patients skull can be instantly determined. This might be used, for example, when you want to plan a trajectory that enters through a patient's previous burr hole.

In movement disorder procedures, target identification usually takes place using either coordinates referential to the ICL, or through the use of coregistered brain atlases (Schaltenbrand and Wahren) [8]. The Stealth-Station software facilitates the use of either method. Formulaic target co-ordinates based on the ICL are preprogrammed, yet modifiable (Fig. 2). The correction of tilt, twist, and rotation of the ICL allows rapid adjustments in relation to the ICL, such as choosing a point that is at the same anterior/posterior and vertical position as that generated by a formula, but that is more lateral or medial in relation to the ICL. Additionally, a fully deformable Schaltenbrand and Wahren atlas resides in the operating software for direct overlay upon axial images, if atlas coregistration is the preferred technique. Of course, a combination approach, or one incorporating direct anatomical targeting (as, for example, of the STN), is easily accommodated. Furthermore, as all axial images are available in the volumetric space, choice of multiple targets in different axial planes is easily done, even in the operating room.

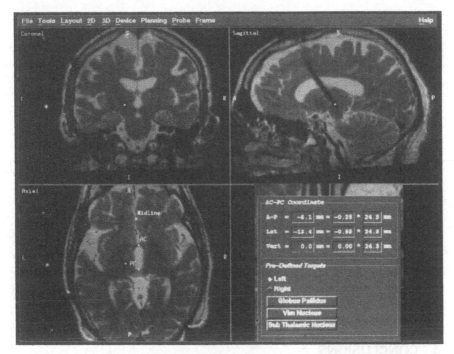

FIGURE 5 The use of the image-guided surgery software to determine the precise location of an implanted DBS lead postoperatively, in relation to the intercommissural line (lower right). In this case, rather than using the "pre-defined targets" function, the cursor was positioned over the tip of the electrode, and the relationship of this point to the intercommissural (AC-PC) line is calculated (under "AC-PC coordinates").

3.3 Trajectory Planning

Once a target is selected, entry points can be determined. Here again computer-assisted image guidance allows a great deal of flexibility in surgical planning. Entry points can be determined preoperatively based on constraints such as the location of sutures, blood vessels, sulci, and ventricles. Moreover, a trajectory that will lead to a particular orientation of a deep brain stimulation (DBS) lead within a target structure can be chosen (for example, double oblique orientation to match that of the STN). The pathway from the entry to the target can be examined in detail using the "planned pathway" or "probe's eye view" options, allowing virtual surgery before the patient is taken to the operating room (Fig. 3).

Entry points constrained by pre-existing scars or burr holes can be determined in the operating room using the Framelink®, which allows the registration of the stereotactic frame to the optic digitizer. The stereotactic coordinates of the frameless pointer are instantly calculated and then easily used in trajectory planning (Fig. 4).

3.4 Intraoperative Use

Frame coordinates corresponding to the desired trajectories are instantly calculated and displayed, allowing trajectory revision to proceed quickly. The Framelink® feature allows the procession of a microelectrode to be tracked as it is introduced into the target structure and projected onto the preoperative image set. The results of micro- or macroelectrode recording and stimulation can be annotated onto the surgical plan to aid in choosing further trajectories. Mirror-imaging of a trajectory from one side to the other is also easily accomplished, as the reformatted dataset is parallel to the ICL. The final position of lesions or implanted deep brain stimulator leads can be saved for comparison to coregistered postoperative image sets (Fig. 5) to confirm the stereotactic accuracy of the implantation or lesion procedure.

4 CONCLUSIONS

Computer-assisted image-guidance systems have the ability to simplify and streamline surgical planning and execution, and accommodate a number of different approaches to stereotactic targeting in movement disorder surgery. The StealthStation is equipped with optical digitizers to allow "frameless" stereotaxy; however, we continue to use rigid frame fixation at our institution to achieve the highest accuracy possible. The StealthStation has reliably allowed safe trajectories to be planned and executed. Lesion and DBS electrode placement have been found to correlate well with planned target locations.

REFERENCES

1. R Meyers. The modification of alternating tremors, rigidity and festination by surgery of the basal ganglia. Res Publ Ass Res Nerve Ment Dis 21:602–665, 1942.
2. EA Spiegel, HT Wycis, M Marks, AJ Lee. Stereotaxic apparatus for operations on the human brain. Science 106:349–350, 1947.
3. J Talairach, H Hecaen, M David, M Monnier, J Ajuriaguerra. Recherches sur la coagulation therapeutique des structures souscorticales chez l'homme. Rev Neurol 91:4–24, 1949.

4. L Leksell. A stereotaxic apparatus for intracerebral surgery. Acta Chir Scand 99: 229–233, 1949.
5. RA Brown, TS Roberts, AG Osborn. Stereotaxic frame and computer software for CT-directed neurosurgical localization. Invest Radiol 15:308–312, 1980.
6. M Kaus, R Steinmeier, T Sporer, O Ganslandt, R Fahlbusch. Technical accuracy of a neuronavigation system measured with a high-precision mechanical micromanipulator. Neurosurgery 41:1431–1436, 1997.
7. J Talairach, M David, P Tournoux, H Corrodor, T Kasina. Atlas d'anatomie stereotaxique. Paris: Masson, 1957.
8. G Schaltenbrand, P Bailey. Introduction to stereotaxis with an atlas of the human brain. Stuttgart: Georg Theme Verlag, 1959.

29

Movement Disorder Surgery with the Leksell System

Ron L. Alterman

The Hyman-Newman Institute for Neurology and Neurosurgery, Beth Israel Medical Center–Singer Division, New York, New York, U.S.A.

1 INTRODUCTION

Lars Leksell introduced his first stereotactic frame in 1949 [1]. Despite numerous modifications over the intervening years, the design and function of the Leksell frame continues to be based on the arc-centered principle [2]. Arc-centered frames position the surgical target in the center of an operating arc. So positioned, the target can be reached from any entry point, as long as the surgical probe is advanced the distance of the radius. This simple yet effective design provides versatility, ease of use, and great accuracy.

The most current Leksell frame, the Model G, is compatible with both magnetic resonance imaging (MRI) and computerized tomography (CT). The G frame may be used for image-guided biopsy or tumor resection, radiosurgery with the Gamma Knife, or so-called "functional" neurosurgical procedures. This chapter discusses the use of the Leksell Model G Frame for performing movement disorder surgery. Space limitations restrict the discussion to a description of the author's technique for performing MRI-guided neuroablative and deep brain stimulation (DBS) procedures. An understanding of the basic use of the Leksell frame is assumed. The uninitiated are referred to a previously published textbook chapter [2] that more fully describes the Leksell system, and the Model G instruction manual, which can be obtained from the manufacturer (Elekta Instruments, Inc., Atlanta, Georgia).

2 TECHNIQUE FOR MOVEMENT DISORDER SURGERY

Ideally, movement disorder patients are awake during surgery to facilitate microelectrode recording (MER) and to permit constant monitoring of the patient's neurological status. If the patient has Parkinson's disease (PD), antiparkinsonian medications are withheld, beginning 12 hours before surgery, also to facilitate MER and to permit assessment of the patient's response to stimulation, ablation, or both. Cessation of levodopa/carbidopa preparations may lead to rebound hypertension, and it is essential that the anesthesiologist maintains strict blood pressure control, keeping the systolic pressure less than 140 mm Hg, to minimize the risk of intracerebral hemorrhage.

2.1 Frame Application

The importance of careful frame application to the success of functional neurosurgical procedures (especially if one foregoes the assistance of an independent stereotactic targeting workstation) is often underestimated. Targeting adjustments are most easily made when the axial targeting images run parallel to the intercommissural (IC) plane and when there is no sideward tilt (roll) or rotation of the frame relative to the head (yaw). Only when the frame is positioned in this manner do adjustments to one frame coordinate translate into anatomical adjustments exclusively in that direction. The ear bars provided with the fame assist greatly toward this end by holding the frame steady relative to the head until it is fixed in place with the skull pins. The ear bars are uncomfortable and the inner ear is difficult to anesthetize; however, the discomfort lasts only for the brief period required to apply the frame (5 to 10 minutes) and is tolerated by most patients. Patients with low pain tolerances or significant head tremor are sedated with propofol for this stage of the procedure.

When targeting with MRI, it is best to use the lowermost pair of holes provided for the ear bars, as this elevates the frame as much as possible from the shoulders, allowing room for the bulky MRI adapter. In addition, skull pins should be selected whose lengths do not extend beyond the margins of the MRI fiducial box. Pins that extend beyond this border may prevent the frame from fitting within the head coil. The manufacturer sells a set of reusable MRI-compatible pins of varying lengths to address this need.

Finally, the frame should be fixed to the head so that the lateral bars of the base ring (i.e., the Y-axis) are parallel to the zygoma, the anteroposterior (AP) angle of which closely approximates that of the IC line. Many human stereotactic atlases employ the IC plane as the central median to which the deep brain structures are related. Therefore, by affixing the frame parallel to the IC line, the acquired axial images will run parallel to the IC plane, and atlas-derived measurements may be more reliably used for MRI-based targeting. Figure 1 demonstrates proper fixation of the Leksell frame.

2.2 The Targeting MRI

The MRI fiducial box and MRI adapter are attached to the frame, and the head is scanned with the frame aligned orthogonal to the scanner axis. A midsagittal T1-weighted MRI is performed and the IC distance is measured. Contiguous 3-mm thick, axial fast spin echo/inversion recovery (FSE/IR)

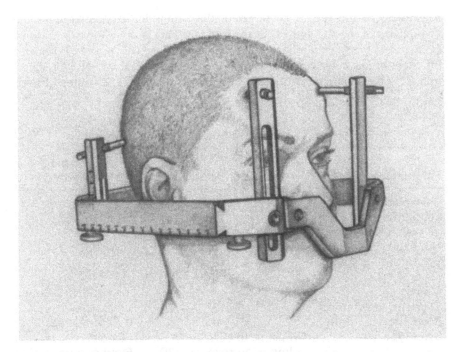

FIGURE 1 Application of the Head Frame. The head frame is secured to the skull with fixation screws at four points. The head is centered in the frame and the frame is aligned in the anteroposterior direction with the zygoma, approximating the angle of the intercommissural plane.

images (Table 1) are obtained through the region of the IC plane. These images beautifully display the deep brain structures and are reported to resist distortion secondary to the magnetic susceptibility effect [3]. After image acquisition, the "inverse video" function generates the image used for targeting (Fig. 2). If the frame is applied correctly, the anterior and posterior commissures (AC and PC, respectively) will be visible on the same or adjacent slices.

The distances between the posterior and middle fiducial markers on the lateral localizing plates are measured to confirm that the axial slices are, in fact, orthogonal to the vertical axis of the frame. The difference between these distances should be no more than 2 mm. If the difference is greater than 2 mm, purely transverse images are not being obtained and the frame should be repositioned in the scanner.

2.3 Determining the Stereotactic Coordinates of the Surgical Target

Regardless of the site to be targeted, the author initially determines the coordinates of the AC and PC at the midline. This is done for two reasons: (1) to assess the degree of head rotation relative to the frame, and (2) because the stereotactic coordinates of functional neurosurgical targets are determined by their known relationship to the commissures. The degree of head

TABLE 1   MRI Scanning Parameters for Stereotactic Targeting

Parameter	Inversion recovery	Coronal T2-weighted
Relaxation time (T_R)	4000	4000
Echo time (T_E)	17	102
Inversion time (T_I)	140	N/A
No. excitations	2	3
Echo train length	8	12
Field of view	24 cm	24 cm
Matrix	256 × 192	256 × 256
Slice thickness (mm)	3	2
Slice interval (mm)	0	0 (interleaved)
Scan type	Fast scan	Fast scan
	Inversion recovery, 2D	Flow compensation

Magnetic resonance image scanning parameters for stereotactic targeting for functional neurosurgical procedures. Scans are performed on a General Electric Echo Speed Scanner (1.5 Tesla).

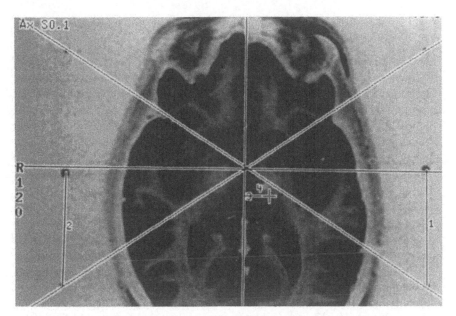

FIGURE 2   Fast Spin Echo/Inversion Recovery Magnetic Resonance Imaging. Axial image at the level of the intercommissural plane demonstrating targeting of the ventrolateral (VL) nucleus of the thalamus. Diagonals connecting the opposing anterior and posterior fiducial markers have been constructed to define the center of the targeting area. Anterior/posterior and right/left axes (Y and X axes, respectively) have been constructed with their origins at the center point. The difference in the distance between the posterior and center fiducial markers on either side of the head (segments 1 and 2) is less than 2 mm. The VL target is 5 mm anterior to and 14 mm lateral to the center point of the posterior commissure, which is clearly visualized.

rotation relative to the frame is represented by the inverse tangent of the difference in the X values of the AC and PC divided by the IC distance

Degree of Rotation = Tan^{-1} ($|\Delta X_{AC\text{-}PC}|$/IC distance

When the frame is properly affixed, $\Delta X_{AC\text{-}PC}$ is negligible (≤ 2 mm).

Once the coordinates of the commissures have been determined, the coordinates of the surgical target are calculated based on the anatomical relationship of the target to the IC plane, as documented in various publications [4–9] and atlases of the human brain.

2.3.1 Targeting the Ventral Lateral Nucleus for Medically Refractory Tremor

The ventral lateral (VL) nucleus can be targeted exclusively with axial FSE/IR images when performing thalamotomy or thalamic DBS lead insertions. The image that best demonstrates the PC is selected. The target for tremor suppression is located 20% to 25% of the IC distance anterior to the PC (typically 5 to 6 mm), and 2 to 3 mm dorsal to the IC plane [4–6]. Target laterality (i.e., the X coordinate) is selected according to the body part that is to be treated. The ventrolateral nucleus of the thalamus is somatotopically organized, medio laterally [4], such that the face is represented medially (10–12 mm lateral of midline), the hand just lateral to the face (13–15 mm), and the leg/foot most lateral, abutting the internal capsule (14–17 mm). The third ventricular and thalamic widths also influence target laterality. When a wide third ventricle is encountered (i.e., >5 mm), laterality should be measured from the ipsilateral wall of the third ventricle and not the midline.

After determining the coordinates for the PC, the target coordinates are calculated as follows:

$X_{VL} = X_{PC} \pm$ 10–17 mm (subtract for a right-sided target; add for left)

$Y_{VL} = Y_{PC} +$ 5 (or 6) mm

$Z_{VL} = Z_{PC}$

Even though the VL target is most commonly located 2 to 3 mm superior to the ventral border of the thalamus [4], the author targets to the depth of the PC to ensure that the surgical trajectory will pass completely through VL. The final depth for lesion or DBS lead placement is based on intraoperative neurophysiology.

2.3.2 Targeting Globus Pallidus Pars Internus (GPi)

The pallidum may also be targeted exclusively with axial FSE/IR images, except that the coordinates for GPi are calculated relative to the mid-commissural point (MCP), the coordinates of which are determined by calculating the means of the coordinates of the commissures. The coordinates for the posteroventral globus pallidus pars internus (GPi) (as originally described by Leksell [7]) are then calculated as follows:

$X_{GPi} = X_{MCP} \pm$ 18–22 mm (subtract for a right-sided placement; add for left)

$Y_{GPi} = Y_{MCP} +$ 2 mm

$GPi = Z_{MCP} +$ 4 mm (i.e. ventral to the IC plane)

When targeting Gpi, one may also obtain coronal T2-weighted or FSE/IR images to examine target depth relative to the optic tract, which lies immediately inferior to GPi.

2.3.3 Targeting Subthalamic Nucleus for Parkinson's Disease

Unlike the thalamus and globus pallidus, the STN is poorly visualized on FSE/IR images; however, the coordinates for STN can be reliably calculated from its relationship with the MCP [9]. Alternatively, the STN may be visualized (although inconsistently), and directly targeted, on thin-cut coronal T2-weighted images (Table 1). Consult the Leksell G Frame manual for instructions on determining target coordinates from coronal MRI.

The coordinates for STN relative to the MCP are calculated as follows:

$$X_{STN} = X_{MCP} \pm 12 \text{ mm (subtract for a right-sided placement;}$$
$$\text{add for left)}$$
$$Y_{STN} = Y_{MCP} - 2 \text{ mm}$$
$$Z_{STN} = Z_{MCP} + 6 \text{ mm (base of STN).}$$

2.4 Operative Technique

After image acquisition and surgical planning, the patient is taken to the operating room and positioned supine on the operating table, which is configured as a reclining chair. The head is immobilized and prepped with bctadine, and the field is sterilely draped.

The MRI-derived coordinates and the surgical trajectory are set on the frame. When targeting VL thalamus or STN, the AP angle of approach is 60° to 70° relative to the IC plane, as this approximates the angle of the ventral intermediate nucleus (the subdivision of VL that is targeted for tremor control) of the STN relative to the IC line. An AP angle of 50° to 60° is used for pallidal procedures. Ideally, the lateral angle of approach for all of these procedures would be 90° (i.e., directly vertical), as this would generate a pure parasagittal trajectory, allowing intraoperative neurophysiological data to be most easily correlated to the parasagittal sections provided in human stereotactic atlases. Moreover, because the somatotopic representation of the contralateral hemibody in the thalamus is oriented in a medial to lateral direction, a pure parasagittal trajectory reduces the risk of crossing representational anatomical planes during a single recording trajectory. Unfortunately, medial trajectories to medial targets such as VL thalamus or STN pass through the ipsilateral lateral ventricle, posing a risk of intraventricular hemorrhage. Therefore, lateral angles that are 5° to 10° lateral of 90° are typically used.

The arc is used to mark the desired entry point on the frontal scalp, anterior to the coronal suture and 2 to 3 cm lateral of the midline. Lidocaine (1%) is administered for local anesthesia. After skin incision and hemostasis, a self-retaining retractor is inserted. A skull perforator (Codman, Inc., Raynham, Massachusetts) is used to make a 14-mm burr hole centered on the entry point. The dura is coagulated and incised in a cruciate fashion.

The author uses a combination of MER and macroelectrode stimulation to physiologically refine the anatomically selected target. The details of micro- and semimicroelectrode recording, as well as macroelectrode stimulation for target localization in the thalamus [4–6, 10], globus pallidus [8,11,12], and subthalamic nucleus [13] have been published elsewhere and are beyond the scope of this report. Once proper targeting is confirmed physiologically, the frame is set up for lesioning or DBS lead insertion.

When performing a neuroablation, the lesioning electrode (Radionics, Inc., Burlington, Massachusetts) is inserted to the physiologically defined

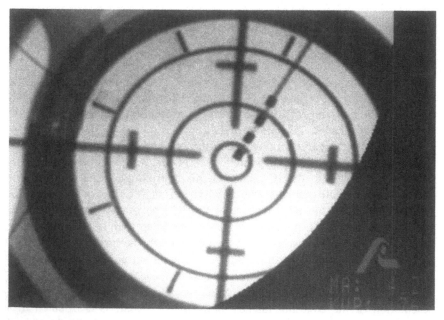

FIGURE 3 DBS Lead Placement. The deep brain stimulation lead is inserted under C-arm fluoroscopic guidance. The circles and cross-hairs are aligned so that a pure lateral image, centered on the target point, is generated.

target and the lesion is made. When ablating GPi, the author performs 4 to 5 lesions along a single trajectory as defined by MER [8]. Thalamotomy lesions are placed at that site where high frequency stimulation (i.e., >130 Hz) arrests tremor without persistent dysesthesia.

Deep brain stimulating leads are inserted under C-arm fluoroscopic guidance (Fig. 3). The manufacturer sells "bomb sites" (i.e., circles and cross hairs) that snap into the rings of the frame and allow the surgeon to generate pure lateral fluoroscopic images that are centered on the frame's target point. When proper placement is confirmed fluoroscopically, the DBS lead is secured at the level of the skull with a burr hole "cap" that is provided with the lead (Model 3387 or 3389, Medtronics, Inc., Minneapolis, Minnesota). The excess lead is encircled around the cap in the subgaleal space. The incision is irrigated with bacitracin saline and closed in a standard fashion.

A postoperative MRI is obtained before proceeding with implantation of the pulse generator. The MRI confirms proper lead placement and demonstrates any hemorrhage related to surgery. If a hemorrhage is found, pulse generator implantation, which is performed under general anesthesia, is delayed. All patients are observed in the neurosurgical observation unit during the evening after lead insertion or neuroablation. Most patients are discharged within 1 or 2 days of surgery.

REFERENCES

1. L Leksell. A stereotaxic apparatus for intracerebral surgery. Acta Chir Scand 99:229–233, 1949.
2. LD Lunsford, D Kondziolka, D Leksell. The Leksell stereotactic system. In: PL Gildenberg, RR Tasker, eds. Textbook of Stereotactic and Functional Neurosurgery. New York: McGraw-Hill, 1998, pp 51–63.
3. Taren JA, Ross DA, Gebarski SS. Stereotactic localization using fast spin-echo imaging in functional disorders. Acta Neurochir Suppl 58:59–60, 1993.
4. PJ Kelly. Contemporary stereotactic ventralis lateral thalamotomy in the treatment of Parkinsonian tremor and other movement disorders. In: MP Heilbrun, ed. Stereotactic Neurosurgery. Baltimore: Williams and Wilkins, 1988, pp 133–148.
5. RAE Bakay, JL Vitek, MR DeLong. Thalamotomy for tremor. In: SS Rengechary, RR Wilkins, eds. Neurosurgical Operative Atlas, Vol 2. Park Ridge, Illinois: American Association of Neurological Surgeons, 1992, pp 299–312.
6. A Lozano. Thalamic deep brain stimulation for the control of tremor. In: SS Rengechary, RR Wilkins, eds. Neurosurgical Operative Atlas, Vol. 7. Park Ridge, Illinois: American Association of Neurological Surgeons, 1998, pp 125–134.

7. E Svennilson, A Torvik, R Lowe, L Leksell. Treatment of parkinsonism by stereotactic thermolesions in the pallidal region. Acta Psychiatr Neurol Scand 35:358–377, 1960.

8. Alterman RL, Sterio D, Beric A, Kelly PJ. Microelectrode recording during posteroventral pallidotomy: Impact on target selection and complications. Neurosurgery 44:315–323, 1999.

9. Starr PA, Vitek JL, DeLong M, Bakay RAE. Magnetic resonance imaging-based stereotactic localization of the globus pallidus and subthalamic nucleus. Neurosurgery 44:303–314, 1999.

10. JO Dostrovsky, KD Davis, L Lee, GD Sher, RR Tasker. Electrical stimulation-induced effects in the human thalamus. In: O Devinsky, A Beric, M Dogali, eds. Electrical and Magnetic Stimulation of the Brain and Spinal Cord. New York: Raven Press, 1993, pp 219–229.

11. A Lozano, W Hutchison, Z Kiss, R Tasker, K Davis, J Dostrovsky. Methods for microelectrode-guided posteroventral pallidotomy. J Neurosurg 84:194–202, 1996.

12. A Beric, D Sterio, M Dogali, R Alterman, P Kelly. Electrical stimulation of the globus pallidus preceding stereotactic posteroventral pallidotomy. Stereotact Funct Neurosurg 66:161–169, 1996.

13. WD Hutchinson, RJ Allan, H Opitz, R Levy, JO Dostrovsky, AE Lang, AM Lozano. Neurophysiologic identification of the subthalamic nucleus in surgery for Parkinson's disease. Ann Neurol 44:622–628, 1998.

30

Movement Disorders Surgery Using the Zamorano-Dujovny Localizing System

Lucía Zamorano and Ramiro A. Pérez de la Torre
Wayne State University, Detroit, Michigan, U.S.A.

1 INTRODUCTION

Movement disorders include essential tremor, chorea, dystonias, and all clinical forms of Parkinson's syndrome. Because of the prevalence of Parkinson's as compared to other movement disorders, as well as its particular neurological consequences, in this chapter we will focus mainly on stereotactic surgical management of Parkinson's disease. Surgical strategies include ablative procedures, such as thalamotomy or pallidotomy; nonablative procedures, such as deep brain stimulation to the ventral intermediate nucleus (VIM), internal globus pallidus (Gpi), and subthalamic nucleus (STN), and neurologically restorative procedures such as brain tissue transplants. We will focus on the first two types.

Stereotactic localizing systems contribute in crucial ways to the surgical options, defining a specific target for the lesioning probe or deep brain stimulator placement, and, just as importantly, help the neurosurgeon avoid critical neurological structures during surgical treatment.

Conceptually, the Zamorano Dujovny (Z-D) stereotactic unit is an arc-centered frame with a carbon fiber base ring as a reference system and a localizer arc. The localizer unit consists of an arc quadrant with three linear scales (a, b, c) and two angular scales (d and e). The first three correspond to the traditional x, y and z axes. The last two (d and e) define the trajectory of the probe.

The carbon fiber head frame, or ring, is placed on the patient and secured in place with pins of varying lengths, depending on ring position. (For an in-depth discussion of ring fixation, please see the chapter titled "Stereotactic Surgery with the Zamorano-Dujovny Frame"). The pins are fixed and secured under local anesthesia with 1% lidocaine and marcaine. The patient's vital signs are monitored, an intravenous line is placed, and supplementary oxygen is provided for the procedure. The head is positioned such that the ring is parallel to the anterior-posterior commissure line (AC-PC line).

2 IMAGE ACQUISITION

Computed tomographic (CT) scans and magnetic resonance imaging (MRI) not only provide clear visualization of the target point, but using a fusion protocol, in which the CT-MRI scans are correlated, provides a comprehensive map of the patient's brain anatomy. In particular, an MRI will show the basal ganglia and the subthalamic nucleus in exquisite detail, which greatly facilitates the preoperative planning process.

2.1 MRI with the Z-D Frame and Localizer

The Z-D frame can be used along with the specific localizer for MRI image acquisition. It is extremely important to generate images parallel to the AC-PC line for use in the planning process. In almost all cases, we recommend CT and MRI scans for image correlation, using skin fiducial markers (IZI Medical Products, Baltimore, Maryland) in several locations on the scalp. The initial step includes taking a T_1-weighted sagittal scout to identify both anterior and posterior commissures and to obtain axial images parallel to that line. A post-contrast CT is taken in 2-mm slice thickness, aligning the gantry to the top of the frame to generate axial parallel images. The image datasets are transferred to the operating room's computer suite through the hospital's network to be used in the planning process.

2.2 MRI Sequences

The specific imaging sequences include post-gadolinium T_1-weighted 2-mm axial and coronal views, and T_2-weighted 2-mm coronal views along with T_1-inversion recovery sequence, axial and coronal. Inversion recovery and

T$_2$-coronals are especially useful for locating the STN, and inversion recovery is extremely helpful for delineating the Gpi.

2.3 MRI and Atlas Fusion

Image processing software is required during the preplanning process to fuse the CT and MRI scans. The ideal software program calibrates an individual patient's imaging studies to three standard neurosurgical atlases, the Talairach, Schaltenbrand, and Watkins, and "warps" the atlases until they reflect the patient's anatomy (Fig. 1). There are nomograms to correct for individual variations in anatomy. This set of images can then be plugged into any or all of several surgical planning modules that provide for comprehensive planning of trajectories, designed to optimize the intervention and minimize damage to uninvolved tissue.

3 PLANNING

Without doubt, target localization is the most important step in movement disorders surgery, the goal of which is to lesion the brain as effectively as

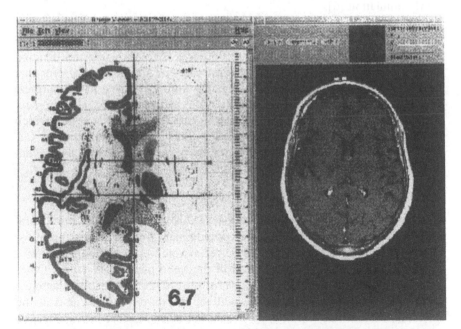

FIGURE 1 Neurological Surgery Planning System (NSPS) functional surgery module showing the correlation between the patient's anatomical imaging study and the Schaltenbrand's stereotactic atlas.

possible or for stimulator placement. There are three methods for target localization: direct and indirect, which are image-guided localizations, and physiological, which includes microelectrode recording, macrostimulation, or both.

3.1   Target Localization (Anatomical)

Target selection depends on the surgeon's preferred surgical method and chosen treatment option. The target site is always contralateral to the predominant symptoms [1]. There are three possible targets for Parkinson's disease, depending on the predominant symptomatology: the motor thalamus, Gpi, and STN [2]. All these structures may be localized indirectly by measuring fixed distances from well-known anatomical structures, such as the internal capsule, third ventricle, the optic tract, or the posterior commissure [3,4].

The VIM of the thalamus [5,6] is the preferred target for thalamotomy, and the internal segment of the Gpi for pallidotomy [7,8]. Subthalamic nucleus stimulation effectively controls contralateral limb tremor in patients with Parkinson's disease, with a success rate similar to that achieved with VIM stimulation [5].

3.1.1   Direct and Indirect Targeting

The direct method of targeting the lesion area involves using the imaging studies to localize the target and generate the specific coordinates for that target. However, *indirect targeting* is more commonly used in the surgical treatment of Parkinson's disease. Basically, all indirect methods rely on measurements taken from the AC-PC line to locate the structures within which lesioning occurs. The imaging modalities include ventriculography, CT, MRI, and fusion CT-MRI. Ventriculography is rarely used since the advent of CT and MRI scans.

3.1.2   VIM, Gpi, and STN Localization

Our suggested target for lesioning at the VIM is located 12 to 17 mm lateral to the midline, 12 to 14 mm for face predominant tremor, 14 to 15 mm for upper extremities, 15 to 17 mm for lower extremities, 4 to 5 mm posterior to the midpoint of AC-PC plane and in the same plane of that line. Other techniques localize the VIM with 25% of the AC-PC distance and anterior to the PC, 11.5 mm lateral to the wall of the third ventricle, and at the intercommissural line [5].

The Gpi is located 18 to 21 mm lateral to the midline of the third ventricle, 2 to 3 mm anterior to the midpoint AC-PC line, and 5 mm below the intercommissural line [9]. The suggested target for the STN is 10 to 12 mm lateral to the third ventricle, 3 to 4 mm posterior to the midpoint AC-PC, and 3 to 4 mm inferior to that line.

4 PHYSIOLOGICAL LOCALIZATION

We strongly encourage electrophysiological monitoring for more accurate delineation of the boundaries of these structures, but anatomical measurements, such as described above, still play a very important role in this surgery.

4.1 Microrecording and Microstimulation

For target localization we start with microrecording. The Z-D frame localizing unit has an adapter for the microdrive. The specific microelectrode is gradually advanced through a guiding cannula until it reaches 20 mm above the level of the desired target (Fig. 2). The microelectrode is connected by short leads to a preamplifier, which increases the signal-to-noise ratio. The signal from the preamplifier is then filtered, amplified, and passed through

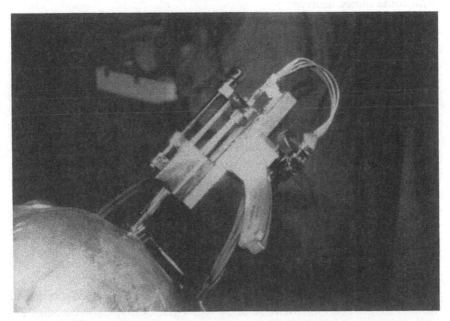

FIGURE 2 Microdrive mounted in the localizing unit of the Zamorano Dujovny (Z-D) frame. The neurosurgeon can change the position of the microelectrode intraoperatively.

a discriminator. The window discriminator is an electronic device that converts action potentials to digital pulses. These digital pulses can then be stored and analyzed off-line. In addition, these pulses can be converted to an audio signal, which is useful for listening to the activity of cells without interference from background neuronal sounds.

4.1.1 Electrophysiological Monitoring in VIM

Once we reach 20 mm above the target, the microelectrode is gradually advanced to record neuronal activity. For the most part, there is a good demarcation between the white matter and the top of the thalamus. The projected extension of the VIM in this place is approximately 11 mm from top to bottom. It is very important to proceed in 2-mm increments until the desired wave form and frequency corresponding to the target has been reached. Rostrally to the ventral caudal (VC) nucleus, the VIM is detected by its moderate high amplitude, noisy behavior, and its kinesthetic response to passive movement of the extremities, again with somatotopic representation with lips and head at the medial edge and lower extremities to the internal capsule. More rostrally there is the ventralis oralis anterior (VOA) and ventralis oralis posterior (VOP) nuclei with tactile neurons intermingled with some motor neurons.

To confirm the location, we proceed with microstimulation through the same microelectrode. The patient should report shock-like sensations in different parts of the body that represent the humunculus of the area. The microdrive allows us to change the location of the microelectrode. The parameters are 0.3 to 1.0 mA, 60 to 100 Hz. Any mismatching in this monitoring mandates repositioning of the microelectrode.

4.1.2 Electrophysiological Recording in Gpi

During pallidotomy, recordings usually proceed from the putamen and external globus pallidus (Gpe) through the Gpi and then close to the optic tract. Neurons in the Gpi of Parkinson's patients have a higher baseline firing rate than neurons in the Gpe (mean 80 Hz). Most commonly, Gpi neurons respond to contralateral movements with an increase in firing rate. In addition, some neurons have been found that respond in synchrony with the patient's tremor.

4.1.3 Recording in the Subthalamus Nucleus

In this region, background noise is high and individual cells are difficult to isolate. Single neurons discharge at 20 to 30 Hz, but typical recordings are of multiple cells, and therefore the discharge frequency is higher. As the microelectrode passes through the inferior border of the STN into the substantia nigra reticulata (SNR), the discharge pattern changes abruptly. The medial and lateral borders of the STN, formed by the lemniscal and corticospinal fibers, are respectively identified by microstimulation-evoked sensory and motor responses [3].

4.2 Macrostimulation

We recommend confirming the location of the target with macrostimulation using the standard stimulator (Neuro50, F. L. Fischer Leibinger, Freiburg, Germany), given the fact that the mere introduction of the needle generates microsignals that can be somewhat confusing. The setup parameters of the stimulator are square waves of 2 to 100 Hz, 1 to 10 mV, 1 ms of duration. Once the accuracy of the target has been confirmed, we proceed with permanent lesioning. In the case of deep brain stimulation, the permanent electrode is left in place and secured, and the corresponding protocol is followed.

5 PROCEDURES

5.1 Ablative Procedures (Lesioning)

When the patient is fitted with the Z-D head ring, given sedation, and the imaging studies are completed, as mentioned previously, he or she is transferred to a preoperative holding area for anesthetic evaluation (the patient's heart rate, blood pressure, and oxygen saturation are continually monitored). Thalamotomics and pallidotomies are usually performed under local anesthesia so that the patient can participate during treatment by performing specific tasks relative to the type of procedure selected.

The setup of the operating suite is crucial to maintaining maximum feedback between the patient and surgical team. Anesthesia staff are positioned on the contralateral side of the surgical approach to be able to monitor the clinical status. The patient is placed in supine position, same as in the imaging scans, to prevent any target shifting. The head is attached to the Mayfield headholder in neutral position. Padding is provided to protect pressure points. Oxygen supply is maintained throughout the procedure to keep optimal saturation levels. Dexamethasone is given intraoperatively along with cefazolin. We avoid mannitol and furosemide because of the possibility of brain shift causing a loss of stereotactic accuracy, especially in these very small targets. A urinary catheter is placed along with an intravenous central line. Shaving is done only in a 4-cm diameter area on the site of the coronal suture.

The localizing arc, along with the instrument carrier, is mounted on the frame to define the entry point on the scalp, selected in the planning process. A small linear incision opens the scalp to the bone, and a burr hole is made to expose the dura mater. This is opened in ordinary fashion, to initiate the electrophysiological monitoring. The final corroboration of the patient's target is the clinical assessment of sensory, motor, and speech areas. The neuropsychologist evaluating the patient must have a comprehensive understanding of complex sensory and speech processing functions. Certain tasks like complex linguistic expressions are encouraged to evaluate the speech apparatus. If the clinical examination excludes potential risk, the next step is permanent lesioning or deep brain stimulator placement. There are a variety of lesioning methods. Because of its reproducibility and precision, radiofrequency is the preferred choice in most medical centers. Once the target is selected, lesioning is subsequently performed using the Neuro50. The usual parameters we follow are 60°C for 60 seconds, three times.

Afterwards, the electrode is withdrawn, and dura covered with Gelfoam. The incision is closed with Vicryl and nylon sutures. The patient is given dexamethasone 10 mg postoperatively every 6 hours, along with antiparkinsonian agents within 24 hours postoperatively, to evaluate the patient before he is discharged from the hospital. An MRI with T_1-, T_2-, and proton densities is done the same day to confirm the lesion location.

6 FOLLOW-UP

Parkinsonian patients are clinically evaluated every 3 months using the Parkinson's clinical scales along with an MRI, usually performed in 6-month intervals. Radiologically, lesioning appears as a hollow space in the target location. Perilesional brain edema around the target is very often observed and implies postgliotic changes. Long-term follow-up is, in fact, recommended for staged bilateral procedures.

7 SUMMARY

The versatility of the Z-D stereotactic frame makes it a suitable system for surgery of patients with movement disorders. The frame is stable enough to support microelectrode recording and to allow passage of lesioning electrodes and is compatible with the Medtronic DBS system. As other techniques, such as transplantation, become available, we anticipate that the Z-D frame will remain an excellent choice for functional neurosurgeons.

ACKNOWLEDGMENT

We wish to extend our gratitude to Julie Bedore for her patience and continued support.

REFERENCES

1. Benabid A, Pollak P, Gao D, Hoffman D, Limousin, Gay E, Payen I, Benazzouz A. Chronic electrical stimulation of the ventralis intermedius nucleus of the thalamus as a treatment of movement disorders. J Neurosurg 84:203–214, 1996.
2. Starr P, Vitek J, Bakay R. Deep brain stimulation for movement disorders. Neurosurg Clin N Am 9:381–402, 1998.
3. Starr P, Vitek J, Bakay R. Ablative surgery and deep brain stimulation for Parkinson's disease. Neurosurgery 43(5):989–1007, 1998.
4. Moriyama E, Beck H, Miyamoto T. Long-term results of ventrolateral thalamotomy for patients with Parkinson's disease. Neurol Med Chir (Tokyo) 39(5): 350–356, 1999.
5. Taha J, Janszon M, Favre J. Thalamic deep brain stimulation for the treatment of head, voice and bilateral limb tremor. J Neurosurg 91:68–72, 1999.
6. Kumar K, Kelly M, Toth C. Deep brain stimulation of the ventral intermediate nucleus of the thalamus for control of tremors in Parkinson's disease and essential tremor. Stereotact Funct Neurosurg 72(1):47–61, 2000.
7. Alterman RL, Kelly PJ. Pallidotomy technique and results: The New York University experience. Neurosurg Clin Am 9(2):337–343, 1998.
8. Sutton JP, Couldwell W, Lew MF, Mallory L, Grafton S, DeGiorgio C, Welsh M, Apuzzo ML, Ahmadi J, Waters CH. Ventroposterior medial pallidotomy in patients with advanced Parkinson's disease. Neurosurgery 36(6):1112–1116, 1995.
9. Laitinen L. Pallidotomy for Parkinson's disease. Neurosurgery Clin N Am 6(1): 105–112, 1995.
10. Benabid A, Pollak P, Hoffman D, Limousin P, Ming D, LeBlas J, Benazzouz A, Segebarth C, Grand S. Chronic stimulation for Parkinson's disease and other movement disorders. In: Gildenberg P, Tasker R, eds. Textbook of Stereotactic and Functional Neurosurgery. New York: McGraw-Hill 1998, pp 1199–1212.
11. Tasker RR. Deep brain stimulation is preferable to thalamotomy for tremor suppression. Surg Neurol 49(2):145–153, 1998.

31

Functional Radiosurgery with the Gamma Knife

Ronald F. Young
Gamma Knife Center, Northwest Hospital, Seattle, Washington, U.S.A.

1 INTRODUCTION

Radiosurgery has been used to treat several functional conditions of the brain. These include (1) chronic pain; (2) trigeminal neuralgia (TN); (3) movement disorders; (4) epilepsy; and (5) psychiatric disorders. With a few minor exceptions, all radiosurgical experience in treating functional disorders has been with the Gamma Knife.

2 CHRONIC PAIN

Chronic pain was among the first conditions treated with the Gamma Knife [1]. In the 1990s, we developed a technique to perform medial thalamotomy using stereotactic magnetic resonance imaging (MRI) localization and the Gamma plan computer dose planning system [2]. The target includes portions of the medial dorsal, intralaminar, center median, and parafascicular thalamic nuclei. Lesions are now made with a single isocenter using the 4-mm secondary collimator helmet of the Gamma Unit and maximum radiosurgical doses of about 140 Gy. These parameters produce, on the average, a spherical lesion of about 90 mm^3 in volume that develops over a period of 3 to 6 months after treatment. Coincident with development of the lesion gradual reduction in chronic pain occurs in the contralateral body and face without any loss of normal sensory function in about two thirds of patients. Nociceptive pain responds better than neuropathic pain to medial thalamotomy. Larger lesions may be made with two or three adjacent isocenters, which results in a higher success rate in terms of pain relief, but also a much higher rate of complications caused by excessively large lesions. We do not recommend multi-isocenter medial thalamotomies any longer.

Radiosurgical cingulotomy or hypophysectomy has been used in a very limited number of patients for treatment of chronic pain with a strong anxiety component or for pain resulting from metastases from prostate or breast cancers.

For cingulotomy, bilateral lesions are made in the cingulum bundle at a point 25 mm posterior to the anterior end of the frontal horns of the lateral ventricles, as determined on stereotactic MRI scans. We have tried both the 4-mm and 8-mm secondary collimator helmets of the Leksell Gamma Unit for making such lesions at various radiosurgical doses. At this point, our experience is not sufficient to make a firm recommendation about radiosurgical dose.

For hypophysectomy, multiple 4-mm isocenters are directed at the anterior pituitary gland. The maximum safe radiosurgical dose is determined by the dose to the optic apparatus, which we believe should generally not exceed 8 Gy.

3 TRIGEMINAL NEURALGIA

Leksell first described radiosurgical treatment of trigeminal neuralgia in 1971 [3]. Our experience now includes more than 450 patients treated for TN with the Gamma Knife [4]. In our treatment protocol, the trigeminal root is identified on axial, coronal, and reconstructed sagittal stereotactic MR images at its point of entry into the pons. Treatment is delivered using the 4-mm secondary collimator helmet of the Gamma Unit. The treatment isocenter is placed over the trigeminal root such that the 50% isodose line is tangential to the pontine surface. A maximum radiosurgical dose of 87 Gy[1] directed to this target results in relief of TN in more than 90% of patients with a latency of 1 day to 6 months after treatment. Long-term follow-up (median 49 months, range 6–108 months) indicates that recurrent pain will reduce the long-term success rate to about 78%. Retreatment of failed initial treatment or recurrences with similar parameters, except for a reduced max-

---

[1] Output factor 0.87 compared with 18-mm collimator output.

imum radiosurgical dose of 45 Gy, will result in pain relief in an additional 80% of patients, for a total relief rate of about 96%. Delayed facial sensory loss has been seen in about 15% of patients and is usually mild or moderate in severity and transient. Permanent, severe loss of facial sensation has been seen in 1% to 2% of treated patients.

For et al. described effective treatment in a series of six patients with severe, uncontrolled cluster headache using a radiosurgical technique identical to that used for the treatment of trigeminal neuralgia [5]. Our limited experience confirms Ford's report. Pollock also reported successful radiosurgical treatment of sphenopalatine neuralgia with the Gamma Knife [6]. Recurrent pain in this patient was successfully treated with a second radiosurgical procedure.

4 MOVEMENT DISORDERS

We have used radiosurgical thalamotomy or pallidotomy to treat the movement disorders of Parkinson's disease, essential tremor, and tremor after stroke, encephalitis, or head injury [7]. For thalamotomy to treat tremor, the target is the ventral intermediate (VIM) thalamic nucleus contralateral to the tremor, which is identified on stereotactic MRI scans. The lesion is created using the 4-mm secondary collimator helmet of the Gamma Unit with a radiosurgical dose maximum of 141 Gy. Tremor is relieved within 6 months of treatment in nearly 90% of patients coincident with development of the thalamotomy lesion. Less than 2% of treated patients have developed side effects from the treatment, such as contralateral sensory loss, weakness, or dysphasia, all of which are usually transient.

Pallidotomy is performed for treatment of bradykinesia, rigidity, and L-dopa induced dyskinesias in patients with Parkinson's disease. The lesion is placed in the internal segment of the globus pallidus (GPi), as identified on stereotactic MRI scans. Lesioning parameters are identical to those for thalamotomy. Short- and long-term follow-up indicates that complete or nearly complete relief of rigidity and bradykinesia was seen in about two thirds of treated patients, with the magnitude of improvement varying from about 20% to 40%. As with radiofrequency pallidotomy, the maximum improvements in rigidity and bradykinesia were seen in the "off state," that is, when the effects of L-dopa were at a minimum. Two patients experienced permanent homonymous hemianiopsias 10 months after pallidotomy. No other complications of any kind were seen.

5 EPILEPSY

Radiosurgical treatment results in marked improvements in the case of so-called "lesional epilepsy" caused by structural lesions, such as tumors or arterior venous malformations. Regis and colleagues have pioneered a Gamma Knife protocol for treatment of nonlesional temporal lobe epilepsy related to mesial temporal sclerosis [8]. Significant reduction in seizure frequency with no significant permanent complications has been reported by Regis' group, but the number of patients so far reported is small and follow-up periods are too limited to make a recommendation about the place of radiosurgery in the surgical treatment of epilepsy.

6 PSYCHONEUROSIS

Kihlstrom et al. described a radiosurgical technique for bilateral anterior capsulotomy for the treatment of obsessive compulsive disorder based on an earlier radiofrequency technique [9]. Once again, the number of patients treated was small and the study was neither randomized nor blinded, so the favorable results are open to question. A cooperative, randomized, prospective study of this technique currently underway at Brown University and Yale University should provide more objective data.

7 SUMMARY

Functional neurosurgery with the Gamma Knife has an established place in the treatment of trigeminal neuralgia. Its role in the treatment of chronic pain and movement disorders is promising, based on preliminary clinical data. Other functional procedures, such as for the treatment of psychoneurosis and epilepsy, should prove amenable to radiosurgical treatment.

REFERENCES

1. Leksell L. Cerebral radiosurgery: Gammathalamotomy in two cases of intractable pain. Acta Chir Scand 134:585–595, 1968.
2. Young RF, Vermeulen SS, Grimm P, Posewitz A. Electrophysiological target localization is not required for the treatment of functional disorders. Stereotact Funct Neurosurg 66(suppl 1):309–319, 1996.
3. Leksell L. Stereotaxic radiosurgery in trigeminal neuralgia. Acta Chir Scand 137:311–314, 1971.
4. Young RF, Vermeulen SS, Grimm P, Blasko J, Posewitz A. Gamma Knife radiosurgery for treatment of trigeminal neuralgia: Idiopathic and tumor related. Neurology 48(3):608–614, 1997.
5. Ford RG, Ford KT, Swaid S, Young P, Jennele R. Gamma Knife treatment of refractory cluster headache. Headache 38(1):3–9, 1998.
6. Pollock BE, Kondziolka D. Stereotactic radiosurgical treatment of sphenopalatine neuralgia. Case report. J Neurosurg 87:450–453, 1997.

7. Young RF, Shumway-Cook A, Vermeulen SS, Grimm P, Blasko J, Posewitz A, Burkhart WA, Goiney RC. Gamma Knife radiosurgery as a lesioning technique in movement disorder surgery. J Neurosurg 89:183–193, 1998.

8. Regis J, Bartolomei F, Metellus P, Rey M, Genton P, Dravet C, Bureau M, Semah F, Gastaut JL, Peragut JC, Chauvel P. Radiosurgery for trigeminal neuralgia and epilepsy. Neurosurg Clin N Am 10:359–377, 1999.

9. Kihlstrom L, Guo W, Lindquist C, Mindus P. Radiobiology of radiosurgery for refractory anxiety disorders. Neurosurgery 36:294–302, 1995.

32

Functional Radiosurgery with a Linac

Robert Smee

Prince of Wales Hospital, Randwick, New South Wales, Australia

1 HISTORY

1.1 Functional Neurosurgery

This concept goes back to 1946 when Spiegal and Wycis treated a patient with Huntington's chorea by injecting alcohol into the globus pallidus and medial thalamus, using their own stereotactic reference system [1]. This provided short-term benefit but enabled the technique to be applied to other functional conditions, such as intractable pain, anxiety, and aggressive disorders, as well as movement disorders.

1.2 Radiosurgery

1.2.1 DXR

The theoretical concept of stereotactic radiation delivery had its genesis in 1951 when Lars Leksell mounted a 280 Kv X-ray source on an arc device so that the source could move along the arc, always being directed at the center of rotation of the arc system (the treatment isocenter) [2]. The first patients treated by this technique had trigeminal neuralgia and the target was the gasserian ganglion.

379

1.2.2   Cyclotron

Leksell then applied the same principal of stereotactic localization using as his radiation source: a 185 MeV cyclotron delivering charged particles (protons) [3]. After some animal experimentation, this treatment approach was applied to a selected group of patients in whom the aim was again to create a small, well-demarcated lesion in the thalamic nuclei for the treatment of movement disorders and intractable pain. In 1959, Kjellberg first considered the concept of pituitary ablation [4] by a focused proton beam from a 186 MeV cyclotron as a form of hormone manipulation for pain relief in women with metastatic breast cancer. This was reported in 1962 by Kjellberg as having good short-term results. Leksell had to abandon the concept of the cyclotron, as the treatment site was 150 K from his neurosurgery center in Stockholm. However, the principle of stereotactic localization and treatment delivery to a functional target was now well and truly established.

1.2.3   Cobalt

Leksell developed his own device, the Gamma Knife, using multiple (initially 170, and then finally 201) cobalt 60 sources arranged around a hemisphere focused on the isocenter [4]. In Spain, Barcia-Salorio rotated a standard cobalt machine under stereotactic conditions to treat patients with acoustic tumors and carotid/cavernous fistulas. In 1985, he described the use of this approach to treat patients with intractable epilepsy [5].

1.2.4   Linear Accelerator

Leksell considered the concept of a linear accelerator (Linac) as his radiation method because of the limited depth dose characteristics with the 280 kV machine; however, problems with collimation and the size of the Linac resulted in abandoning that approach. Betti, in 1983 [6], provided the first description of stereotactic radiosurgery (SRS) performed using a linear accelerator, where the machine remained stationary with the patient being rotated through the various arcs in a rotating chair. Colombo [7] and Hartman [8], both in 1985, reported the technique of isocentric rotation of the Linac gantry around the patient, as is the standard now. This concept has been further modified with miniature linear accelerators being either attached to a robotic arm (the CyberKnife, Ch. 10), or on a rotating gantry as is used in computed tomography (CT).

2   PATIENT SELECTION

The majority of patients with some type of functional condition will be managed surgically. However, some patients will have persistent problems despite surgery or for medical or personal reasons, will decline the surgical approach. As the benefits of a radiosurgery approach become better publicized, patients and clinicians will become more aware of this approach and may select it as the primary mode of treatment for certain conditions. For example, in patients with movement disorders, the open surgical approach would still be preferable, as radiofrequency stimulation of the target region, with feedback from the awake patient, provides the best demonstration of the target site. However, with trigeminal neuralgia, the argument for a primary radiosurgery approach becomes more attractive, given that the trigeminal nerve is surrounded by cerebrospinal fluid and is readily visualized on high-resolution magnetic resonance imaging (MRI).

3 DOSE AND COLLIMATOR SIZE

Doses used for functional stereotactic radiosurgery have traditionally been high and the volume small [9]. This has stemmed from two concepts: (1) a high dose is needed to create a well-defined lesion with an area of necrosis with a short time-frame to benefit, and (2) the nerve tracts to be treated are usually small in diameter and, consequently, in volume. Kihlstrom, in reporting the Karolinska experience [10], of SRS for obsessive compulsive and anxiety neuroses, noted that when using a dose of 186 Gy marginal dose (typically 50% of the maximum dose), the use of the 8-mm collimator has resulted in significant edema, not seen when the 4-mm collimator is used. Thus Kondziolka [11] advocates that when using a 4-mm collimator with the Gamma Knife, a marginal dose of 128 Gy can be safely delivered, whereas if the 8-mm collimator is used, necrosis is evident from 50 Gy upward. Therefore, the standard dose for treatment of trigeminal neuralgia is 70 Gy to the target margin, with good to excellent benefit rates of 50% to 90% reported. Interestingly, in the treatment of intractable epilepsy, Barcia-Salorio used doses as low as 10 Gy [5], Regis [12] used 25 Gy, and in both series the majority of patients reportedly gained benefit. The difficulty in defining the epileptic focus in these two series may have been the main determinant of the doses used.

4 LINAC EXPERIENCE

Functional SRS will constitute only a very small proportion of the treatments rendered in any Linac-based radiosurgery program. Few articles has been published on it over the last 5 years in the English literature [13]. In our own experience of more than 530 cases in 8 years, we have treated six patients for primary trigeminal neuralgia (TN) (excluding those whose presentation related to, for example, a petrous ridge meningioma). Thus, the description of treatment procedure will focus on that for TN. However, the principles enable the method to be extrapolated to other functional conditions.

5 IMAGING

5.1 MRI

Referrred patients come with a diagnostic scan that excludes any type of tumor condition that could be causing the patient's pain. For image planning, all patients have a T1-weighted, gradient echo MR scan [MP Rage magnetization prepared rapid acquisition gradient echo] on a Siemens 1.5 Tesla Vision scanner. Images are acquired in three dimension and reconstructed in 1-mm thick axial and coronal slices with 1 mm separation. This scan is downloaded onto an optical disc and transferred to the planning computer, although ethernet transfer, if available, is also appropriate. For best demonstration of the course of the trigeminal nerve, a CISS MR scan is also performed [CISS (constructive interference with the steady state) a fine slice three-dimensional volume T2-weighted scan] in axial planes.

5.2 CT

After application of the Radionics BRW headring, we obtain a noncontrast helical CT scan with 1-mm slice thickness through the upper posterior fossa and 3-mm slice thickness through the remainder of the brain.

6 DOSE PLANNING

6.1 Target Localization

All CT and MR data are loaded onto a workstation for planning using the Radionics program X Knife-4. Before planning, CT and MR datasets are registered using Radionics Image Fusion software. After registration, outlines drawn on the MR scans are automatically transformed to the coordinate system of the CT dataset, which is stereotactically defined through the BRW frame. It is our standard practice that the optic chiasm and brainstem are outlined as critical structures and, consequently, dose volume histograms allow assessment of the dose given to these structures. The root entry zone of the trigeminal nerve into the pons is chosen as the site of treatment delivery. A point within that structure thus becomes the isocenter.

6.2 Collimator Size

We initially used a 5-mm collimator for treatment delivery; however, concern about the inaccuracies (including imaging, headring localization, planning, and delivery) prompted introduction of a 6.5-mm collimator for this purpose. Furthermore, dose homogeneity near the isocenter is higher with the 6.5-mm collimator, as an increasing degree of electronic disequilibrium results at these small collimator sizes.

6.3 Arc Selection

The dose-limiting structure is the brainstem, along with the constraint imposed by the dose rate of the Linac. Thus, to give 70 Gy with a maximum of 10 MU (monitor units) per degree of arc and less than 1 cGy per MU at isocenter, a total of more than 700° of arc rotation is required. This results in multiple short arcs [7–10], given the small collimator size. Some of the arcs may need to be treated more than once because of the large MU per degree required. This situation is exacerbated by the low output of the small cone. As each start point of an arc needs to be reset within the room, the duration of the procedure is lengthened by the requirement to re-enter the room on multiple occasions. This can be overcome by two means: first, some Linacs offer a high dose rate "research" mode, and second, gantry rotation may be able to be reset from the Linac console. These modifications are available only on certain modern accelerators.

7 MACHINE PREPARATION

7.1 Floor Stand

A nondedicated Linac is available at the end of its normal treatment day. The floor stand to which the headring is attached is screwed onto the base plate of the arc rotation system at a predetermined point. The isocenter will be determined from the planning computer, and by matching with the BRW phantom base, the x,y, and z coordinates on the floor stand will be set. Having a floor stand prevents full arc rotation underneath the couch, thus limiting the way structures in the posterior fossa can be treated. The floor stand provided greater rigidity of fixation and accuracy than earlier couch-mounted systems. However, currently available couch mounts are as accurate as floor mounts and are the preferred method.

7.2 Ball Film Check

This is performed with a double-exposure radiograph film with a 1-cm lead ball at the isocenter of the gantry rotation. Eight radiographs are taken with the machine gantry and couch rotated at various angles. The projection of the circular collimator on the film should be concentric with the projection of the ball, indicating that the X-ray source is focused on the isocenter throughout gantry rotation. Unsatisfactory performance would be indicated by any significant asymmetry in any direction.

7.3 Record and Verify

While machine preparation is taking place, all the parameters relating to dose delivery (e.g., start and stop angle, the arcs, position of the arcs, monitor units per degree of arc, etc.) are downloaded onto the record and verify (R and V) system for that Linac. All the parameters for the treatment are independently checked by a physicist, along with all the data entered onto the R and V system.

7.4 Isocenter Setup

The angiogram localizer box is attached to the floor stand and the computed isocenter for treatment is set and verified by laser lights. When the headring (and patient) are "docked" to the floor stand, the angiogram localizer box is reattached and positioning verified with the laser lights. Any variation will then be from patient movement. Patient position is adjusted then to ensure that the laser lights realign to the initially designated isocenter.

8 TREATMENT

8.1 Accelerator

All single-dose treatment is delivered on a Varian Clinac 1800 (Varian, Palo Alto, USA), with 6 MV X-rays the designated energy.

8.2 Headring Check

With the patient lying supine, the treatment couch is raised and the headring is "docked" to the floor stand, making the patient as comfortable as possible. Using the arc attachment of the BRW headring, the check is then performed using four points at 45° intervals away from the pin sites to ensure that the headring has not moved, as all measurements are in relationship to the ring, not to the patient's head.

8.3 Isocenter Check

Double-exposure radiographs are taken of the patient's head with the angiogram localizer box attached to the headring, using a 1-cm collimator. Anteroposterior (AP) and right lateral radiographs are taken of the patient's head and the respective fiducial marks on the box then digitized to obtain AP, lateral, and vertical coordinates. This verifies that the isocenter set-up for treatment corresponds to the planned isocenter. Typical variations between the two sets of coordinates would be less than 0.5 mm.

8.4 Beam On

As the point of fixation of the BRW headring to the floor stand is by two posteriorly located couplings, there is the possibility that the patient may "rock" on the floor stand during the 50 to 60 minutes it takes for treatment. Thus, an independent fixation device secures the anterior point of the headring through a T-shaped coupling to the couch. This prevents any inadvertent headring movement. For couch-mounted systems where the attachment of the ring to the couch is through two laterally based fixation points, this may not be necessary. During the multiple short-arc treatment procedure, the patient is constantly monitored. At least twice through the procedure, the angiogram localizer box is reattached to the BRW headring, and the laser lights are used to verify headring alignment. Two of our patients, who were mildly demented, required the procedure to be done under a general anesthetic (GA). Thus, while each couch movement was taking place, the anesthetic equipment also needed to be moved, ensuring that the monitors could be viewed through the closed circuit television while the anesthetist sat at the control panel during beam-on time.

9 POST TREATMENT

Once treatment is concluded, the headring is removed. The patient is advised to use ice packs to the anterior pin sites two times per day for the ensuing 48 hours. As the area postrema would have received a small dose during the treatment, a precautionary standard dose of dexamethasone 4 mg is given to all patients. With this, there has been no significant nausea or vomiting after the procedure. All patients other than those who are having a GA for the procedure are treated as outpatients and are able to go home immediately after the procedure.

10 FOLLOW-UP

All patients are seen about 4 weeks after the procedure. The response typically is that there is no change for the first 1 to 2 weeks, then 1 to 2 weeks of some improvement, after which intensity and frequency of attacks are reduced. Only one of the patients so treated has gained no benefit; it is relevant that she had had seven prior surgical procedures before being referred. One patient, for the first time in many years, was totally pain free for 3 months but had recurrence of the pain. The patient was retreated, with a dose of 60 Gy being given to a different point along the nerve.

REFERENCES

1. EA Spiegel, HT Wycis. Stereoencephalotomy. Part 1. New York: Grune & Stratton, 1952.
2. L Leksell. Stereotaxic radiosurgery in trigeminal neuralgia. Acta Chir Scand 137:311–314, 1971.
3. L Leksell. Stereotaxis and Radiosurgery: An Operative System. Springfield, IL: Charles C. Thomas, 1971.
4. RN Kjellberg, AM Koehler, WM Preston, WH Sweet. Stereotaxic instrument for use with the Bragg peak of a proton beam. Confin Neurol 22:183–189, 1962.
5. JL Barcio-Salario, H Roldant, G Hernandez. Radiosurgical treatment of epilepsy. Appl Neurophysiol 48:400–405, 1985.
6. O Betti, V Derechinsy. Irradiation stereotaxique multifasceaux. Neurochirurgie 29:295–298, 1983.
7. F Colombo, A Benedetti, F Pozza. External stereotactic irradiation by linear accelerator. Neurosurgery 16:154–160, 1985.
8. G Hartmann, W Schegel, V Sturm. Cerebral radiation surgery using moving field irradiation at a linerar accelerator facility. Int J Radiat Oncol Biol Physiol 2:1185–1192, 1985.
9. C Lindquist, L Kihlstrom, E Hellstrand. Functional neurosurgery: A future for Gamma Knife? Stereotact Funct Neurosurg 57:72–81, 1992.
10. L Kihlstrom, WY Guo, C Lindquist. Radiobiology of radiosurgery for refractory anxiety disorders. Neurosurgery 36:294–302, 1995.
11. D Kondziolka, B Perez, JC Flickinger, LD Lunsford. Gamma Knife brain surgery. Prog Neurol Surg 14:212–221, 1998.
12. J Regis, JC Peragut, M Rey. First selective amygdalohippocampic radiosurgery for mesial temporal lobe epilepsy. Stereotact Funct Neurosurg 64(suppl) 193–201, 1995.
13. AA De Salles, WW Buxton, T Solberg, P. Medin, V Vassilev, C Carbatan-Awang. Linear accelerator radiosurgery for Trigeminal neuralgia. Radiosurgery 1997. Radiosurgery 2:173–182, 1998.

33

Classification of Pain

Zvi Israel

Hadassah University Hospital, Jerusalem, Israel

Kim Burchiel

Oregon Health and Science University, Portland, Oregon, U.S.A.

"They can rule the world while they can persuade us
our pain belongs in some order.
Is death by famine worse than death by suicide,
than a life of famine and suicide . . .?"

Adrienne Rich (b. 1929), U.S. poet. [1]

1 INTRODUCTION

Many difficulties hinder a unifying nosology of pain. Among these is the
fact that pain is of interest to many disciplines, each approaching pain management with its own biases, different viewpoints, and languages, such that
no single classification will satisfy all. In fact, many major textbooks of pain
management do not even attempt such classification. The multidisciplinary
committee on the taxonomy of pain of the International Association for the
Study of Pain (IASP) went some way to solving this problem in 1986 [2].

2 CLASSIFICATION

One useful way for neurosurgeons to classify pain is based on inferred neurophysiological mechanisms (Fig. 1). Such a classification is practically use-

387

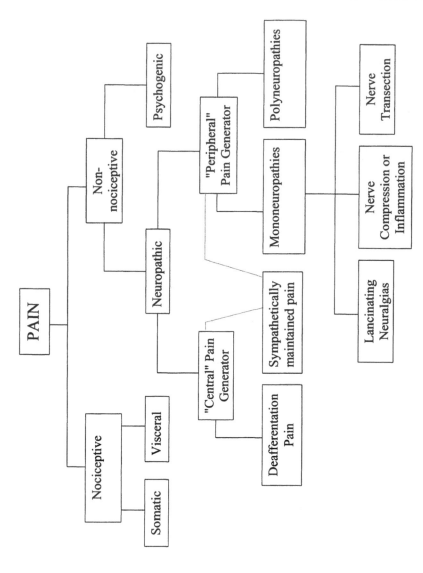

FIGURE 1 A simplified classification of pain.

ful because it tends to promote a uniform approach to pain management. Pain can be further described in terms of etiology, the region of the body affected, or its temporal aspects.

2.1 Nociceptive Pain

When pain is considered to be compatible with tissue damage associated with an identifiable somatic or visceral lesion or injury, it is known as nociceptive. Nociceptive pain originating from somatic structures (skin, muscle, connective tissue) is typically well localized, sharp, aching, or throbbing. In contrast, visceral pain is generally less well localized but may have a specific referral pattern. If a hollow viscus is obstructed, the pain may be gnawing or cramping in nature, whereas if an organ capsule or mesentery is involved, it may be sharp and throbbing.

Nociception is conveyed through primary afferent neurons responsive to noxious stimuli. Nociceptive pain usually will respond to intervention that ameliorates or denervates the offending peripheral lesion and to analgesic medication, especially opioids.

2.2 Neuropathic Pain

In contrast, neuropathic pain is believed to be associated with sustained activity at a site of aberrant somatosensory processing in the peripheral or central nervous system resulting from neural injury or irritation. Typically, neuropathic pain persists long after the precipitating event.

Neuropathic pain is clinically diverse. Patients may describe unfamiliar burning, electric shock-like or shooting dysesthesias, which may be spontaneous or evoked by movement. Examination may reveal allodynia, hypalgesia or hyperalgesia, hypesthesia or hyperesthesia, or hyperpathia. There may be other focal neurological deficits, including weakness or autonomic changes, such as swelling or vasomotor instability. Trophic changes in the form of alterations of skin, subcutaneous tissues, hair, and nails may also occur. However, neuropathic pain is not always dysesthetic. The neurological deficit may be very subtle, thus the diagnosis is not always straightforward.

Neuropathic pain may result from a variety of central and peripheral mechanisms that can interact in complex ways. The observation that some patients with neuropathic pain have disorders that appear to be primarily sustained by processes within the central nervous system (e.g., pain precipitated by stroke) and others by peripheral processes (e.g., a painful peripheral neuroma) allows an extended classification based on inferred pathophysiology. Neuropathic pain syndromes are usually refractory to traditional analgesics. "Adjuvant" analgesics are often prescribed, such as anticonvulsants or antidepressants. Chronic narcotic usage has been especially controversial;

however, it is now clear that a significant proportion of neuropathic pain patients with diverse diagnoses do indeed respond to systemic or intrathecal narcotics.

2.2.1 Deafferentation Pain

The response characteristics of central neurons in the pain pathway may change if the peripheral input is partially or completely damaged. This is known as "central sensitization" and is essentially the result of abnormal signal amplification, such that nonnoxious stimuli can now trigger pain. The neural pathways that lead to the sensation of pain have not been clearly delineated. The mechanistic substrate is thought to involve both functional and structural changes at the cellular level and is poorly understood. Examples of specific central deafferentation syndromes include central pain, pain associated with plexus avulsion injuries, spinal cord injuries, post-herpetic neuralgia, and phantom pain.

"Central pain" generically includes a large number of deafferentation pain syndromes that can occur after injury to the central nervous system. These include thalamic pain, post-stroke pain, pain caused by multiple sclerosis, parkinsonism, and syringomyelia. Phantom pain is the neuropathic pain that may occur after the amputation of *any* body part (limb, breast, tooth).

Certain of these syndromes can be successfully treated by ablative procedures (paradoxically accentuating the deafferentation), notably plexus avulsion, and some spinal cord injury (SCI) pain syndromes by dorsal root entry zone ablation (DREZ procedure).

2.2.2 Sympathetically Maintained Pain

Sympathetically maintained pain (SMP) is a subtype of neuropathic pain that appears to be sustained by release of norepinephrine caused by efferent activity in the sympathetic nervous system. There is controversy concerning the mechanisms involved, which pain syndromes may be included in this category, and even whether such an entity truly exists. Furthermore, there has been considerable confusion between the diagnosis of SMP and complex regional pain syndrome (CRPS). Sympathetically maintained pain may also simultaneously exist with sympathetically independent pain.

Both peripheral and central mechanisms have been implicated in the generation of SMP. Campbell considers SMP to be a *complication* of a neuropathic pain trigger, rather than an entity in itself [3]. Sympathetically maintained pain may be diagnosed by way of a sympathetic ganglion block or by intravenous administration of the α-adrenergic antagonist, phentolamine. These tests may also give an indication of whether pharmacological sympatholysis or surgical sympathectomy is likely to palliate the pain syndrome.

Complex regional pain syndrome is a term adopted by the IASP to refer to disorders that have the clinical characteristics of reflex sympathetic dystrophy (RSD), (CRPS type I) or causalgia (CRPS type II). Patients with CRPS are assumed to have neuropathic pain that may or may not have an SMP component. Similarly, a patient with SMP may or may not meet the criteria for CRPS. Thus, although there is a clear association between CRPS and SMP, they are considered to be independent entities.

2.2.3 Peripheral Nerve Pain

Both central and peripheral mechanisms contribute to neuropathic pain, and CNS changes can be demonstrated secondary to peripheral nerve pathology; however, a predominant peripheral generator may be implicated for certain entities. Peripheral nerve disease is associated with loss of function (motor, sensory, or both) and is typically nonpainful. Certain neuropathic diseases however, characteristically are associated with pain. Most painful polyneuropathies are axonopathies. These may be associated with diabetes or with nutritional deficiencies of thiamine, niacin, pyridoxine, or others. For the most part these have little neurosurgical relevance. Painful mononeuropathies are thought to be always associated with a peripheral nerve injury.

Lancinating neuralgias. Dysesthetic pain associated with lancinating neuralgias is typically short-lived and shock-like. An attack may consist of a single 'shock' or several runs of variable duration. Occasionally this is associated with a more constant background burning pain or dull ache in the same distribution. Pain may be spontaneous or triggered by benign sensory or motor stimuli in the receptive field of the affected nerve. Patients may experience pain-free periods of days, weeks, or months and will usually initially respond well to an anticonvulsant such as carbamazepine or gabapentin.

Most commonly affected are the trigeminal, glossopharyngeal, vagal (superior laryngeal branch), and geniculate nerves. One inferred mechanism involves compression of these nerves by a tortuous vascular loop, such that decompression is curative or significantly palliative.

For intercostal neuralgia and ilioinguinal neuralgia, a nerve injury is usually implicated. The mechanism responsible for occipital neuralgia remains essentially unknown. Invasive therapies often afford significant palliation. Decompression and electrical stimulation are preferred over ablative procedures, such as rhizotomy or ganglionectomy.

Nerve compression. "Entrapment neuropathy" implies compression of a nerve in a specific location as determined by local anatomy (bony or fibrous tunnel), changes in tissue consistency (metabolic disease), trauma (accidental or occupational), or congenital anatomical variations. The neuropathy is thought to occur as a result of decreased neural blood supply.

A diagnosis of nerve compression or entrapment should be entertained whenever no other pathological lesion is found in a patient with chronic pain. Often the pain will follow a classic distribution associated with a specific nerve, but occasionally pain is referred and may involve an entire limb. Pain tends to be a constant deep "nerve" ache. It may vary according to position or movement. Typically, the severity of the pain is disproportionate to the relatively trivial extent of any neurological impairment; however, care must be taken not to miss a subtle neurological deficit, as this is often a key to the diagnosis. Local tenderness is often accompanied by a Tinel's sign over the point of compression, thought to represent ectopic excitability of the nerve in response to the slowing of axonal transport.

Electrodiagnostic tests are useful adjuncts to the clinical syndrome. Treatment is by surgical decompression.

Peripheral nerve trauma. The normal reaction to any peripheral nerve injury involving axonotmesis (disruption of axonal continuity) or worse, involves some degree of neuroma formation. Neuroma formation cannot be prevented. Neuromas are bulb shaped and consist of scar tissue intermingled with neuronal elements. Fortunately only a minority of neuromas are painful, and this seems to occur when the neuroma is easily or repeatedly traumatized in a subcutaneous position or near a joint. However, when they *are* painful, they may be exquisitely allodynic. A Tinel's sign over the neuroma is characteristic. There is an accompanying neurological deficit associated with the dysfunctional nerve.

Infiltrating around the neuroma with local anaesthetic in the outpatient clinic gives a good indication as to the utility of surgery for any individual case. The goal at operation is to remove the neuroma and implant the cut nerve deep within muscle or bone, away from scar tissue or a joint. If the neuroma is in-continuity and some crucial motor function remains, the situation is more problematic. External neurolysis is probably the best initial option before considering excision of the neuroma with grafting.

REFERENCES

1. Rich A. The Dream of a Common Language, pt. 1, "Hunger." (1978). From: The dream of a common language: Poems 1974–1977 by Adrienne Rich. W. W. Norton & Company, Inc., New York, 1978.

2. Merskey H. Classification of chronic pain, descriptions of chronic pain syndromes and definition of pain terms. Pain Suppl 3, S10–S11, S13–S24, S217, 1986.
3. Campbell JN. Peripheral nerve injury and sympathetically maintained pain: Mechanisms and surgical approach. In: Levy RM, North RB, eds. Neurosurgical Management of Pain. New York, Springer-Verlag, 1997.

34

Percutaneous Techniques for Trigeminal Neuralgia

Edward J. Zampella

Chatham Neurological Associates, Summit, New Jersey, U.S.A.

Jeffrey A. Brown

Wayne State University School of Medicine, Detroit, Michigan, U.S.A.

Hooman Azmi

New Jersey Medical School, Newark, New Jersey, U.S.A.

1 INTRODUCTION

Nicholas Andre recognized trigeminal neuralgia as a definite clinical entity in 1756 [1]. In 1773, John Fothergill described 14 cases of what he termed tic douloureux [2]. He noted that the pain in these patients was paroxysmal and sudden in its onset, the condition was more common in men than in women, and that it occurred more often in older people. His description of the symptoms is still used to make the diagnosis of trigeminal neuralgia. Despite various advances in neuroimaging and clinical electrophysiology, this remains a clinical diagnosis in which the patient's history is the most important factor.

Characteristically, the patient with trigeminal neuralgia suffers from severe facial pain that occurs suddenly and is brief, at the most lasting a few minutes. The pain is very often described by the patient as knifelike, and may also be likened to an electrical shock. Some patients may develop an additional constant aching component upon which the knifelike pain is then superimposed. The pain is unilateral in more than 95% of cases, is confined to one or more of the distributions of the trigeminal nerve, and involves the lower face (second or third division) more frequently than the eye or the forehead. Bilateral trigeminal neuralgia may occur, but more often the patient will have symptoms first on one side of the face and then the other, rather than having simultaneous bilateral pain. The onset of pain may be set off by stimulation of a trigger point, or sometimes by the mere movement of, or any contact with, the skin over the face or mouth. The patient may experience symptom-free intervals between paroxysmal periods of pain. Women are affected more often than men and the disease is most commonly seen in patients older than age 50.

2 TREATMENT

A single, completely satisfactory method of treating trigeminal neuralgia in all patients has yet to be described. In all cases the initial therapy should be medical. Carbamazepine (Tegretol) and phenytoin (Dilantin) are the two drugs that have traditionally shown the greatest promise for patients with trigeminal neuralgia. Baclofen (Lioresal) may be useful in the treatment of patients whose pain has become refractory to treatment with carbamazepine or phenytoin [3]. Treatment with gabapentin (Neurontin) in recent years has become common in patients with trigeminal neuralgia, even though there are no large scale controlled studies of this drug's efficacy in this disease [4]. When control of the patient's symptoms is no longer possible with nontoxic levels of drugs, operative management should be considered.

The surgical treatment of patients with trigeminal neuralgia can be either nondestructive or destructive. The nondestructive procedure most frequently used is microvascular decompression of the trigeminal nerve root entry zone. The modern procedure, developed by Peter Jannetta, is based on observations made by Walter Dandy that in patients with trigeminal neuralgia, vascular compression of the trigeminal root at the pons is the etiology of the pain. By elevating the vessel off the nerve root entry zone, the procedure aims to produce pain relief without causing dysfunction of the trigeminal nerve. Microvascular decompression is a very effective treatment giving long-term pain relief in more than 90% of patients who undergo the procedure. It may not be appropriate, however, for patients in poor health or in elderly patients who would not tolerate a craniotomy. It is also not appropriate in patients whose symptoms are caused by multiple sclerosis.

The goal of the destructive procedures is partial disruption of the sensory pathway to eliminate painful input. Peripheral neurectomy, retrogasserian neurotomy, and trigeminal tractotomy have, for the most part, been surpassed by the percutaneous procedures. These include retrogasserian glycerol rhizolysis, retrogasserian radiofrequency zhizotomy, and percutaneous compression of the gasserian ganglion. All three of these procedures can be performed percutaneously and meet the goal of modern surgical therapy, that is, long-term pain relief, minimal neurological deficit, and negligible morbidity.

3 INDICATIONS

A percutaneous ablative approach is indicated for patients with trigeminal neuralgia who no longer benefit from medical therapy or for whom the side effects of such medical therapy are no longer tolerable.

Glycerol rhizolysis or balloon compression may be indicated for patients with multidivisional pain. Selective radiofrequency rhizotomy may be indicated, especially in patients with isolated third division pain because it is possible to limit the nerve injury to the region of the jaw. Balloon compression, because it selectively injures large myelinated fibers, can be helpful for patients with first division pain.

The advantage of a percutaneous procedure over a craniectomy for microvascular decompression is that it is usually performed as an outpatient procedure. The risk of injury to the brain, other cranial nerves, or intracranial blood vessels is much less. The total hospital cost is less. Balloon compression and glycerol rhizolysis require less of an investment in equipment than radiofrequency rhizotomy. Balloon compression does not require the patient to be awake, whereas radiofrequency rhizotomy, and to some extent, glycerol rhizolysis, do require cooperation. Elderly patients in discomfort and under some sedation may find it difficult to provide such cooperation, and thus may be better candidates for balloon compression.

4 PREOPERATIVE STUDIES

Imaging studies performed before any of the percutaneous procedures should include a magnetic resonance imaging (MRI) (with and without contrast) of the brain and skull base to exclude a skull base tumor, and a submentovertex view of the skull, to ascertain any anomalous anatomy and the relative size of the foramen ovale. Serum clotting studies (prothrombin time, partial thromboplastin time, International Normalizing Ratio (INR), and platelet count) should be performed preoperatively, as abnormalities of clotting are contraindications to the percutaneous procedures.

5 PROCEDURES

5.1 Approach: General Technique

Local infiltration anesthesia combined with intravenous (I.V.) sedation should be adequate for all of the percutaneous techniques. In the past, short-acting barbiturates, such as Brevitol, have been recommended. Diprivan administered as a continuous infusion may also be reliable in obtaining a controlled and adequate sedation. Supplemental O_2 is administered by nasal cannula. Cardiovascular monitoring with I.V. access is essential as significant increase in blood pressure and bradycardia are often seen with stimulation of the trigeminal root fibers.

Intraoperative fluoroscopy (lateral) is required for localizing the tip of the rhizolysis needle. Biplane fluoroscopy [anterior-posterior (AP)/lateral] with a submentovertex projection allows the surgeon to both direct the needle toward the foramen ovale and gauge its course without repositioning the patient or the unit.

Ablative percutaneous procedures directed at the retrogasserian fibers share a common approach. This approach has been previously described by Hartel [5]. The usual site of needle insertion is approximately 2.5 cm lateral to the corner of the mouth on the symptomatic side. The entry site is more lateral and inferior for first division pain and more medial for third division lesions. Two additional landmarks are marked on the skin before starting the procedure. The first of the additional landmarks is a point directly beneath the midpoint of the ipsilateral pupil with the eyes looking straight ahead; the second is a point one third of the distance along the line drawn from the external auditory canal to the lateral canthus of the eye (Fig. 1). The intersection of the parasagittal and coronal planes drawn through these points is the approximate location of the foramen ovale and is the target of the needle tip (Fig. 2). The needle or cannula is directed to a point on a plane with the zygomatic arch, 2.5 cm anterior to the external auditory canal, and with the medial aspect of the pupil. Fluoroscopic guidance is always used when penetrating the foramen ovale. When the neurosurgeon is using the lateral view, the needle is directed just inferior to the lateral pterygoid wing. The surgeon should place a finger in the mouth to assure that the oral mucosa is not punctured. On the lateral radiograph the needle is seen to be directed toward the radiographic intersection of clivus and petrous bone. It is possible to puncture the internal carotid artery with this approach, as the artery is only protected by thinned bone at the skull base.

Once the foramen is entered, an anterior-posterior image can be obtained. With this image, the petrous bone is positioned in the radiographic center of the orbit. The trigeminal nerve forms a groove in the petrous bone as it enters Meckel's cave. The radiofrequency electrode, balloon catheter, or spinal needle must be directed toward this groove to create a lesion in the retrogasserian fibers. When seen on a lateral view, the needle is directed at the radiographic intersection of the clivus and petrous bone.

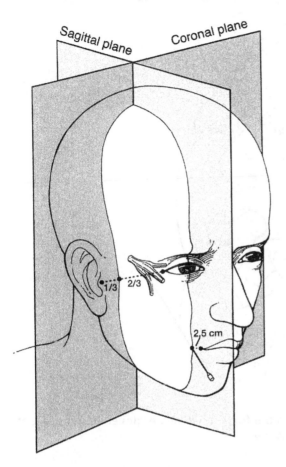

FIGURE 1   Surface landmarks for penetration of the foramen ovale: needle of entry 2.5 cm lateral to the mouth, directed to the intersection of midpupillary line and a point one third of the distance from the tragus to the lateral canthus.

5.2   Retrogasserian Glycerol Rhizolysis

Results from the first series of patients treated by glycerol rhizolysis were published by Hakanson in 1981 [6]. Previously, glycerol was used in mixtures containing ethanol or phenol for the rhizotomy procedure. The observation that glycerol alone was effective for the treatment of trigeminal neu-

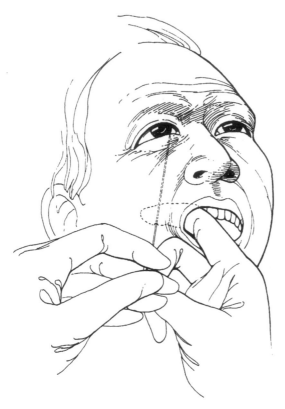

FIGURE 2   Point of needle in the foramen ovale. A gloved finger prevents penetration of the oral mucosa.

ralgia eliminated the need for other substances in the procedure. Glycerol is a demyelinating agent that reduces sensory input to the trigeminal system [7].

It may be easier to perform glycerol rhizotomy with the patient positioned on the transport stretcher rather than the operating room table (thereby decreasing the risk of displacing the glycerol during transfer of the patient from the table to the stretcher). Before starting the procedure, as a matter of patient comfort, the patient's buttocks should be aligned with the fold in the table (as the patient will be in a sitting position for approximately 4 hours after injection).

An 18-gauge/4-inch Quincke needle with a 22-degree bevel and trocar (Popper and Sona, New Hyde Park, NY) is used after noting the above landmarks. After prepping the skin with an antiseptic solution, with the patient in the supine position, the entry point is anesthetized and the rhizotomy needle is used to puncture the skin of the cheek. The index finger of the surgeon's gloved hand is placed in the patient's mouth to guide the needle through the soft tissues of the cheek, taking care not to puncture the oral mucosa.

As the needle tip punctures the foramen, a slight contraction of the masseter muscle is often felt as a gentle bite on the surgeon's gloved finger. Intravenous sedation is given for this step. As the trocar is removed from the needle, cerebrospinal fluid may drip from its lumen, but this finding is not essential for correct placement and may occur even if the needle is lateral to the intended target. Indeed if glycerol has been previously injected, cerebrospinal fluid may not flow from the trigeminal cistern at all.

The foramen ovale is entered while the patient is positioned supine. The location of the needle tip in the foramen ovale may be confirmed by instilling a small bolus of nonionic radiopaque contrast slowly under continuous fluoroscopy, with the patient in the semisitting position (Fig. 3). The volume of the contrast that can be instilled before overflow can be used as a rough estimate of the volume of Meckel's cave. The average volume is 0.24 ml (0.1–0.5 ml). An X-ray is taken at this time for inclusion in the patient's record. With the needle in place, the patient is moved from semi-sitting to supine position then back to the operative position (to spill the contrast out of Meckel's cave). At this point if glycerol rhizolysis is the intended technique, the patient should be placed in as close to a 90-degree sitting position as possible; he or she may be moved to a stretcher if need be, so that head movement after injection is minimized. A small volume (0.25–0.75 cc) of sterile anhydrous glycerol is injected slowly and the needle subsequently withdrawn.

With injection of the glycerol, many patients have marked blood pressure elevation. Tearing of the ipsilateral eye and a flushing of the skin of the cheek may also be seen. Depending on the level of sedation, patients may complain of pain during and immediately after the injection. They should be reassured that this is normal. After the needle is withdrawn, the patient is transported to the recovery room in a sitting position where he or she remains for 2 to 4 hours. To minimize movement and reduce the risk of displacing the glycerol, the patient's head may be taped to the stretcher with a pillow folded in half behind it.

Selective lesioning of the trigeminal branches may be obtained by positioning the patient's head. When the head is in a neutral position (chin on the horizon), a lesion of the second and third division of the trigeminal nerve can be produced. With the head slightly flexed (chin below the horizon), first division lesions can be produced. Partial filling of the trigeminal cistern can also cause selective damage. For third division pain, half the cistern is filled. For second and third division pain, two thirds is filled.

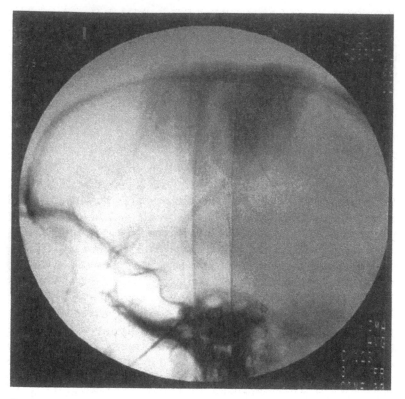

FIGURE 3 Lateral fluoroscopic projection: needle in the trigeminal cistern.

Glycerol may be "floated" on top of iodine contrast for selective injury of the first division.

Glycerol rhizolysis will produce pain relief in a high percentage of patients within hours of injection. Diminished sensation in the involved root distribution is not essential for relief of pain, but its presence often correlates with a longer duration of the pain-free period. A few patients may not experience relief after glycerol rhizolysis. For these patients who do not respond within 7 to 10 days, the procedure may be repeated or other techniques may be used.

Jho and Lundsford reported 90% early pain relief with 55% of patients pain free without need for medication [8]. Other reports indicate a 30% to 50% recurrence rate over 2 to 10 years. Moderate to severe sensory deficit has been reported in 19% of patients, more often in patients who underwent multiple procedures. It is a matter of concern that it is difficult to predict the degree of sensory loss for each patient [9].

5.3 Selective Radiofrequency Rhizotomy

Radiofrequency trigeminal rhizotomy depends on a differential vulnerability of pain and touch fibers to thermocoagulation. The A-delta and C fibers that relay pain are more susceptible to injury than the A-alpha and beta fibers that carry touch sensation. There are two electrode types. Either a thin cordotomy-type electrode or a larger, curved electrode with temperature monitoring capabilities are available [10,11]. Thermistor controlled radio-frequency lesion generators are available from several sources (Radionics, Burlington, MA). Lesions are made sequentially with a temperature-monitoring electrode at 60 degrees to 90 degrees. The temperature is increased by 5-degree intervals, and the patient is re-examined after each lesion. When using a cordotomy-type electrode, the lesion is made at 10 V and 60 mA for 20 seconds, increasing gradually toward a maximum of 18 to 20 V and 90 to 100 mA [12].

The technique of needle placement is essentially the same as for glycerol rhizolysis but upon entering the foramen, sedation is stopped, as it is necessary for the patient to be awake for the prelesioning testing. The first-division fibers are located superomedially, as seen on both the lateral and AP views. Third division fibers are located in the lateral portion of the entrance to Meckel's cave on the AP view, with the electrode just short of the edge of the petrous bone. On the lateral view, the electrode should be seen lying parallel to the petrous bone. It may be necessary to reposition the needle entry site to redirect the electrode tip appropriately. Third-division fibers are reached by redirecting the electrode curve inferiorly, with its tip lying 5 mm proximal to the clival line [13].

An insulated electrode is passed through the needle, and stimulation at approximately 50 Hz is used when adjusting the position of the electrode. Optimum position of the electrode is ascertained when a nonpainful paresthesia is produced in the distribution of the intended trigeminal division at a low threshold (0.2–0.3 volts). If masseter muscle contraction is observed at less than 0.5 volts, the electrode is too close to the motor root and the needle should be repositioned laterally. An initial radiofrequency lesion can be made at 60 mA for 10 seconds, followed by a 20-second and then a 30-second lesion. It is important to test the patient in between each of the lesions.

If insufficient sensory loss is determined, the current can be increased by 10 to 70 mA and a series of three lesions made again. This can be repeated to a maximum of 110 mA. If a lesion cannot be produced by a maximum of 110 mA for 30 seconds, the needle is not in the appropriate position, and the procedure should be either terminated or the needle repositioned. The endpoint of lesion production is deep hypalgesia in the division or divisions of the trigeminal nerve where the pain arises. The patient should experience the prick of a safety pin as touch but not as pinprick.

5.4 Retrogasserian Balloon Compression

Balloon compression of the trigeminal ganglion was described by Mullan and Lichter in 1983 [14]. Balloon compression is performed under general anesthesia and does not require patient cooperation, yet it can selectively treat pain limited to specific divisions [14–17]. Compression is especially helpful in first-division pain because the unmyelinated fibers that mediate the blink reflex are preserved by the mechanical injury generated by the balloon. Compression is also helpful for multidivisional pain. It is relatively inexpensive, with disposable units costing less than $500.

The balloon catheter is introduced through a #14-gauge blunt cannula that is directed to the foramen ovale. Straight or curved guiding stylets (Cook, Inc., Bloomington, IN) are positioned within the entrance to Meckel's cave 18 mm beyond the foramen ovale. Anterior-posterior and lateral fluoroscopic views provide guidance. The catheter is then directed to the site where the trigeminal nerve traverses the edge of the petrous bone through a small elliptical opening in the dura. The balloon is inflated for 1 minute to a pressure of 1.3 to 1.6 atmospheres, as measured by an insufflation syringe with an attached transducer (Merit Medical, Inc., Salt Lake City, UT). Alternatively, approximately 0.5 to 0.7 ml of radiopaque contrast is placed through the needle and the balloon distended.

When properly positioned, the tip of the balloon compresses the retrogasserian trigeminal nerve against the petrous bone and the firm medial edge of the dura. Radiographically, the balloon will have a "pear" shape caused by its position at the Meckel's cave entrance. The balloon is allowed to remain full for approximately 1 minute and subsequently, the balloon is deflated and the entire needle catheter assembly removed as a unit to avoid shearing off the tip of the catheter. During inflation, a significant trigeminal reflex response causes bradycardia. This indicates appropriate compression. If this is a concern, especially in the more elderly or medically unstable patient, the patient may be fitted with an external pacemaker set to trigger should the heart rate drop below 40 beats/minute.

By adjusting the angle at which the balloon catheter is inserted and the position of the catheter tip in the "porus trigeminus," the entrance to Meckel's cave, selective divisional injury can be obtained. By using a curved stylet to direct the catheter tip toward the medial portion of the porus, the first division is favored. Directing the catheter toward the lateral porus and angling the cannula so that it lies parallel to the petrous ridge favors third-division fibers.

Balloon compression has a higher incidence of masseter and pterygoid muscle weakness than other percutaneous techniques. This weakness usually resolves, but patients may experience temporomandibular joint discomfort until it does. This discomfort may be treated with anti-inflammatory medication. The recurrence rate for balloon compression is comparable to that in other percutaneous techniques, and the procedure can be repeated for recurrence without greater technical difficulty.

5.5 Complications and Recurrence

Complications seen from percutaneous ablative therapy for trigeminal neuralgia have been extensively documented. The oral mucosa may be penetrated during the approach, resulting in bacterial meningitis or brain abscess. A carotid-cavernous fistula may result from injury to the internal carotid artery. There is a possibility of otalgia from eustacian tube dysfunction, or temporomandibular joint tenderness along with jaw weakness. Aseptic meningitis has been reported, as well as intracranial hemorrhage from acute hypertension. Other reported complications are bradycardia with subsequent hypotension, neurokeratitis, temporary diplopia, optic nerve injury, subdural hematoma, postoperative herpes simplex activation, bothersome facial sensory loss and dysesthesias, and anesthesia dolorosa [18,19]. These potential morbidities need to be discussed with patients as part of the preoperative meeting even though the risk of their occurrence is 2% or less.

As long as the surgical endpoint selected is mild to moderate hypesthesia, there will be a recurrence rate of 20% to 25%, depending on the time elapsed after surgery, with recurrence rates being twice as high for trigeminal neuralgia associated with multiple sclerosis. Recurrent pain occurs either because of regeneration of injured myelin or from progression of the disease to include untreated trigeminal sensory divisions.

Each of these ablative procedures can be safely repeated for recurrence, as long as the goal remains the creation of mild to moderate hypesthesia. There is no evidence to suggest that patients who have undergone a percutaneous ablative procedure are at any disadvantage should they later undergo microvascular decompression for recurrence. However, the success rate for treatment by a repeat procedure is lower than that for a primary procedure and the recurrence rate is higher.

6 DISCUSSION

Glycerol rhizolysis, radiofrequency rhizotomy, and balloon compression of the trigeminal ganglia are all effective, simple, and attractive techniques for treating trigeminal neuralgia in patients for whom medical therapy has become ineffective or drug-related toxicity has occurred; patients in whom a craniotomy and microvascular decompression is contraindicated because of age or poor health; patients who have been previously treated with microvascular decompression and have now experienced recurrence of pain; and a select group of patients with trigeminal neuralgia secondary to multiple sclerosis or nerve injury distal to the dorsal root ganglion. All of the procedures share the risk of complications related to needle placement. As a general rule, however, the incidence of complications is low. Satisfactory relief of pain should be obtained in more than 90% of patients for periods extending from 6 months to several years with these techniques. In cases in which pain relief is not satisfactory with a single procedure, a second attempt at that procedure or a different technique may be performed. It is important to remember that most patients can gain relief at the hands of a persistent surgeon.

REFERENCES

1. André N, cited in Stookey B, Pansohoff J. Trigeminal Neuralgia: Its History and Treatment. Springfield, IL, Charles C. Thomas, 1959, pp 13–23.
2. Fothergill J. Of a painful affection of the face. Med Observat Inquir 5:129–142, 1773.
3. Fromm GH, Terrence DF, Chatha AS. Baclofen in the treatment of trigeminal neuralgia: Double blind study and long term follow-up. Ann Neurol 15:240–244, 1984.
4. Sist TC, Filadora VA, Miner M, Lema M. Experience with gabapentin for neuropathic pain in the head and neck: Report of ten cases. J Pharmacol Exp Ther 282:1242–1246, 1997.
5. Hartel F. Veben die intracariella injektions behandlung der toxigeminus neuralgie. Med Klin 10:582–584, 1914.
6. Hakanson S. Trigeminal neuralgia treated by the injection of glycerol into the trigeminal cistern. Neurosurgery 9:638–646, 1981.
7. Lundsford LD, Bennet MH, Martinez AJ. Experimental trigeminal glycerol injection: Electrophysiological and morphological effects. Arch Neurol 42:146–149, 1985.
8. Joh HD, Lunsford LD. Percutaneous retrogasserian glycerol rhizotomy. Current technique and results. Neurosurg Clin N Am 8:63–74, 1997.
9. Sweet WH, Polletti CE. Problems with retrogasserian glycerol in the treatment of trigeminal neuralgia. Appl Neurophysiol 48:252–257, 1985.
10. Nugent GR. Technique and results of 800 percutaneous radiofrequency thermocoagulations for trigeminal neuralgia. Appl Neurophysiol 45:504–507, 1982.
11. Nugent GR. Radiofrequency treatment of trigeminal neuralgia using a cordotomy-type electrode. A method. Neurosurg Clin N Am 8:41–52, 1997.

12. Taha JM, Tew JM Jr. Treatment of trigeminal neuralgia by percutaneous radiofrequency rhizotomy. Neurosurg Clin N Am 8:31–39, 1997.
13. Taha JM, Tew JM Jr. Comparison of surgical treatments for trigeminal neuralgia: Reevaluation of radiofrequency rhizotomy [see comments]. Neurosurgery 38:865–871, 1996.
14. Mullan S, Lichtor T. Percutaneous microcompression of the trigeminal ganglion in trigeminal neuralgia. J Neurosurg 59:1007–1012, 1983.
15. Lichtor T, Mullan JF. A 10-year follow-up review of percutaneous microcompression of the trigeminal ganglion. J Neurosurg 72:49–54, 1990.
16. Brown JA, McDaniel MD, Weaver MT. Percutaneous trigeminal nerve compression for treatment of trigeminal neuralgia: Results in 50 patients. Neurosurgery 32:570–573, 1993.
17. Brown JA. Direct carotid cavernous fistula after trigeminal balloon microcompression gangliolysis: Case report [letter; comment]. Neurosurgery 40:886, 1997.
18. Sweet WH, Poletti CE. Complications of percutaneous rhizotomy and microvascular decompression operations for facial pain. In: Schmidek HH, Sweet WH, eds. Operative Neurosurgical Techniques: Indications, Methods and Results. Third ed. Philadelphia: W.B. Saunders Company, 1995, pp 1543–1546.
19. Linderoth B, Hakanson S. Retrogasserian glycerol rhizolysis in trigeminal neuralgia. In: Schmidek HH, Sweet WH, eds. Operative Neurosurgical Techniques. Third ed. Philadelphia: W.B. Saunders Company, 1995, pp 1523–1536.

35

Percutaneous Surgery for Atypical Facial Pain

G. Robert Nugent
Robert C. Byrd Health Sciences Center,
Morgantown, West Virginia, U.S.A.

1 INTRODUCTION

Without question, the treatment of atypical facial pain can only be addressed by defining the term. It means different things to different people. Under this heading there are: atypical facial neuralgia; pain from damage to the trigeminal nerve, often from trauma, dental, and ear, nose, and throat (ENT) procedures; trigeminal neuropathy; atypical trigeminal neuralgia; anesthesia dolorosa; as well as a host of other ill-defined face pain problems. In general, it is prudent to think long and hard before making permanent sensory deficits (lesions proximal to the gasserian ganglion) in this group of patients. whose problem may be difficult to define or understand.

"Atypical facial neuralgia," or "facial pain not fulfilling criteria of previously described groups," as described in the International Headache Society classification, to most is a pain that is psychogenically determined. The pain may be considered to be a "somatization disorder," a "conversion disorder," the result of "hypochondriasis," or a "body dysmorphic disorder." [1] The pain is usually constant ("I've had this pain day and night for 3 years"), often bizarrely described, migrates, and has a predilection for women. It radiates beyond the trigeminal distribution, is frequently associ-

409

ated with depression, and the underlying psychopathology is often obvious. The Minnesota Multiphasic Personality Inventory (MMPI) is often strikingly abnormal in these patients and *no surgical intervention is indicated.* My approach to this problem is to sympathetically inform the patient that as a surgeon I can do nothing to help them and to guide them, when possible, to psychotherapeutic workers. If they are not already on narcotics or have had no surgery, it is important to counsel and warn them of: (1) the frequency and hazards of drug addiction, and (2) the often unnecessary surgery that well-meaning but misguided clinicians may recommend.

Trigeminal neuralgia is a classic and stereotyped clinical entity and usually easily diagnosed, but there are occasions when certain atypical features creep into the picture, raising the question of whether one is dealing with true trigeminal neuralgia. If true trigeminal neuralgia is *not* the underlying problem, creating permanent sensory deficit in the face may make the matter worse, because the pain is not relieved and now the patient has an unwanted numb face. In this case, peripheral radiofrequency (RF) blocks may be helpful in clearing the air [2]. If it is not true tic, the sensory deficit will fade in months to a year—or more if a dense block is obtained, and no bridges have been burned. It is important to inform the patient that the sensory deficit from these extracranial blocks is usually more dense than that obtained from retrogasserian RF blocks and that he or she will most likely be happier with the central lesions should that be the ultimate approach.

The third division can be blocked by the subzygomatic approach, reaching the mandibular nerve as it exits from the foramen ovale. It is better to block the mandibular nerve with radiofrequency than with alcohol because of the reported spread of the alcohol up into the ganglion and cerebrospinal fluid with sometimes disastrous results. Furthermore, the use of a small cordotomy-type electrode, which is bent at its tip, facilitates the localization of the nerve by directing and redirecting the electrode to the lowest threshold for stimulation. When the electrode is on the nerve, the stimulation threshold is usually around 0.1 volt. A thin-walled 18-gauge lumbar puncture (LP) needle is used with a marker set on the needle at 5 cm. The landmark for needle introduction under local anesthesia is a point 2 cm anterior to the ear canal with the needle oriented below the zygoma perpendicular to the skull in the anteroposterior dimension and angled 115 degrees superiorly (Fig. 1). The LP needle usually slides across the base of the middle fossa impinging on the mandibular nerve at a depth of 5 cm. When the electrode is on the nerve, the patient is put to sleep with 35 to 40 mg of methohexital (Brevital). A maximal lesion is made, the current gradually raised until boiling occurs as evidenced by a sudden drop in the voltage reading. If the nerve is not readily reached, a submento-vertex radiograph may help in orientation by

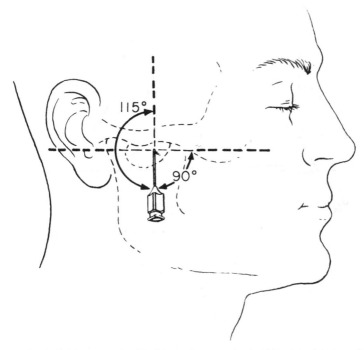

FIGURE 1   The needle orientation for a subzygomatic block of the mandibular nerve at the foramen ovale. From B. Stookey and J. Ransohoff. Trigeminal Neuralgia. Its History and Treatment, 1959. Courtesy of Charles C. Thomas, Publisher, Ltd., Springfield, Illinois.

revealing the foramen ovale. Remember that the search is in an anteroposterior direction with the nerve passing straight inferiorly at this point.

The maxillary nerve usually has to be blocked more centrally in the pterygomaxillary fissure. The approach here is to place the marker on the LP needle at 6 cm and introduce the needle beneath the zygoma 3 cm anterior to the ear canal. The orientation is 110 degrees anteriorly and 115 degrees superiorly (Fig. 2). The needle usually strikes the pterygoid plate at about 5 cm. It is then walked anteriorly until it falls into the fissure. The maxillary nerve is usually right there. In a small percentage of patients, anatomical variation prevents the maxillary nerve from being reached by this approach. Remember that the search here is in a superior-inferior direction, as the nerve is passing horizontally in the fissure. A lesion is made, as described above.

A frequent atypical face pain problem seen by the neurosurgeon is the pain resulting from an injury to the trigeminal nerve, whether it is from

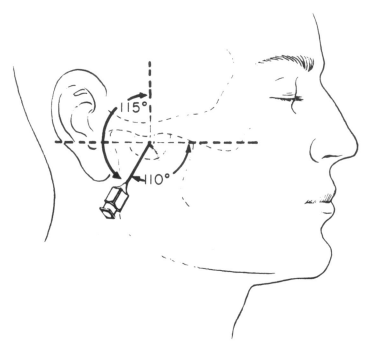

FIGURE 2 The needle orientation for a subzygomatic block of the maxillary nerve in the pterygomaxillary fissure. From B. Stookey and J. Ransohoff. Trigeminal Neuralgia. Its History and Treatment, 1959. Courtesy of Charles C. Thomas, Publisher, Ltd., Springfield, Illinois.

trauma, sinus disease, or surgical procedures on the face. Some refer to this as "trigeminal neuropathic pain" [3]. This pain is localized to this nerve, most often in the second division and is the result of injury to the nerve peripherally. There may be no overt sensory loss and usually there is no relief from anticonvulsants such as carbamazepine. This injury may, in time, lead to the development of central self-generating and self-perpetuating neuronal discharges that are perceived as chronic face pain [4]. That this central mechanism may be at play is supported by the observation that destructive lesions proximal to more peripheral lesions, which could be reasoned to interrupt afferent discharges, are often ineffective in relieving the pain. Therefore, although extracranial RF blocks, as described above, can easily be performed, they should only be attempted if the neurosurgeon sees the patient early after the onset of the pain and before central mechanisms become established. Unfortunately, this is rarely the case and the neurosurgeon more often first sees the patient many months or years after the onset. Thorough informed consent is necessary if RF blocks are to be used in these patients. An alternative and nondestructive approach to be considered in these patients is the use of chronic electrical stimulation of the gasserian ganglion by the percutaneous insertion of electrodes by way of the foramen ovale. Approximately 50% of patients so treated obtain good relief with acceptable complications. Several reports outlining the results and technique are available [5–7].

The stereotaxic approach to the nucleus caudalis has been used to treat with RF various atypical face pain problems [8]. This is a complicated technique not used by many at this time and the complications of ataxia and severe dysesthesias have dissuaded many from its general use. Similarly, RF mesencephalic tractotomy should be reserved for those familiar with the technique and aware of the significant complications: oculomotor dysfunction and 5% mortality. These techniques are best for those with chronic face pain from cancer, not for the "garden variety" of atypical face pain. The same can be said regarding the use of RF thalamotomy, which has primarily been used to treat post-herpetic neuralgia and anesthesia dolorosa, often with inconsistent results.

Akin to trigeminal neuropathic pain is the pain limited to areas of the trigeminal nerve that is unrelated to peripheral injury. It is of unknown origin and spontaneous in onset. This is a most difficult area to understand or treat, and the best advice would be to avoid any RF destructive procedures.

A difficult and atypical pain problem refractory to analgesic medication is chronic ocular pain, usually secondary to glaucoma, penetrating injury, or previous retinal detachment surgery. Radiofrequency lesions to the retrogasserian first-division fibers were successful in immediately and completely relieving this pain in all nine patients [9].

To treat these patients, the retrogasserian rootlets are approached by the previously described techniques for RF thermocoagulation [2,10,11]. Using this approach, graded incremental lesions in the first division can be made by treating the first division fibers while the patient is awake. It is important to appreciate that RF lesions in the first division are often associated with little, or sometimes no discomfort, facilitating treatment in the awake patient but, at the same time, providing no clue to the surgeon that he is indeed making a lesion. Corneal sensation can be lost if the awake patient is not constantly monitored while the lesion is being made. The lesioning is accomplished by making multiple incremental thermocoagulations of increasing voltage (and milliamperage) while constantly observing the eyelash blink reflex. This reflex is tested by flicking the eyelash with the twisted corner of a single layer of facial tissue. As the lesion creeps into the first division, there is first a diminution of the consensual blink followed by a decrease in the direct blink. With this technique, the lesioning can then be stopped when there is some loss of corneal sensation but with preservation of the corneal reflex. It would appear that this treatment for this clinical entity is largely unknown and underutilized.

Although not properly an atypical facial pain, chronic migrainous neuralgia, a form of cluster headache, can be intractable and unresponsive to medical therapy. These patients may be desperate for relief. The pain is usually centered and most severe in the region of the eye. Radiofrequency thermocoagulation has been used to treat patients with this syndrome. The results were excellent in eight patients in a University of Minnesota series [12]. Seven of these eight patients had an analgesic or hypalgesic cornea. In a Mayo Clinic series, the results were excellent in 11 and good in two of 24 patients in who analgesia of the first division was obtained [13]. The results were poor in seven patients in whom little sensory deficit was obtained in V_1, and two patients with 75% loss of sensation had a poor result. In a third series of 27 patients with this disorder, RF retrogasserian rhizolysis produced excellent results in 15 patients, very good in 2, good in 3, fair in 1, and poor in 6 [14]. The complications were mild and transient and the benefits of surgery far outweighed the discomfort from the complications. Thus, if sensory deficit in the first division can be obtained, RF treatment of this difficult entity may offer lasting relief. This treatment is also probably underutilized.

It is important to appreciate that an anesthetic cornea only rarely leads to serious complications, keratitis in particular. A review of 100 patients with anesthetic corneas as the result of alcohol injections into the trigeminal sensory root found that only five patients became blind [15]. One of these patients was "mentally not normal," one was an alcoholic, one had preexisting corneal scarring, and one was "a rather simple man" who did not seek early treatment. The fear of blindness from keratitis would seem to be somewhat overrated and should not deter the patient or surgeon from pursuing RF treatment when indicated. Early treatment of keratitis is most important.

In summary, the use of destructive RF thermocoagulations to treat atypical facial pain is limited and the surgeon must prudently and cautiously heed the advice of those with experience in this area and suppress the compulsion to pursue a seemingly sound, but misguided, course of treatment.

REFERENCES

1. Fiorini F. Headache and Facial Pain. Stuttgart-New York: Thieme, 1999, p 259.
2. Nugent GR. Percutaneous techniques for trigeminal neuralgia. In: AH Kaye, P McL Black, eds. Operative Neurosurgery. London: Churchill Livingstone, 2000, pp 1615–1616.

3. Burchiel KJ. Trigeminal neuropathic pain. Acta Neurochir (suppl)58:145–149, 1993.
4. Anderson LS, Black RG, Abraham MD, Ward AA Jr. Neuronal hyperactivity in experimental trigeminal deafferentation. J Neurosurg 35:444–452, 1971.
5. Meyerson BA, Hakanson S. Suppression of pain in trigeminal neuropathy by electric stimulation of the gasserian ganglion. Neurosurgery 18:59–66, 1986.
6. Young RF. Electrical stimulation of the trigeminal nerve root for the treatment of chronic facial pain. J Neurosurg 83:72–78, 1995.
7. Taub E, Munz M, Tasker RR. Chronic electrical stimulation of the gasserian ganglion for the relief of pain in a series of 34 patients. J Neurosurg 86:197–202, 1997.
8. Schvarcz JR. Stereotaxic trigeminal nucleotomy for dysesthetic facial pain. Stereotact Funct Neurosurg 68:175–181, 1997.
9. Rosenberg M, Hoyt CS, King JS, Jay WM. Treatment of chronic ocular pain by selective thermocoagulation of the trigeminal ganglion. Am J Ophthalmol 91:526–529, 1981.
10. Nugent GR. Surgical treatment: Radiofrequency gangliolysis and rhizotomy. In: Fromm GH, Sessle BJ, eds. Trigeminal Neuralgia: Current Concepts Regarding Pathogenesis and Treatment. London: Butterworth-Heinemann, 1991, pp 159–184.
11. Nugent GR. Trigeminal neuralgia treatment by percutaneous electro-coagulation. In: Wilkins RH, Rengachary SS, eds. Neurosurgery. 2nd ed. New York: McGraw-Hill, 1996, pp 3945–3951.
12. Maxwell RE. Surgical control of chronic migrainous neuralgia by trigeminal gangliorhizolysis. J Neurosurg 57:459–466, 1982.
13. Onofrio BM, Campbell JK. Surgical treatment of chronic cluster headache. Mayo Clin Proc 61:537–544, 1986.
14. Mathew NT, Hurt W. Percutaneous radiofrequency trigeminal gangliorhizolysis in intractable cluster headache. Headache 28:328–331, 1988.
15. Davies MS. Corneal anaesthesia after alcohol injection of the trigeminal sensory root. Brit J Ophthalmol 54:577–586, 1970.

36

Epidural Spinal Cord Stimulation: Indications and Technique

Konstantin V. Slavin
University of Illinois at Chicago, Chicago, Illinois, U.S.A.

1   INTRODUCTION

Spinal cord stimulation (SCS) is probably the most commonly performed surgical procedure for pain treatment in the United States, although the exact mechanism of its action remains largely unknown [1]. Several theories have been proposed to explain the pain suppressive effect of SCS. The most commonly accepted of these is the well-known "gate-control" theory of Melzack and Wall [2], which postulates the existence of a "gate" mechanism in the central nervous system that controls the processing and transmission of sensory information, including the nociceptive input. According to this theory, the impulse transmission in the nociceptive afferent pathway is modulated by activity in large-caliber myelinated non-nociceptive A-fiber afferents. Therefore, electrical stimulation of these large fibers anywhere along their course in the peripheral nerves or in the dorsal columns of the spinal cord can block central pain signaling.

An alternative theory explains the suppression of pain by a frequency-related conduction block that takes place at the branching point of the primary myelinated afferents into dorsal horns and dorsal column fibers [3]. In addition, clinical and experimental studies indicate that SCS may inhibit ischemic pain by improving regional blood flow [4] or decreasing tissue oxygen demands [5].

Whatever the underlying principle of SCS, the stimulation of the dorsal columns of the spinal cord produces pain relief in certain subsets of patients, and its success seems to correlate well with the production of stimulation-related paresthesias in the painful region [6].

2 INDICATIONS

The generally acceptable indication for SCS is neuropathic pain caused by injury to the nervous system either at or distal to the spinal cord (Table 1). This includes pain originating from peripheral nerve injury, neuropathies, postamputation stump pain, or complex regional pain syndromes (CRPS) types 1 and 2 (previously known as reflex sympathetic dystrophy and causalgia, respectively). Pain originating from the nerve roots, as in arachnoiditis or radiculopathies, also responds well to SCS. Patients with endzone pain after spinal cord injury and those with intercostal neuralgias may benefit from SCS as well.

However the main group of patients considered to be candidates for SCS are those with a combination of neuropathic and nociceptive pain, a condition that is usually referred to as "failed back surgery syndrome." Practical experience suggests that patients with predominantly radicular pain radiating to one or both legs respond better to SCS than those with predominantly axial low back pain.

A separate set of indications consists of pain syndromes resulting from

TABLE 1 Indications for Spinal Cord Stimulation

Common indications
  Failed back surgery syndrome
  Chronic arachnoiditis
  Painful peripheral neuropathy
  Postamputation stump pain
  Complex regional pain syndromes (types 1 and 2)
  Radiculopathy
  Spinal cord injury pain
Questionable indications
  Intercostal neuralgia
  Phantom limb pain
Additional indications
  Peripheral vascular disease
  Intractable angina

---

tissue ischemia. Two conditions—lower extremity pain caused by occlusive vascular disease and intractable angina—appear to respond so well to SCS that they have become the primary indications for SCS in Europe. Interestingly, SCS does not mask the pain of acute myocardial infarction, making this therapeutic modality safer [7].

In regard to the general selection of patients for SCS, the basic rules of pain surgery apply: patients should have failed less invasive therapeutic approaches and should have favorable psychological evaluations (ruling out somatization, major depression, and other psychological and psychiatric abnormalities). Also, in most cases one would prefer to know the exact diagnosis and underlying medical problem, although this may not be possible in some patients (eg, CRPS type 1). General contraindications to surgery or implantation of hardware, such as generalized infection, coagulation abnormalities, and serious concurrent medical diseases that would prevent even the brief general anesthesia necessary for the system implantation, need to be considered before the operation. Relative contraindications, such as advanced age, relatively short life expectancy, history of drug abuse, and the presence of other implanted electronic devices (eg, pacemakers), should also be taken into consideration. A separate condition for SCS surgery is the patient's ability to perceive paresthesias in the painful area; this limits SCS use in patients with painful anesthesia. The final decision about permanent implantation of the SCS system depends on the results of the SCS trial; this will be further discussed in this chapter.

3 TECHNICAL CONSIDERATIONS

Spinal cord stimulation technology has evolved from the relatively simple monopolar electrodes used in the original studies during the mid-1960s [8,9] to sophisticated multielectrode arrays for monopolar, bipolar, and tripolar stimulation that may be attached either to a completely implantable system for impulse generation or to a radiofrequency-coupled system with an implantable receiver and externally attached antenna controlled by a battery-powered impulse generator (Table 2).

The configuration of the electrode determines the ability to vary stimulation parameters, the position of the active electrode, and the direction of the stimulation. Therefore, more contacts are generally better, allowing more freedom in the selection of stimulation paradigms. However, the programming process may become cumbersome, and standard implantable generators may not be able to handle complex electrode configurations, which raises the second (and opposing) principle of "the simpler the better." In most cases, the choice between the somewhat simpler, easier-to-use quadripolar electrodes and the more complicated, but also more versatile, 8- or

TABLE 2   Spinal Cord Stimulation System
Components

Electrodes
  Percutaneous
    Four-contact leads
      Verify (temporary) (Medtronic 3862)
      Pisces-Quad (Medtronic 3487A)
      Pisces-Quad Compact (Medtronic 3887)
      Pisces-Quad Plus (Medtronic 3888)
      Quatrode (ANS)
    Eight-contact leads
      Octad (Medtronic 3898)
      Octrode (ANS)
  Laminectomy (paddle) electrodes
    Four-contact leads
      Resume II (Medtronic 3587A)
      Resume TL (Medtronic 3986)
      TTL lead (Medtronic)
      SymMix (Medtronic 3982)
    Eight-contact leads
      Lamitrode-8 (ANS)
      Specify (Medtronic 3988)
    Sixteen-contact electrodes
      Lamitrode-88 (ANS)
Implantable impulse generators
  ITREL-II (Medtronic 7424)
  ITREL-3 (Medtronic 7425)
  Genesis (ANS)
  Synergy (Medtronic 7427)
  Synergy Versitrel (Medtronic 7427V)
Radiofrequency receivers
  Renew (ANS, MNR908/MNR916)
  X-trel (Medtronic 3470)
  Mattrix (Medtronic 3271/3272)

The equipment listed in this table is manufactured by
Medtronic, Inc., Minneapolis, MN, and Advanced Neuromodulation Systems (ANS), Inc., Plano, TX

16-contact leads depends on each particular patient's symptoms, pain distribution and patterns, and the results of prior treatments with SCS.

Selection of electrode type may also be affected by prior surgical interventions and individual anatomical variations. Percutaneous electrodes are
easier to insert, but they have a greater tendency to migrate in the epidural

space. Laminectomy (paddle or plate) electrodes require a larger surgical opening and allow less freedom in axial placement, but their rate of displacement is definitely smaller compared to that of the percutaneous (wire) electrodes. In addition to that, they seem to require less energy to achieve the same results as the wire electrodes, as their metal contacts face only the dura and are isolated from the posterior epidural space, whereas percutaneous electrodes are in circumferential contact with the surrounding tissues.

When it comes to choosing the power supply and programming equipment, here again each option has its own pitfalls and benefits. Fully implantable devices [implantable pulse generators (IPG)] are more convenient for patients because the entire SCS system is placed inside the patient's body and the need for external attachments is eliminated. Patients can swim or shower without stopping the stimulation and do not have to worry about poor contact between the antenna and receiver. Implantable pulse generator systems, however, have only limited internal battery power, and, therefore, must be replaced every several (1–7) years, depending on the system usage and stimulation parameters. This obviously increases the long-term cost of the hardware. Also, the currently available IPGs have only limited options for electrode configurations and generally provide only single-channel stimulation. Patients with IPGs have fewer options for adjusting their stimulation parameters; however, this feature makes the devices somewhat safer.

Radiofrequency (RF)-coupled devices may, at least theoretically, serve forever without additional surgical interventions. The receiver is implanted subcutaneously and connected to the electrode(s). The power source/programming module is usually worn externally and communicates with the receiver through an externally applied flexible pancake-shaped antenna that is placed over the receiver. The battery change process is extremely simple, and the programming module is significantly more versatile than that of an IPG. In addition to the ability to change some or all of the stimulation parameters, some modules have integrated computer chips that memorize certain electrode configurations and stimulation paradigms and change from one to another with a simple push of a button. Most RF-coupled systems allow operations with two or more independent channels and are capable of covering 4, 8, or 16 electrode contacts. This becomes especially important in patients with complex pain patterns and in those cases where pain areas change with time. On the other hand, RF-coupled systems require a significantly higher degree of patient participation, which may be difficult for some patients. In addition, some patients develop dermatitis or other local skin reactions that prevent them from wearing the antennas for extended periods. Also, some patients state that having a permanent external device limits their freedom, and the are often willing to trade some of the benefits of RF-coupled systems for a completely implantable system.

Over the next few decades, technological advances will allow us to overcome most of these pitfalls. The SCS system of the future will combine all of the benefits mentioned here in one smaller and more versatile unit.

4 SCS TRIAL

Once the decision of whether to proceed with SCS is made, the surgeon must determine the type of the electrode and length of the SCS trial. There are two general approaches to SCS trials, each with its own advantages.

The first route assumes that the lead used for the trial will have to be discarded, regardless of the trial results. The trial starts with insertion of the screening electrode (which is usually less expensive but otherwise very similar to a permanent percutaneous electrode). The insertion does not require an incision and can be done in the doctor's office; the lead is removed and discarded before the final implantation. An X-ray image of the temporary electrode is usually taken before its removal so the landmarks for permanent electrode insertion can be identified. This decreases the infection rate. The procedure can be done on an outpatient basis with a minute amount of local anesthetic, but there are some obvious drawbacks. First, there is the cost of the discarded electrode. Second, one has to enter the epidural space twice, even if the first electrode was placed perfectly and provided excellent pain relief. In addition, the surgeon must be confident that the second electrode will be inserted into the same position as the first, allowing a comparable degree of pain relief without an additional trial (as the second part of the surgery is usually done under general anesthesia). The idea of "screening" is, however, attractive, and many surgeons use this technique to evaluate the general responsiveness of the patient to SCS or as a prelude to the insertion of a laminectomy ("surgical") lead.

Another approach assumes that the electrode used for the trial will subsequently be connected to the rest of the SCS system. The initial insertion of the electrode is performed so that it can be internalized, thereby eliminating the need for reinsertion. To minimize the risk of infection, the electrode is connected to a temporary extension wire, which in turn is tunneled under the skin and brought to the surface a few inches from the original incision. This extension wire is subsequently discarded, whereas the electrode itself stays in place and is connected to the permanent extension wire during internalization. To minimize the risk of displacement, the electrode is anchored to the fascia with nonabsorbable sutures. A radiographic image is obtained after the initial insertion and then again during internalization to rule out inadvertent electrode displacement. An obvious advantage of this method is that the final electrode position is tested before system internalization, allowing the second stage of surgery (IPG/receiver implantation and passage of the long extension wires) to be done under general anesthesia. On the other hand, the initial insertion has to be done in the operating room and if the trial fails, the patient has to be returned to the operating room to have the electrode removed.

5 ELECTRODE IMPLANTATION TECHNIQUE

The procedure of electrode implantation for SCS is fairly straightforward. Percutaneous (wire) electrodes are inserted through a needle. A standard 18-Ga Tuohy needle is supplied with the electrode and comes with a stylet. The needle is inserted into the epidural space under fluoroscopic guidance after the tissues are infiltrated with a local anesthetic solution. Usually, a slightly paramedian entry point is preferred to avoid midline placement of the fragile electrode, where it may be damaged by the hard spinous processes. The aim of needle insertion is usually a point just below the spinous process one or two levels cephalad to the point of skin penetration. This allows the electrode to be placed in the central posterior epidural space and guides the needle at about 5° to the skin surface, making the electrode passage somewhat easier. Entrance into the epidural space is best confirmed by the well-known "loss-of-resistance" technique: resistance against injection of air or sterile water through a glass syringe suddenly disappears when the needle penetrates the ligamentum flavum and enters the epidural space.

The level of electrode placement is chosen preoperatively based on the patient's pain distribution. Previous experience shows that maximal paresthesias from SCS follow a somatotopic distribution. Positioning the active electrode at the T11-12 level results in paresthesias in the foot; T10-11, the anterior thigh; T4-5, the abdomen; C7-T1, the upper chest; and C4-6, the forearm and hand [10,11]. The low back region is probably the least responsive to SCS; the optimal position of the electrode to produce paresthesias in this region is usually at the T8-11 vertebral level [11].

Once the epidural space has been entered, the percutaneous electrode is introduced through the needle and then advanced in a cephalad direction under fluoroscopic guidance (Fig. 1). The electrode becomes relatively rigid with the guidewire inside; it is possible to manipulate the electrode inside the epidural space and advance it up to the desired level by gently pushing and rotating the electrode shaft. A slight curve of the guidewire tip allows minimal steering, which is especially important when passing through stenotic levels or epidural scar tissue. It is generally advisable to place the percutaneous electrode one level higher than the final target and then optimize the electrode position based on the intraoperative trial by pulling the electrode down.

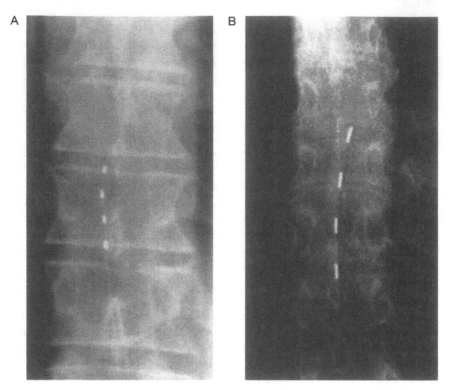

FIGURE 1 Intraoperative images of percutaneously inserted spinal cord stimulation electrodes. Each electrode has four contacts that may provide stimulation with a variety of configurations, including monopolar and bipolar stimulation modes. **A**, Pisces-Quad electrode (Medtronic); **B**, Pisces-Quad Plus (Medtronic).

If the subarachnoid space is entered during needle manipulation (manifested by cerebrospinal fluid outflow from the needle hub), the procedure does not need to be aborted. Most surgeons prefer to withdraw the needle and change the level of insertion so the electrode does not accidentally enter the dura through the hole made by the needle. In these cases, the patient should be warned of the possibility of spinal headaches and advised to stay flat for several hours and consume extra fluids, but the need for additional intervention, such as epidural blood patching, is rare.

The goal of the intraoperative trial is not to eliminate the pain nor to quantify the degree of pain relief, but to test the location of paresthesias and adjust the electrode position for optimal coverage. The electrode is connected to the screening device either directly or through a temporary extension wire, and the various electrode configurations are tested while the patient is asked about his/her sensations. The use of multiple contacts allows one to move the active (negative) contact along the electrode without actually repositioning the device. Stimulation-induced paresthesias follow the general somatotopic map; induction of paresthesias superior (cephalad) to the desired area requires repositioning of the electrode more inferiorly (caudal) and vice versa. It may also be necessary to shift the laterality of the electrode depending on the patient's pain patterns and paresthesia thresholds. This is usually accomplished by carefully pulling the electrode one or two levels down and then advancing it with some rotational steering using the guidewire curvature. Obviously, when it comes to axial advancement, the percutaneous electrodes provide much more freedom to manipulate, with their flexibility and ease of insertion up to six or seven levels from the target location.

Once the intraoperative trial is completed, a fluoroscopic image of the electrode position is obtained and saved on the screen so it may be later compared with the final electrode position. The electrode is then anchored to the overlying fascia. This is done through small incisions above and below the point of needle insertion. The needle itself is removed after the incision is made but before the anchoring procedure. The electrode kit usually contains several anchors; some of them are soft and flexible, with lower profiles and less tensile strength. Others are made of hard plastic; these have higher profiles, but are more reliable for holding the electrode in place. It is advisable to place the anchor as close as possible to the point where the electrode passes through the fascia so that movement of the electrode is minimized. After that, a temporary extension wire is passed subcutaneously and brought to the skin surface 10 to 15 cm from the original incision. The entire path of the extension wire and the site of its exit through the skin is infiltrated with local anesthetic. Advance consideration of the final position of the implanted system allows the surgeon to tunnel the temporary wires on the side opposite the final position of the IPG/receiver, so the track of the permanent extension wires does not cross that of the temporary ones. The connection between the electrode and the temporary extension wire is then secured with all four screws and covered with a silicone sleeve. If this connection is placed close to the midline, it is easy to identify during the internalization procedure. The excess wire is usually coiled above the fascia but below the connection with the temporary wire to protect the electrode during internalization or revision.

The incision is then irrigated with antibiotic solution and closed in standard fashion. It is not necessary to place an additional suture at the site where the temporary wire exits. Coiling of the wire on the skin surface and adhesive dressing may be sufficient to prevent dislodgement, but one may still want to add a purse-string stitch to minimize the risk of infection. In general, however, long tunneling of the temporary wire, short duration (1 week or less) of the outpatient trial, and careful observation of sterile technique during all stages of surgery may lower the infection rate to zero. The general rules for electrode handling are listed in Table 3.

In some patients who have undergone prior surgical interventions and have extensive epidural fibrosis or a multilevel posterior fusion, it may be very difficult to enter the epidural space or manipulate inside it. In these instances, the open approach—surgical exposure of the epidural space and insertion of laminectomy electrodes—may be the only choice even at the trial stage.

The procedure for laminectomy electrode insertion is similar to the percutaneous placement, but the opening of the epidural space is done by a limited laminectomy immediately below the target level for stimulation. The generally accepted approach involves a midline opening of the spinal canal with removal of the spinous process, visualization and transection of the ligamentum flavum, and identification of the underlying dura mater. A special plastic template and curvilinear spacer are used to dissect the epidural plane and prepare the area for electrode insertion. Once again, intraoperative fluoroscopy is used to monitor electrode advancement and position (Fig. 2). It is also possible to insert the laminectomy-type electrodes through a unilateral spinal exposure. With this method, a small hemilaminotomy is per-

TABLE 3 Considerations for SCS Lead Implantation

- Avoid bending or kinking the lead. If there is any excess lead body, create gently coiled loops of no less than 2 cm.
- Use fingers or a rubber-tipped bayonet forceps when handling the lead.
- Do not tie a suture directly to the lead body. Use the anchor supplied in the lead kit.
- Avoid placing tension on the lead during surgery. Leave the lead body as loose as possible after connecting the extension to avoid unnecessary tension on the lead.
- Do not force the lead up the epidural space. Use the guidewire packaged in the lead kit to clear a path for the lead.
- Be extremely careful with sharp instruments around the lead.
- Should any system component become damaged during implant, remove it and replace it with another component for permanent system implantation.

Reprinted with permission from "Spinal Cord Stimulation. Percutaneous Lead Implantation Guide." Medtronic, Minneapolis, 1997.

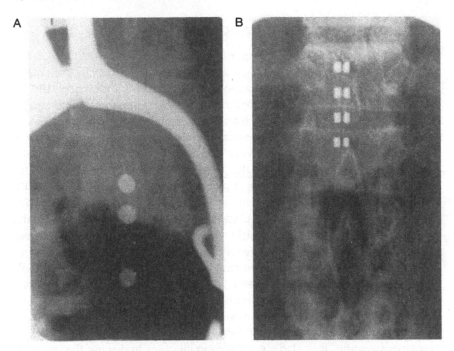

FIGURE 2 Intraoperative images of surgically implanted laminectomy electrodes (courtesy of Dr. Kim J. Burchiel, Portland, Oregon). **A**, Resume four-contact electrode (Medtronic). **B**, Specify eight-contact electrode (Medtronic). Specify electrode allows for either simultaneous stimulation with identical configuration of contacts using an implantable generator or independent stimulation with different configuration of contacts using radiofrequency-coupled systems.

formed immediately lateral to the spinous process, and the root of the spinous process is undercut with rongeurs. This approach minimizes surgical trauma and is better tolerated by the patients, which is particularly important as most procedures are done under local anesthesia.

The surgical lead may be placed either above or below the laminectomy/laminotomy level and the position of the lead is adjusted based on the intraoperative trial results. The procedure for anchoring and tunneling the surgical lead is essentially identical to that for percutaneous electrodes, except in some cases the lead may be anchored to the interspinous ligament before layer-by-layer closure of the incision. It is important to note that sometimes surgical leads may be hard to remove, especially after they have been in the epidural space for a long time, and therefore it may be necessary to remove the wire but leave the paddle inside.

6 ELECTRODE INTERNALIZATION

If the stimulation trial is satisfactory, achieving at least 50% pain relief without intolerable side effects such as unpleasant paresthesias, the patient is prepared for electrode internalization. The final system selection (IPG vs RF receiver), which depends on optimal stimulation parameters and patient preferences, can be made before internalization. The internalization procedure is usually performed under general anesthesia, as IPG/receiver insertion and especially wire tunneling are very painful and poorly tolerated by awake patients. It is possible to implant the generator/receiver in the superior gluteal area, but most surgeons prefer to place it in the anterior abdominal wall. Posterior placement allows the patient to remain in the prone position for internalization, whereas anterior placement is usually performed with the patient in the lateral decubitus position, which permits access to both lumbar and anterior abdominal regions. For SCS systems that focus on the cervical or upper thoracic spinal cord (as in cases of arm pain or intractable angina), the IPG or receiver may be implanted in the subclavicular area, as is done with pacemakers or deep brain stimulators. When placing RF receivers, one must consider the patient's convenience in applying the antenna and avoid areas that are covered with body hair or that may subject the antenna to excessive sweating. It is also a good idea in all cases to discuss the insertion site with the patient before the surgery and to avoid the belt line, which may irritate subcutaneously placed hardware.

The internalization procedure starts with cutting the temporary extension wire with sterile instruments at the skin level after the entire area has been disinfected and sterilized. Both the lumbar and the anterior abdominal areas are prepped and draped in standard fashion after the patient is placed in the lateral decubitus position (with the operative side up) and padded/secured with a deflated "bean bag." The original incision is then reopened, taking care to avoid cutting the electrode lying above the fascia. The connection of the electrode and the temporary extension wire is exposed, the silicone sleeve is removed, all screws are unscrewed, and the remainder of the temporary extension wire is discarded. A second incision is then made in the anterior abdominal area, taking care to ensure that the IPG/receiver will not overlay the bony structures (ribs, iliac crest). A pocket for the IPG or receiver is made above the fascia, but not too far under the skin, because the thick layer of tissue above the IPG/receiver may interfere with programming or RF coupling. Generally, RF receivers should be placed within 1 cm of the skin's surface to maintain a good connection with the external antenna.

Once the pocket is prepared, a permanent set of extension wires is passed subcutaneously using a special passer that usually comes sterilely prepacked with an appropriate extension wire kit. In most cases, it is necessary to move the passer in a posterior-to-anterior direction, so the extension wire can be brought from the abdominal incision to the lumbar one. The connection between the extension wire and the electrode is secured with all four screws, an additional silicone sleeve, and several nonabsorbable sutures. The electrode is coiled under the connection site so it will be better protected from accidental damage if the patient requires electrode revision. Anteriorly, the extension wire is connected to the IPG/receiver, and the connection is secured with built-in screws. The IPG or receiver needs to be secured to the underlying fascia with one or more nonabsorbable sutures. Excess extension wire is coiled behind the IPG/receiver, not only for cosmetic reasons but also to avoid interference with programming or RF coupling. It also allows easy identification of the IPG when it needs to be revised/replaced (ie, when the battery is exhausted).

After the implantation is complete, both incisions are irrigated with antibiotic solution and closed in a standard layer-by-layer fashion. Sterile dressings are placed over the incisions and changed during the postoperative period as necessary. Sutures are removed after all incisions are healed.

7 POSTIMPLANTATION PROGRAMMING

The programming of the SCS system may be performed soon after the patient's awakening from the general anesthesia. Obviously, stimulation parameters similar to those that were tested during the trial may be used. Some electrode configurations, however, are technically impossible during the stimulation trial. The best example is "monopolar" stimulation, when one of the electrode contacts is active and the IPG case serves as a reference. This mode allows for a lower stimulation voltage compared with the bipolar configurations and should be tried first when a completely internalized system is used.

Stimulation settings need to be checked regularly during the postoperative period. It is often necessary to adjust not only the amplitude of the stimulation, but also the frequency and the pulse width and even the electrode configuration, months or years after system implantation. This may be explained in part by the dynamic character of pain syndromes and by the development of tolerance to the stimulation or possible movement of the electrode in the epidural space.

Patient education is extremely important and should be started before surgical implantation. Patients with fully implanted SCS systems must understand how to use the handheld programmer or the magnet to turn the stimulator on and off and to change certain stimulation parameters. Patients with RF-coupled systems should be even more carefully educated about the power source/programming module because it allows more freedom in adjusting the stimulation parameters. In all cases, patients need to clearly understand the signs of system malfunction and should be able to contact the neurosurgeon (or other implanting physician) or their clinical personnel at any time. Spinal cord stimulation is unlikely to cause life-threatening complications (except perhaps a systemic infection); however, these patients must be closely followed, both to check the SCS status and functionality and to monitor response to SCS therapy.

ACKNOWLEDGMENT

The author wishes to thank Ms. Amy Akers for her assistance in preparing this chapter.

REFERENCES

1. Linderoth B, Foreman RD. Physiology of spinal cord stimulation: Review and update. Neuromodulation 2:150–164, 1999.
2. Melzack R, Wall PD. Pain mechanisms: A new theory. Science 150:971–978, 1965.
3. Campbell JN, Davis KD, Meyer RA, North RB. The mechanism by which dorsal column stimulation affects pain: Evidence for a new hypothesis. Pain 5:S228, 1990.
4. Linderoth B, Fedorcsak I, Meyerson BA. Peripheral vasodilatation after spinal cord stimulation: Animal studies of putative effector mechanisms. Neurosurgery 28:187–195, 1991.
5. Mannheimer C, Eliasson T, Andersson B, Bergh CH, Augustinsson LE, Emanuelsson H, Waagstein F. Effects of spinal cord stimulation in angina pectoris induced by pacing and possible mechanisms of action. BMJ 307:477–480, 1993.
6. North RB, Kidd DH, Zahurak M, James CS, Long DM. Spinal cord stimulation for chronic, intractable pain: Experience over two decades. Neurosurgery 32: 384–395, 1993.
7. Andersen C, Hole P, Oxhoj H. Does pain relief with spinal cord stimulation for angina conceal myocardial infarction? Br Heart J 71:419–421, 1994.
8. Shealy CN, Mortimer JT, Reswick J. Electrical inhibition of pain by stimulation of the dorsal column: Preliminary clinical report. Anesth Analg 46:489–491, 1967.
9. White JC, Sweet WH. Pain and the neurosurgeon. A forty-year experience. Springfield, IL: Charles C. Thomas, 1969, pp 900–901.
10. Barolat G, Massaro F, He J, Zeme S, Ketcik B. Mapping of sensory responses to epidural stimulation of the intraspinal neural structures in man. J Neurosurg 78:233–239, 1993.
11. Holsheimer J, Barolat G. Spinal geometry and paresthesia coverage in spinal cord stimulation. Neuromodulation 1:129–136, 1998.

37

Thalamic Stimulation Versus Thalamotomy

Krishna Kumar and Denny Demeria
University of Saskatchewan and Regina General Hospital,
Regina, Canada

1 INTRODUCTION

Chronic pain is a debilitating affliction whose successful treatment continues to challenge physicians and surgeons alike. Its damaging effects are pervasive, affecting both the socioeconomic and psychological status of an individual. Chronic pain treatments are often refractory to pharmacological and other nonsurgical treatments. Thalamotomy can deliver modest pain relief but is often associated with various undesirable side effects, like dysarthria, gait disturbance, and cognitive dysfunction, especially if performed bilaterally. This led to the development of stimulating techniques. The current interest in the field is derived from pioneer animal stimulation studies by Reynolds [1] and Mayer [2], and subsequent perfection of these techniques in humans by Adams [3], Richardson and Akil [4], Hosobuchi [5], and Turnbull [6]. Deep brain stimulation (DBS) effectively mimics a lesion but is reversible in nature.

The exact mechanism by which DBS achieves pain control is not well understood. There is evidence of increased concentrations of β-endorphins and met-enkephalins in the cerebrospinal fluid (CSF) after periventricular gray (PVG) stimulation [7–9]; this effect, however, is not seen with sensory thalamic nucleus (STh) or internal capsule (IC) stimulation [7]. This suggests an opioid-mediated mechanism of pain relief with PVG stimulation. The pain relief on STh or IC stimulation is hypothesized to be achieved by depolarizing blockage or jamming of the neurons, the axonal tracts, or both.

2 INDICATIONS AND PROGNOSTIC FACTORS

The conditions that respond favorably to DBS include failed back syndrome, causalgia, radiculopathies, peripheral neuropathies, trigeminal neuropathies, and phantom limb pain [10–12]. Conditions that respond poorly to DBS include paraplegic pain, thalamic pain syndromes, and postherpetic neuralgia. In general, nociceptive pain responds more favorably to PVG stimulation, whereas neuropathic pain responds to STh stimulation. Patients with pain syndromes who have had multiple operations to a given body area experience a greater degree of benefit than those without prior surgical intervention. Gender and age do not statistically affect the degree of pain relief. Depression is a very common accompaniment to chronic pain syndromes and needs to be treated before undertaking definitive surgery. We have found that patients who did not require therapy for depression had a better prognosis than those who did.

3 PATIENT SELECTION

Before being considered for DBS, patients are funneled through a multidisciplinary pain clinic setting where the conservative methods for pain control were initially tried but failed. They are assessed psychologically and treated for anxiety, depression, and somatization. Patients should meet the following basic criteria to be considered for DBS: (1) known organic cause of pain; (2) failure of conventional pain management methods; (3) absence of major psychiatric pathology or secondary gain; (4) ability to provide informed consent; (5) cessation of inappropriate drug use; (6) a favorable response to a morphine-naloxone test, which is helpful in evaluating nociceptive pain, thus aiding in target site selection [12,13]. These are not an absolute criteria for patient selection, they have a positive predictive value of 0.8, thus increasing the confidence in PVG stimulation [12]. We continue to favor its use.

3.1 Clinical Evaluation

For the purpose of evaluating the benefits of DBS or thalamotomy, a McGill Pain Questionnaire [14] and visual analog scale [15], are used both pre- and postoperatively to quantify pain levels. The use of a disinterested third party aids in eliminating bias when evaluating results.

4 TARGET SELECTION

The sites commonly selected for DBS include PVG, specific STh, and IC. The type of pain a patient presents with dictates the anatomical target selection. Nociceptive pain, which is usually diffuse, midline, deep, boring, and may be bilateral with one side being more painful than the other, responds best to PVG stimulation. Neuropathic pain, which is usually characterized as being localized, burning, and felt on the surface, often unilateral, is amenable to STh stimulation. Deafferentation pain of thalamic origin, where little viable thalamic tissue is available for stimulation, is treated by IC stimulation.

5 EQUIPMENT AND PROCEDURES

5.1 Electrode Use

Until 3 years ago, a four-contact Schreiver-type electrode (Fig. 1A) was used, which required a unique carrier for its introduction. Today, a four-contact coaxial lead (Medtronics, Inc., MN; model 3387) is used (Fig. 1B).

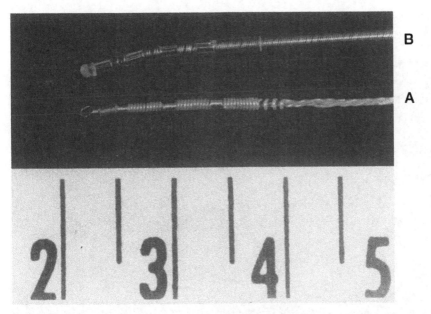

FIGURE 1   Electrodes used for deep brain stimulation. **A,** Schreiver-type four-contact point electrode. **B,** Coaxial electrode. (Courtesy of Medtronic, Inc.)

Each stimulating contact is cylindrical, made of a platinum-iridium alloy, 1.5-mm long and spaced 3.0 mm apart. The multipolar organization of the electrode allows for a number of bipolar combinations to be explored intra-operatively and during the subsequent trial period.

5.2 Surgical Technique

For the purposes of implantation of a deep brain electrode, any of the several commercially available stereotactic frames can be used. In North America today, the most popular stereotactic frames are CRW (Radionics, Burlington, MASS) and Leksell (Electa, Atlanta, GA). The procedure is completed in two stages. The initial stage is dedicated to implanting an electrode at the desired target site, and at a second stage, after a trial stimulation, the system is internalized using a fully programmable and implantable pulse generator (Fig. 2).

The first stage is performed under local anesthesia where a stereotactic frame is fixed to the patient's head. The frame should be applied such that it is parallel to the line joining the anterior (AC) and posterior commissures (PC). For this purpose, a line extending from the external auditory meatus

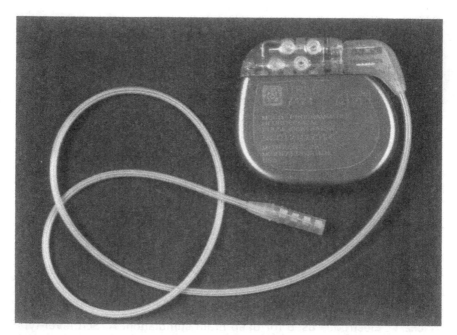

FIGURE 2 Fully implantable and programmable pulse generator, Itrel-II with its extension cord. (Courtesy of Medtronic, Inc.)

to the lateral canthus will approximate this AC-PC line. The patient is then submitted either to computed tomography (CT) or magnetic resonance imaging (MRI), with an appropriate localizer box. Coordinates for the target are acquired from appropriate computed tomographic or magnetic resonance imaging slices. Atlases that are commonly used for plotting target sites include those compiled by Emmers and Tasker [16], or Schaltenbrand and Wahren [17]. Until the advent of high-resolution CT scanners or MRI, ventriculography was used for target localization. Currently, MRI is the preferred imaging technique.

5.2.1 Anatomic Target Localization

The target site for PVG stimulation is 2 mm anterior to the posterior commissure on the line joining the anterior and posterior commissures, and 2 to 3 mm lateral to the posterior third ventricle, within the parafascicularis-center-median complex (Fig. 3).

Sensory thalamus electrodes are implanted in the region where the medial lemniscus enters the sensory thalamus. The final location for electrode placement is determined by the anatomical location of the pain—for instance, for facial pain, the nucleus ventralis posterior medialis (Vpm) is used; for arm, upper, or lower extremity and trunk pain, the nucleus ventralis posterior lateralis (Vpl) is chosen. The Vpm is located 8 to 10 mm lateral to the midline, and 8 to 10 mm posterior to the midpoint of the line joining the anterior and posterior commissures. The Vpl nucleus is located 14 to 16 mm lateral to the midline and 10 to 12 mm posterior to the midpoint of the line joining the anterior and posterior commissures.

For patients selected for internal capsule implantation, the target site is located within the posterior limb of the IC, located approximately 25 mm lateral to the midline, and 12 to 14 mm posterior to the midpoint of the intercommissural line.

5.2.2 Surgical Procedure

After the coordinates of the target site have been determined, the patient is returned to the operating room, where the stereotactic frame is fixed to the operating table, with the help of a Mayfield clamp. Under local anesthesia, a burr hole is made 3 cm parasagittally, at the level of the coronal suture, on the side contralateral to the maximum pain. The dura is coagulated and incised in a cruciate fashion. The pial surface is also coagulated and incised, avoiding surface vessels. The target coordinates, which have been selected, are then mounted and a search probe with a tip diameter of 1.1 mm (Radionics) is introduced into the brain parenchyma, to a point 5.0 mm proximal to the chosen target. Physiological localization is commenced at this time, with the aim of correlating physiological and anatomical findings. Physio-

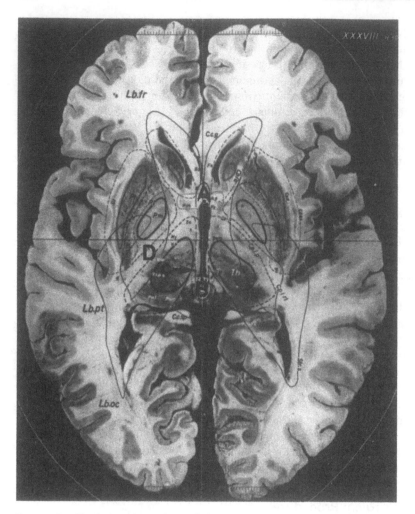

FIGURE 3   Horizontal section of the brain at the level of the intercommissural line. **A**, Anterior commissure; **B**, Posterior commissure; **C**, Periventicular gray; **D**, Internal capsule; **Th**, Thalamus. (Reproduced from Schaltenbrand G. Wahren W: Atlas for Stereotaxy of Human Brain. 2nd ed. Stuttgart: George Thieme, 1977). By permission.

logical correlation can be achieved either with microelectrode recording and stimulation, or macrostimulation. Microelectrode stimulation is more precise, as it provides definitive physiological identification of receptive fields and neural firings. However, it is time consuming and requires special training in neurophysiology. Macrostimulation is rapid and requires minimal equipment. For treatment of pain patients, macrostimulation serves equally well.

The probe is then advanced toward the target site in increments of 1.0 mm. For physiological confirmation, stimulation is initiated 5.0 mm above the target and is continued to 3 to 5.0 mm below the target. Final electrode placement is determined by a positive physiological response. For PVG stimulation, a warm or cold feeling, felt contralaterally or over the body generally, during intraoperative stimulation, is considered a favorable prognostic sign. These feelings are described as relaxing, pleasurable, and likened to a post-orgasmic state. Because of the proximity of the Edinger-Westphal and third cranial nerve nuclei to the target area, the patient may experience blurred vision at the initiation of stimulation. At greater amplitudes, this may progress to oscillopsia, nystagmus, or upward-gaze deficits. This tends to disappear when the amplitude is decreased or stimulation is ceased. A few patients may experience contralateral paresthesia on the face, which is attributed to current spreading to the medial lemniscus. Patients often report pain reduction after 10 minutes of successful intraoperative stimulation. Anterior placement of the electrode more than 3.0 mm could lead to sympathetic responses, such as anxiety and fear, whereas posterior and deeper placement in the periaqueductal gray matter or brainstem could cause adverse responses such as vertigo, smothering, or nausea.

For IC or STh implantation, lower voltage stimulation at 100 Hz will yield paresthesia in the area encompassing the entire painful region, when the proper target site is reached.

5.2.3 Implantation of the DBS Electrode

Once the physiological confirmation of the target site is achieved, the search probe is removed and replaced by the stimulating electrode. To confirm the final position and trajectory of the DBS electrode, the use of intraoperative fluoroscopy is mandatory. This ensures that during subsequent manipulations, the lead does not migrate dorsally or ventrally from its intended position. Once final electrode placement has been achieved, trial stimulation is initiated with a handheld pulse generator device (Screener, Medtronics). If the physiological confirmatory signs are reproduced, the stylet of the electrode is removed and the stem of the electrode is then fixed to the skull with the help of a burr hole ring and cap (Medtronics). External percutaneous lead extensions are connected to the distal end of the deep brain electrode, which is brought out through a separate stab incision, and the wound is closed.

6 TRIAL STIMULATION

Trial stimulation begins 2 to 3 days after implantation and continues for 5 to 7 days. During this period, the neuromodulation team ascertains the best electrode combination, frequency, pulse width, and amplitude for optimal pain control. Periventricular gray stimulation yields best results with a frequency of 50 to 75 Hz, voltages from 1 to 5 V and a pulse width of 120 to 210 μs. Conversely, STh stimulation is optimized at 75 to 100 Hz, 2 to 8 V, and 210 to 330 μs.

7 PULSE GENERATOR IMPLANTATION
AND PROGRAMMING

Those patients achieving greater than 50% pain relief as compared to presurgical levels have their systems internalized under general anesthesia. Those patients who do not achieve this degree of pain control have their electrodes removed.

   The distal end of the deep brain electrode is connected to an implantable and programmable pulse stimulator (Itrel II or III, Medtronic), which is placed in a subcutaneous pocket in the infraclavicular region. For this purpose, a connector cord has to be tunneled through the subcutaneous tissues in the neck and scalp. The proximal female end of the connector cord is connected to the distal end of the deep brain electrode. The distal end of the connector cord, which has two pins, is inserted in the proper sockets of the pulse generator and is secured by tightening the Allen screws. The pulse generator is returned to the infraclavicular subcutaneous pocket, and the wounds are closed. The pulse generator is activated the next day, and the optimum stimulator parameters are programmed using a command module. The patient can also activate or deactivate the unit by holding a magnet over the pulse generator for 3 seconds.

   Sensory thalamus implant patients require more stimulation per day as compared to PVG implant patients. To prolong battery life, the pulse generators are used in a cycling mode. The PVG implants have an "on" period for 40 to 50 seconds every 10 to 15 minutes. Sensory thalamus stimulators are activated for at least 60 seconds every 10 minutes.

8 COMPLICATIONS

Hardware-related issues are the most common complications (9.4%) [12]. These include electrode fracture, electrical leakage at connector sites or resulting from insulation breaks, and hardware malfunction. These are corrected by replacement of the appropriate part. Wound infections, when superficial, are treated with antimicrobial therapy, and failing this, may require removal of the system. Other complications include seizures and intracerebral hematomas. Bendok and Levy [18] report a meta-analysis of 649 DBS patients, in which the incidence of intracerebral hemorrhage was 1.59% to 4.1%. Fourteen of 649 patients suffered neurological deficits as a result of intracranial hematoma. Stimulation can induce migraine-like headaches, which has been reported to have an incidence of 8.6 to 23% [19,20]. It has been observed to occur more frequently in PVG stimulation, although it has been reported in STh stimulation as well.

During the follow-up period, tolerance may develop. Tolerance is a major cause of loss of pain control in the follow-up period and is defined as a progressive loss of effective pain control in spite of a functioning stimulation program. It is much more frequent with PVG stimulation [21,22], although it has been reported in STh implants as well [12,23]. Tolerance is treated initially by a 3- to 4-week stimulation holiday, introduction of pharmacotherapy, such as amitryptiline, and if this fails, contralateral hemispheric electrode implants will alleviate tolerance in PVG implants, but not STh implants [11,12].

9 DISCUSSION

Thalamotomy has been used for the alleviation of chronic pain [24,25]. When used in the treatment of chronic benign pain, it has a low success rate of approximately 30% [25]. Bilateral procedures have a serious drawback of producing ataxia, dysarthria, and cognitive deficits. Tasker's [26] review of medial thalamotomy cases for central and deafferentation pain gives an average success rate of only 29%, but produced cognitive disturbances in 54.2% of patients with unilateral medial thalamotomy and in 75% of patients with bilateral lesions. Dorsal median thalamotomy is preferred for the treatment of chronic malignant pain, in which early pain relief reported by up to 80% of patients [27]. However, it has the serious disadvantages of producing profound changes in personality and depression. In spite of low success rates and high complication rates, there may be a place for lesions in the medial thalamus in the treatment of central and deafferentation pain, especially for allodynia and hyperpathia, when chronic electrical stimulation of the ventral caudal nucleus fails [26].

The leading advantage of DBS is that it is adjustable and reversible and allows for maximum efficacy while minimizing complications. The stimulation program achieves an average long-term success rate of 59% for nociceptive pain when treated by PVG stimulation [18]. The long-term benefits in STh stimulation for neuropathic pain achieve 56% long-term success [18].

The major concern in neurostimulation programs is the cost of the equipment implanted. In the United States, the total cost of the implantable equipment is approximately $11,000 (the breakdown of costs being approximately: lead $2,000; pulse generator Itrel-II or III $8,000; extension cord, burr hole ring and cap, etc. $1,000). To this, one needs to add the costs associated with screening the patient pre- and postoperatively, and the cost of regulating and optimizing the pulse generator in the postoperative period. The battery life of the pulse generator varies from 4 to 5 years depending on usage. As the pulse generator is a sealed unit, it will require replacement at the end of its life.

In spite of these costs, neurostimulation is superior to ablative surgery, both in terms of degree and duration of pain control. The complications are few and acceptable with little by way of cognitive deficits. Thus, it remains the treatment of choice for chronic benign pain in a select group of cases.

It is regrettable that this procedure has not yet received approval by the Food and Drug Administration for use in the United States, but is approved in Canada and European countries.

10 CONCLUSIONS

Our combined success rates involving PVG and STh nuclei stimulation approaches 63%, in a mean follow-up period of 78 months [12]. Properly placed electrodes have acceptable complication rates, with few cognitive deficits. It is recognized that the cost of this modality could be an inhibiting factor, but it is far superior to the destructive procedure of thalamotomy, as this can lead to cognitive deficits, especially when bilateral lesions are made. Deep brain stimulation is a viable alternative for patients with benign chronic pain in whom conventional measures have failed.

REFERENCES

1. Reynolds DV. The surgery in the rat during electrical analgesia induced by focal brain stimulation. Science 164:444–445, 1969.
2. Mayer DJ, Wolfe TL, Akil H, Carder B, Liebeskind JC. Analgesia from electrical stimulation in the brain stem of the rat. Science 174:1351–1354, 1971.
3. Adams JE, Hosobuchi Y, Fields HL. Stimulation of internal capsule for relief of chronic pain. J Neurosurg 41:740–744, 1974.
4. Richardson DE, Akil H. Pain reduction by electrical brain stimulation in man. J Neurosurg 41:178–194, 1977.
5. Hosobuchi Y, Adams JE, Rutkin B. Chronic thalamic stimulation for the control of facial anesthesia dolorosa. Arch Neurol 29:158–161, 1973.

6. Turnbull I, Shulman R, Woodhurst W. Thalamic stimulation for neuropathic pain. J Neurosurg 52:486–493, 1980.
7. Hosobuchi Y, Rossier J, Bloom PE, Guillemin R. Periaqueductal gray stimulation for pain suppression in humans. In: Bonica JJ, Liebeskind JC, Albe-Fessard DG, eds. Advances in Pain Research and Therapy. Vol. 3. New York: Raven Press, 1979, pp 515–523.
8. Young RF, Flemming WB, van Norman AS, Yaksh TL. Release of beta-endorphin and methionine-enkaphalin into cerebrospinal fluid during deep brain stimulation for chronic pain: Effects of stimulation locus and site of sampling. J Neurosurg 79:816–825, 1993.
9. Dionne RA, Mueller GP, Young RF, Greenberg RP, Hargreaves KM, Gracely R, Dubner R. Contrast medium causes the apparent increase in beta-endorphin levels in human cerebrospinal fluid following brain stimulation. Pain 20:313–321, 1984.
10. Kumar K, Wyant GM. Deep brain stimulation for control of intractable pain in humans. Transplant/Implant Today 4:40–46, 1987.
11. Kumar K, Wyant GM, Nath RK. Deep brain stimulation for control of intractable pain in humans, present and future: A ten-year follow-up. Neurosurgery 26:774–782, 1990.
12. Kumar K, Toth C, Nath RK. Deep brain stimulation for intractable pain: A 15-year experience. Neurosurgery 40:736–747, 1997.
13. Hosobuchi Y. Subcortical electrical stimulation for control of intractable pain in humans. J Neurosurg 64:543–553, 1986.
14. Carlsson AM. Assessment of chronic pain: Aspects of reliability and validity of visual analog scale. Pain 16:87–101, 1983.
15. Hukkison S. Visual analog scale. In: Melzack R, ed. Pain Measurement and Assessment. New York: Raven Press, 1983, pp 33–40.
16. Emmers R, Tasker RR. The Human Somesthetic Thalamus with Maps for Physiological Target Localization during Stereotactic Neurosurgery. New York: Raven press, 1975.
17. Schaltenbrand G, Wahren W. Atlas for Stereotaxy of the Human Brain. New York: Thieme, 1977.
18. Bendok B, Levy RM. Brain stimulation for persistent pain management. In: Textbook of Stereotactic and Functional Neurosurgery. New York: McGraw-Hill, 1998, pp 1539–1546.
19. Veloso F, Kumar K, Toth C. Headache secondary to deep brain implantation. Headache 38:507–515, 1998.
20. Raskin NH, Hosobuchi Y, Lamb S. Headache may arise from perturbation of brain. Headache 24:416–420, 1987.
21. Hosobuchi Y, Lamb S, Bascom D. Tryptophan loading may reverse tolerance to opiate analgesics in humans: A preliminary report. Pain 9:161–169, 1980.
22. Hosobuchi Y. The current status of analgesic brain stimulation. Acta Neurochir Suppl (Wien) 30:79–84. 1980.
23. Young RF, Chambi VI. Pain relief by electrical stimulation of the periaqueductal and periventricular gray matter: Evidence for a non-opioid mechanism. J Neurosurg 66:364–371, 1987.

24. White JC, Sweet WH. Pain and the neurosurgeon. A forty-year experience. Springfield, IL: Thomas, 1969, p 854.

25. Voris HC, Whisler WW. Results of stereotaxic surgery for intractable pain. Confin Neurol 37:86–96, 1975.

26. Tasker RR. Thalamotomy. In: Friedman WA, ed. Neurosurgery Clinics of North America. Vol. 1. Philadelphia: Saunders, 1990, pp 854–864.

27. Gildenberg PL. Functional neurosurgery. In: Schmidek HH, Sweet WH, eds. Operative Neurosurgical Techniques. Indications, Method and Results. Vol. 2. New York: Grune and Stratton, 1983, pp 1001–1016.

38

Intrathecal Narcotics: Spinal and Intraventricular

Konstantin V. Slavin

University of Illinois at Chicago, Chicago, Illinois, U.S.A.

Angelyn M. Solko

Harborview Medical Center and University of Washington School of Pharmacy, Seattle, Washington, U.S.A.

1 INTRODUCTION

A scientific basis for the application of intrathecal opioids was first laid in 1970s when highly specific opioid receptors were discovered in the nervous system of rats and primates [1]. Subsequently, opioid receptors were identified in the substantia gelatinosa of the dorsal root entry zone of the human spinal cord [2]. Clinical effectiveness of intrathecal morphine was demonstrated by Wang [3] in 1979 and since then, the idea of intrathecal drug delivery for pain control has gained wide acceptance in medical circles.

Chronic pain is estimated to affect 15% to 30% of the general population of the United States, which translates into considerable healthcare expenditures. Ten years ago, low back pain alone was estimated to cost $25 billion a year in medical care expenses. Although staggering, this figure still fails to include the loss of productivity of affected individuals and the decrease in their quality of life (and that of their families). All this makes it very important to evaluate the array of available therapeutic options to maximize patient comfort while minimizing adverse effects.

The best example of a constructive approach in pain management is an algorithm suggested by the World Health Organization (WHO) for treatment of cancer-related pain [4]. This straightforward, three-step ladder approach advocates progressively stronger analgesic combinations until the patient is free from pain. Application of WHO guidelines may well control more than 80% of cancer-related pain syndromes. Intraspinal regimens are not currently included in the guidelines, but many authors have proposed the addition of a fourth step to incorporate the use of intrathecal opioids and surgical interventions [5].

2 INDICATIONS

Clinical and experimental data show that the analgesic effect of neuraxial opioids is achieved through action at spinal and supraspinal receptors with minimal influence on motor, sensory, or sympathetic reflexes. The exclusive location of opioid receptors involved in nociception and pain transmission within the central nervous system results in the ability to achieve similar analgesic action (equianalgesia) with the use of significantly lower doses of the opioid medication when administered directly into the cerebrospinal fluid. Secondary to this, equianalgesic doses of intrathecally administered opioids produce fewer side effects than systemic administration.

A patient's responsiveness to pain management modalities frequently depends on the type(s) of pain that he or she experiences [5]. Nociceptive pain that arises from actual or potential tissue injury may be generally divided into visceral and somatic. Visceral nociceptive pain is seen in patients with pancreatic, lung, and liver cancers; it is described as a constant, dull, aching pain, diffuse in nature and often difficult to localize. Somatic nociceptive pain may be pain that is observed, for example, in patients with bone metastases and muscular injury; it also can be constant and aching but takes on a more localized and throbbing nature. Neuropathic pain originates from injury to the nervous system itself and represents a pathological phenomenon that, as far as we know, does not carry any useful or protective function. This type of pain is characterized as a burning, shooting pain. Traditionally, intraspinal narcotic therapy for neuropathic pain has been considered less effective, but recent studies have proven its validity as a more conservative therapeutic option compared with irreversible neuroablative surgery. Mixed neuropathic and nociceptive pain is also a possibility and often requires a combination of narcotic and adjunctive medications.

Intrathecal opioids were originally limited to pain from a cancer etiology, but their use in pain of nonmalignant origin is rapidly gaining acceptance [6]. Some of the current "benign" (non-cancer-related) disease states treated with intraspinal administration of opioids include failed back surgery syndrome [7], postherpetic neuralgia [8], phantom limb pain [9], lumbar

arachnoiditis, multiple sclerosis, rheumatoid arthritis, amyloidosis polyneuropathy [10], reflex sympathetic dystrophy, and vertebral collapse caused by
osteoporosis.

3 PATIENT SELECTION

A patient with chronic pain that is expected to persist for more than 6 months
should be considered for intrathecal opioid therapy. The ideal candidate is
one who has already failed conventional narcotic treatment, experienced
intolerable side effects, or failed other pain management modalities such as
spinal cord stimulation.

A thorough physical assessment, psychological evaluation, and test
dose trial must be performed before scheduling the actual surgery for pump
placement. Medical history, physical assessment, and appropriate imaging
tests allow one to determine the type of pain that the patient is experiencing.
Baseline pain rating can be assessed with a visual analogue scale (VAS),
numerical pain rating, verbal pain scale, patient and caregiver questionnaires,
and pain drawings.

Disease states that would preclude pump implantation should also be
identified. Contraindications to implantation generally consist of aplastic
anemia, systemic infections, allergies to the metal or plastics used in the
pump or catheter, active intravenous drug abuse, and coagulopathies [11].
Psychological contraindications can be identified by commonly used tests,
such as the McGill Pain Questionnaire, Minnesota Mutiphasic Personality
Inventory (MMPI-2), and the Beck Depression Inventory. Formal psychiatric
consultation should be considered.

A trial of intraspinal opioid, either epidural or intrathecal, is used as a
mechanism to predict long-term success. A positive response is usually defined as a 50% reduction in baseline pain scores without the presence of
intolerable side effects. The trial can be performed by a bolus injection or
as a continuous infusion. The exact technique generally depends on the
clinician's comfort level and judgment. One of the most common techniques
involves insertion of an epidural catheter and gradual titration of continuous
morphine infusion until the desired effect is achieved. A trial with continuous
infusion mimics a pump more closely. Because the epidural route is associated with larger dosing requirements and more extensive systemic uptake,
an intrathecal trial may result in fewer side effects. However, so far there is
no evidence that either approach (epidural vs intrathecal, continuous vs bolus
administration, opioid only vs placebo controlled) results in higher predict-
ability of subsequent treatment success [12].

4 PUMP SELECTION AND SURGICAL TECHNIQUE

There are many different techniques for long-term intrathecal drug administration (Table 1). The simplest methods include external and tunneled catheters and subcutaneous ports. These are often inserted by anesthesiologists and serve best for intra-axial trials and short-term management of intractable pain. Neurosurgeons may be called to help with insertion of these catheters if patients have complicated spinal anatomy and need laminectomy for intraspinal access. More commonly, however, neurosurgeons use intra-axial drug administration techniques that involve implantation of the drug pump system. The pumps that are used for intrathecal drug administration are divided into continuous flow and programmable types, and each type has its own benefits and disadvantages.

Pumps with continuous flow can deliver opiates and other medications intrathecally and epidurally at a fixed preset rate. These pumps are connected to standard intraspinal catheters and require refilling every few weeks, depending on pump volume and flow rate. Medication refills are performed by percutaneous access of the pump reservoir. The flow rate is maintained by constant pressure of compressed freon gas onto reservoir bellows. The delivered dose of medication may be adjusted by changing the concentration of the injected solution. The reservoir holds between 30 and 50 ml of fluid, and the flow rate is calibrated and preset at 1.0 ml to 6.0 ml per day [13]. Some pumps in this category have sideports that allow bolus injections using special needles. The most commonly used fixed flow rate pump in earlier clinical studies was the Infusaid® Model 400, manufactured by Infusaid Corp. [14]. Other models include IP 35.1 made by Anschütz, and model 4000 manufactured by Therex Corp. [15]. Currently, Arrow International manufactures and markets a 30-ml constant flow implantable pump with bolus safety valve (model 3000) and similar 16-ml pump (model 3000-16). Both models are available with high-, medium- and low-flow infusion rates.

TABLE 1 Types of Intrathecal Drug Delivery Systems

1. Short-term intraspinal (epidural or intrathecal) catheters
2. Long-term tunneled catheters (externalized)
3. Intraspinal catheters connected to implantable (injection/infusion) port
4. Intraspinal catheters with implanted bag/reservoir and manual pump
5. Implanted systems with constant flow-rate pumps
6. Implanted systems with programmable pumps

A programmable variable rate pump provides multiple options that are not available with other systems. This system is also fully implantable and is refilled percutaneously. The programmable pump is manufactured by Medtronic, Inc.; it contains an 18-ml collapsible drug reservoir with a center fill port equipped with self-sealing silicone septum and a needle stop. A battery-driven miniature peristaltic pump delivers medication from the reservoir to the intrathecal catheter through a 0.22-μm bacterial retentive filter. The rate of infusion may be changed using a pump programmer that communicates with the pump through a two-way radiofrequency link. The telemetry process also allows assessment of battery status and remaining volume of medication inside the reservoir, adjustment of the infusion mode, and setting alarms for low battery power and low drug volume. In addition to this information, the electronic module of the pump stores the date and time of latest prescription change, patient identification, name and concentration of medication, infusion parameters, and alarm settings. Available infusion modes include continuous, complex continuous, single bolus, and periodic bolus modes. Infusion rates may vary between 0.1 and 1.5 ml/day. Programmable pumps have gained wide popularity during the last 15 years primarily because of their versatility and reliability.

All types of intrathecal delivery systems require the presence of an intrathecal catheter. Such a catheter is usually made of silicone and can tolerate a certain degree of kinking without obstructing its lumen. The technique of catheter insertion into the intrathecal space is similar for all system types. For catheters that are connected to the implantable pump, we recommend anchoring the catheter to the lumbar fascia before catheter tunneling. For this purpose, a vertical incision is performed to accommodate the anchor and to expose the fascia. For short-term catheters, anchoring is not needed because it may interfere with catheter removal.

If the insertion is performed in the operating room, fluoroscopic control using a C-arm is recommended. Midlumbar placement of the needle is preferred. A standard 16-gauge Tuohy needle may be inserted paramedially at the L3-4 level, aiming slightly in a cephalad direction. Once the dura is penetrated, the needle stylet is removed, and cerebrospinal fluid backflow confirms subarachnoid position of the needle tip. After that, an intrathecal catheter with a guidewire in it is inserted through the needle and carefully advanced in a cephalad direction under fluoroscopic guidance. Absence of resistance during advancement of the catheter usually indicates correct positioning in the intrathecal space. Slight rotation of the spinal needle may help in guiding the catheter.

After the catheter is advanced to the desired level, the guidewire and the spinal needle are removed and patency of the catheter is checked by observing flow of the cerebrospinal fluid from the catheter tip. If the catheter is intended for connection to an implantable pump, it needs to be anchored to prevent its dislodgement. Variously shaped anchors are usually supplied with intrathecal catheters. They may be sutured to the underlying fascia with nonabsorbable sutures before the tunneling of the catheter. After the anchoring, the catheter is tunneled toward the pump pocket using a special tunneling rod that is passed subcutaneously from the pocket to the lumbar incision.

Pumps for intrathecal drug administration are usually inserted into the anterior abdominal wall, most commonly into the left upper quadrant. The exact location of the pump is chosen after consideration of the patient's belt line, wheelchair arms, prostheses, other implantable devices (e.g., spinal cord stimulators), scars from previous surgical interventions, ostomies, etc.

A straight skin incision is made over the planned pump site. The subcutaneous pocket is created so that the pump is covered by a soft tissue layer no more than 2.5 cm in thickness. The pump is fitted into the pocket and appropriate enlargement of the pocket is performed so that neither the central reservoir port nor the sideport rests under the skin incision. Meticulous hemostasis is a must.

Once the intrathecal catheter is tunneled to the pump pocket using a tunneling rod, the catheter is connected to the pump attachment. The connection is covered with a silicone sleeve and secured with nonabsorbable sutures. Pump attachments are available in straight and right-angle configurations that fit different pump models.

Before the attachment of the catheter to the pump, the pump needs to be tested and filled with medication. The programmable pump needs to be interrogated using a pump programmer. The calibration constant is checked and compared to the pump label. Pump settings are then changed from factory preset slow continuous infusion to a complete "stop." A small "purge" bolus is started so that the internal tubing of the pump may be cleared. At the same time, the alarms are turned on and the residual volume of the pump reservoir is checked. Once the purging bolus is completed, the pump reservoir is entered with a noncoring needle and emptied by gentle aspiration of the fluid from the reservoir using a 20-ml syringe. It is usually possible to aspirate 14 to 16 ml of fluid from an 18-ml pump and 6 to 8 ml from a 10-ml pump. The prescribed medication is then injected into the reservoir through the central refill port. Detailed instructions for pump preparation and filling are typically supplied with the pump. For a fixed rate pump, the rate of infusion has to be checked by observing the flow from the silicone extension tubing that is an integral part of the pump. A drop of fluid should form at the tubing tip if a filled pump is kept at temperature of 90° to 95° F (32°–35° C) for 10 minutes.

Once the pump is tested and its reservoir is filled, the catheter is attached to the catheter connector or extension tubing of the pump. All tubing connections are secured with nonabsorbable sutures. The pump is then placed into its subcutaneous pocket, and excess catheter tubing is coiled behind the pump. Suturing of the pump to the underlying fascia is performed with nonabsorbable sutures that are passed either through metal loops on the pump surface or through a Dacron sock that is supplied with the programmable pump. After additional irrigation, final hemostasis is achieved and incisions are closed in standard fashion.

5 INITIATING INTRATHECAL THERAPY

Morphine is the most commonly used intrathecal medication for pain relief and is currently the only drug approved by the U.S. Food and Drug Administration (FDA) for intrathecal pain therapy. Its long duration of action, predictable receptor affinity, and well-studied dosage titration and side effect profile make it the ideal narcotic to start with when initiating intraspinal analgesia in the majority of patients. The patient's average daily dose of narcotics from all sources needs to be converted to an equianalgesic intravenous morphine dose (Table 2). From there the epidural dose is one tenth of the intravenous dose and the intrathecal dose is one tenth that of the epidural dose. Therefore, a patient that requires 300 mg of continuous release oral morphine each day would need approximately 100 mg intravenously, 10 mg epidurally, and only 1 mg intrathecally per day.

Drug properties, such as receptor affinity and lipophilicity, and patient factors, such as age, pain severity, and the presence of neuropathic pain, can make predicting the effects of the preliminary infusion rate challenging. To avoid overdosing, only 50% of the calculated dose should be programmed when initiating therapy, changing to other narcotics, or adding adjunctive medications. Breakthrough narcotics with a short onset of action, adminis-

TABLE 2 Approximate Equianalgesic Dose

	Oral	Parenteral
Morphine	30 mg	10 mg
Hydromorphone	7.5 mg	1.5 mg
Levorphanol	2 mg	4 mg
Methadone	20 mg	10 mg
Oxycodone	30 mg	15 mg
Codeine	200 mg	120 mg

tered orally, should be continued until intrathecal therapy is effective. Dose increases of 20% to 30% are generally made every 5 to 7 days. A specific ceiling dose has not been defined, but hyperanalgesic syndrome can occur at high intrathecal doses (more than 25 mg per day of morphine) [16]. These high-dose-related symptoms include acute severe pain, hypersensitivity, autonomic abnormalities in the lower extremities, myoclonus, and piloerection. The morphine metabolite morphine-3-glucuronide is thought to be responsible. It binds to the glycine receptor producing strychnine-like effects on the spinal cord. Therefore, caution is necessary at high doses because of the unpredictability of this syndrome.

6 ALTERNATIVE DRUGS

6.1 Opioids

When intrathecal morphine has been titrated to ceiling effect levels or when other intolerable side effects arise, switching treatment to another opiate may prove advantageous (Fig. 1). Although not FDA approved for use in the United States, hydromorphone is the second narcotic of choice for intrathecal installation. It is a mu agonist that is five to ten times more potent than morphine [17]. Hydromorphone has less rostral spread in the cerebrospinal fluid (CSF), causing less stimulation at the chemoreceptor trigger zone, which may translate into less nausea and vomiting.

Meperidine, a phenylpiperdine derivative, has been used in intrathecal pumps as well. It is more lipid soluble than morphine or hydromorphone and has a quicker onset of action. However, one of meperidine's metabolites, normeperidine, is associated with neurostimulant side effects, such as psychosis and seizures. More data on its use may prove beneficial, as meperidine has displayed some additional, local, nonopioid receptor-dependent, anesthetic properties [17].

Intrathecal methadone is approximately 18 times less potent than intrathecal morphine [17]. The subsequent need for frequent refills and this drug's high side effect profile make its use limited. Both sufentanil and fentanyl have been tried, but more studies are needed.

6.2 Adjunctive Anesthetics

Synergistic antinociceptive activity has been displayed by the addition of local anesthetics to intraspinal opioids. They act by different mechanisms, primarily blunting neuroexcitability within the spinal cord. Bupivacaine is most frequently used because of its long duration of action, but tetracaine [18] and lidocaine also have been studied. The addition of bupivacaine not only improves pain control but can decrease morphine requirements, thereby

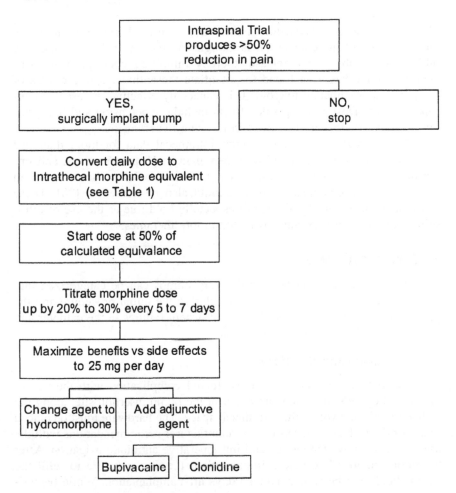

FIGURE 1 Initiating intrathecal therapy.

reducing side effects and the need for frequent pump refills [19]. High doses of bupivicaine (e.g., more than 30–60 mg per day) have been associated with sensory deficits, motor complaints, autonomic dysfunction, and neurotoxicity [17].

6.3 Adjunctive Alpha Agonists

When the use of the spinal anesthetics in a patient with chronic pain is ineffective or intolerable, changing the adjunctive therapy to an alpha-2-adrenergic agonist may prove successful [18]. Within this drug class, clonidine, tizanidine, and dexmedotomidine have been used, but clonidine is the most common of these agents. It is thought to produce analgesic effects by inhibition of substance P release, thereby inhibiting nociceptive neurons [18]. Clonidine has been found to potentiate the antinociceptive effects of morphine approximately fivefold. It is especially effective in cases of neuropathic pain. Dose-limiting side effects include hypotension and bradycardia. Abrupt withdrawal may result in rebound hypertension.

It is important to analyze future intrathecal data for more than just efficacy. Without proper attention to osmolality, pH, preservatives, and impurities, many substances used may result in neurotoxicity. The stability and compatibility of combination drugs should also be addressed [20]. These pharmacological considerations will especially hold true as the use of intraspinal administration expands to include more therapies.

7 COMPLICATIONS

Complications of intrathecal drug delivery pumps can be categorized into three areas: surgical complications both during the initial procedure and the postoperative healing phase, technical or system failures in the catheter and the pump itself, and medication-related.

7.2 Surgical Complications

Infection risks are probably the most feared complication with the use of intraspinal opioids. Infection can occur at the pump insertion site, along the catheter track, and within the intrathecal space. The hardware must be placed under sterile technique according to manufacturer recommendations with the use of perioperative antibiotics and intraoperative antibiotic irrigation. After the initial pump filling before implantation, the first puncture to refill the pump should not be earlier than 10 days after implantation. While bacteriostatic filters are present in the pump and the catheter tubing, great care should be taken by trained practitioners to not introduce bacteria during subsequent refills. Meningitis, although rare, should be suspected in the presence of fever, headache, stiff neck, rigors, and photophobia. If an infection develops, normal skin flora, such as *Staphylococcus aureus* and *S. epidermidis*, are the most common offenders.

Excessive bleeding is another surgical complication. The procedure does not involve highly vascular areas, but the blind nature of the tunneling rod and catheter placement may prove problematic. Postsurgical formation of a small epidural hematoma can create a medium for bacterial growth; a large clot can compress the spinal cord or cauda equina. As mentioned above, if patients have bleeding disorders or are anticoagulated, these represent an absolute contraindication to pump placement.

Tissue damage resulting in neurological sequelae such as radiculitis, myelitis, paralysis, and incontinence may also occur [16]. Intrathecal granuloma formation at the catheter tip can present as intractable pain or weakness and have devastating effects [21]. Cerebrospinal fluid leakage and the formation of CSF hygromas is also possible.

7.3 Drug Delivery System Complications

Complications involving the intrathecal hardware itself are most often related to the catheter, and pump malfunction is rare. The catheter can become kinked, obstructed, dislodged, or disconnected, and it can leak or break [22]. Interestingly, some data indicate that the majority of catheter system complications are related to implantation technique at the time of surgery and not the catheter tubing itself [22]. The patient who reports a sudden loss of pain relief or acute withdrawal symptoms should be evaluated radiographically for a catheter dysfunction. Patients who exhibit signs of narcotic overdose, either secondary to pump malfunction or miscalculation during refills, should also have the reservoir drained and scanned. It is important to use only radiocontrast agents that have been approved for use intraspinally to avoid additional adverse effects. Naloxone, an opiate antagonist, may also be required to reverse the analgesic.

The rapid acceptance of implantable pumps can likely be linked to the improvements in the technology of the pumps themselves. Side ports accessible by small 25-gauge needles, batteries with longer half-lives (36 to 60 months), and catheters reinforced with a titanium coil, have decreased the likelihood of problems and have made intrathecal pump placement a more feasible alternative.

Typical narcotic side effects include pruritus, nausea, vomiting, urinary retention, constipation, sexual dysfunction, and respiratory depression. The exact mechanism of pruritus is unclear. Histamine release is not thought to be the etiology, but antihistamines, such as diphenhydramine, are often effective. Nausea and vomiting are common with intrathecal opioids. It is thought that the side effects result from interaction with opioid receptors in the area postrema. Nausea could also be caused by unresolved constipation. These symptoms tend to be dose-related and are usually relieved by antiemetics, such as metoclopramide, prochloroperazine, and ondansetron. Urinary retention is an adverse effect most commonly found in elderly men with enlarged prostates. It is not a dose-related phenomenon, but rather a drug interaction with opioid receptors in the sacral spinal cord. Their stimulation causes detrusor muscle relaxation and an increase in bladder capacity. Adjunctive treatment with terazosin may be helpful. Constipation from opioids is caused by decreased gastric motility and prolonged intestinal transit time. To increase gastrointestinal motility, stimulant laxatives, such as bisacodyl, are beneficial. Increased retention time allows for greater fluid extraction and stool softeners, such as docusate, or bulk-forming laxatives, such as psyllium, counteract these effects. Sexual dysfunction is another adverse effect that should be monitored in both men and women. Levels of thyroid functioning, cortisol, and testosterone or estrogen should be obtained and followed if loss of libido, difficulty achieving or maintaining an erection, or amenorrhea develops. Some patients may require hormone replacement and the use of steroids.

Respiratory depression occurs most often in the opioid-naïve after initiation or dose increase. It can occur early (within hours) or late and is the result of interaction at the medullary respiratory center within the brain. Caution should be exercised with coadministration from any route of other central nervous system depressants. Tolerance to this side effect develops with continued narcotic exposure.

7.4 Tolerance/Addiction

Many practitioners are hesitant to resort to intrathecal opioid administration because of unrealistic fears of tolerance, physical dependence, or addiction development. Analgesic tolerance is defined as a situation in which exposure to the opioid itself causes higher dosages to maintain the same level of analgesic effect. Early intrathecal animal models have shown that after only 7 days of repeated bolus doses of intrathecal morphine in primates, no effects of the drug could be seen [23]. Clinical practice, however, does not exhibit such rapid tolerance. In fact, it is difficult to distinguish opiate tolerance from increased pain requirements resulting from disease progression.

Physical dependence and addiction, although often referred to interchangeably, are actually very different. Physical dependence occurs after chronic use of narcotics by all routes of administration. The term refers to signs of withdrawal upon abrupt discontinuation of opioids. Addiction, on the other hand, is a psychological dependence on narcotics, displayed by drug-seeking behavior without regard to harm to self or others. The likelihood of development of addiction in a person with no history of drug abuse is low. Narcotic abuse represents a relative contraindication to pump placement; however, the dose cannot be altered without an external programmer. A thorough patient history and common sense must be used to determine the best course of action.

8 INTRAVENTRICULAR OPIOID ADMINISTRATION

The presence of intracerebral opioid receptors forms the scientific basis for direct administration of opioid analgesics into the cerebral ventricles for control of intractable pain [24]. The clinical experience indicates that intraventricular administration of morphine is most useful for cancer patients with pain in the upper body, particularly the head and neck, and for patients with diffuse pain [25].

Medication may be administered into the temporal horn of the lateral ventricle or into the cisterna magna, but the most commonly used route involves catheterization of the lateral ventricle or the third ventricle using a precoronal burr hole [25]. The intraventricular catheter is connected to a reservoir placed into the subcutaneous space. Both standard Ommaya reservoirs (2-ml capacity) and smaller pediatric miniports with self-sealing elastomer membrane have been used for intraventricular access ports [25].

Through these implantable access ports, intraventricular morphine is administered by regular injections of sterile preservative-free morphine solution percutaneously into the reservoir. The injections are usually done daily, but in some cases maximal analgesia was achieved by dividing the total daily dose of morphine into two equal doses administered every 12 hours. This technique provided good results in several clinical series with duration of treatment up to 40 months [25]. Continuous infusion of morphine by means of externally worn battery-powered infusion pumps connected to a ventricular reservoir was also described [26].

It is also possible to administer intraventricular morphine using an implanted pump. Both fixed rate pumps and programmable pumps have been used for this purpose. The pump is usually connected to a convertible Ommaya reservoir attached to the intraventricular catheter [27].

The main side effect of intraventricular opioid administration is nausea requiring regular use of antiemetics. Other side effects include drowsiness, somnolence and mental clouding, visual hallucinations, miosis, headache, dizziness, pruritis, diaphoresis, urinary retention, and constipation [25]. Drug overdose results in respiratory depression [28] that may be reversed with naloxone. Infections occur with both implanted ports and pumps, sometimes necessitating removal of hardware with systemic or intraventricular antibiotics. Additional reported complications include intracerebral hemorrhages from chronic reservoir use, reservoir leakage, and epileptic seizures [29].

From published experience with more than 450 patients with intraventricular morphine administration [25,29], it appears that this modality may be highly effective and is relatively safe for the treatment of head, neck, upper body, and diffuse pain of neoplastic origin.

9 CONCLUSION

The effective care of a patient with chronic pain may often prove challenging. However, with intraspinal and intraventricular opioid therapies, this patient population may achieve exceptional pain control with a minimal degree of adverse effects. Development of new drug delivery technologies and new analgesic agents will make chemical neuromodulation a better means of pain management, with further decrease and possible elimination of neurodestructive procedures in the future.

REFERENCES

1. Yaksh TL, Rudy TA. Analgesia mediated by a direct spinal action of narcotics. Science 192:1357–1358, 1976.
2. Snyder SH. Opiate receptors and internal opiates. Sci Am 236(3):44–56, 1977.
3. Wang JF, Nauss LA, Thomas JE. Pain relief by intrathecally applied morphine in man. Anesthesiology 50:149–151, 1979.
4. World Health Organization Expert Committee. Cancer relief and palliative care. World Health Organization Technical Report Series 804:1–73, 1990.
5. Deer T, Winkelmüller W, Erdine S, Bedder M, Burchiel K. Intrathecal therapy for cancer and nonmalignant pain: Patient selection and patient management. Neuromodulation 2:55–66, 1999.
6. Doleys DM, Coleton M, Tutak U. Use of intraspinal infusion with noncancer pain patients: Follow-up and comparison of worker's compensation vs. nonworker's compensation patients. Neuromodulation 1:149–159, 1998.
7. de Lissovoy G, Brown R, Halpern M, Hassenbusch SJ, Ross E. Cost-effectiveness of long-term intrathecal morphine therapy for pain associated with failed back surgery syndrome. Clin Ther 19:96–112, 1997.
8. Dahm P, Nitescu P, Appelgren L, Curelaru I. Continuous intrathecal infusion of opioid and bupivacaine in the treatment of refractory pain due to postherpetic neuralgia: A case report. Neuromodulation 1:85–89, 1998.
9. Dahm P, Nitescu P, Appelgren L, Curelaru I. Long-term intrathecal infusion of opioid and/or bupivacaine in the prophylaxis and treatment of phantom limb pain. Neuromodulation 1:111–128, 1998.
10. Lundborg CN, Nitescu PV, Appelgren LK, Curelaru ID. Long-term intrathecal (IT) administration of opioid and bupivacaine relieved intractable pain in a patient with familial amyloidosis polyneuropathy: A case report. Neuromodulation 1:199–208, 1998.
11. Krames ES, Olson K. Clinical realities and economic considerations: Patient selection in intrathecal therapy. J Pain Symptom Manage 14:S3–S13, 1997.
12. Fanciullo GJ, Rose RJ, Lunt PG, Whalen PK, Ross E. The state of implantable pain therapies in the United States: A nationwide survey of academic teaching programs. Anesth Analg 88:1311–1316, 1999.
13. Johnston J, Reich S, Bailey A, Sluetz J. Shiley Infusaid pump technology. Ann NY Acad Sci 531:57–65, 1988.
14. Krames ES, Gershow J, Glassberg A, Kenfick T, Lyons A, Taylor P, Wilkie D. Continuous infusion of spinally administered narcotics for the relief of pain due to malignant disorders. Cancer 56:696–702, 1985.

15. Winkelmüller M, Winkelmüller W. Long-term effects of continuous intrathecal opioid treatment in chronic pain of nonmalignant etiology. J Neurosurg 85: 458–467, 1996.
16. Schuchard M, Lanning R, North R, Reig E, Krames E. Neurologic sequelae of intraspinal drug delivery systems: Results of a survey of American implanters of implantable drug delivery systems. Neuromodulation 1:137–148, 1998.
17. Mercadante S. Problems of long-term spinal opioid treatment in advanced cancer patients. Pain 79:1–13, 1999.
18. Hassenbusch SJ, Garber J, Buchser E, Du Pen S, Nitescu P. Alternative intrathecal agents for the treatment of pain. Neuromodulation 2:85–91, 1999.
19. Dario A, Marra A, Marra P, Dorizzi A. Intrathecal administration of different drugs by programmable infusion device in chronic pain. A case report. Neuromodulation 1:107–110, 1998.
20. Johnson CE, Christen C, Perez MM, Ma M. Compatibility of bupivacaine hydrochloride and morphine hydrochloride. Am J Health System Pharm 54: 61–64, 1997.
21. Bejjani GK, Karim NO, Tzortzidis F. Intrathecal granuloma after implantation of a morphine pump: Case report and review of the literature. Surg Neurol 48: 288–291, 1997.
22. Follett KA, Naumann CP. A prospective study of catheter-related complications of intrathecal drug delivery systems. J Pain Symptom Manage 19:209–215, 2000.
23. Yaksh T. Analgesic actions of intrathecal opiates in cats and primates. Brain Res 153:205–210, 1978.
24. Lazorthes Y, Verdie JC, Bastide R, Lavados A, Descouens D. Spinal versus intraventricular chronic opiate administration with implantable drug delivery devices for cancer pain. Appl Neurophysiol 48:234–241, 1985.
25. Lazorthes YR, Sallerin BAM, Verdié JCP. Intracerebroventricular administration of morphine for control of irreducible cancer pain. Neurosurgery 37:422–429, 1995.
26. Lobato RD, Madrid JL, Fatela LV, Sarabia R, Rivas JJ, Gozalo A. Intraventricular morphine for intractable cancer pain: Rationale, methods, clinical results. Acta Anesth Scand 31(Suppl 85):68–74, 1987.
27. Dennis GC, De Witty RL. Long-term intraventricular infusion of morphine for intractable pain in cancer of the head and neck. Neurosurgery 26:404–408, 1990.
28. Langlade A, Serrie A, Sandouk P, Thurel C, Cunin G. Levels of morphine and metabolites in CSF during respiratory depression after intraventricular morphine injection. Pain 44:175–178, 1991.
29. Karavelis A, Foroglou G, Selviaridis P, Fountilas G. Intraventricular administration of morphine for control of intractable cancer pain in 90 patients. Neurosurgery 39:57–62, 1996.

39

Cordotomy for Pain

Yücel Kanpolat
University of Ankara School of Medicine, Ankara, Turkey

1 INTRODUCTION

Cordotomy is a procedure based on sectioning of the lateral spinothalamic tract (LST). Edinger first identified the LST in 1889, and in 1905, Spiller reported that pain and temperature sensations ascend in the anterolateral spinal cord based on autopsy findings of tuberculoma patients at the thoracic level of the spinal cord [1,2]. In 1910 Schüller sectioned the anterolateral tract in monkeys and named the procedure "chordotomie" [3]. The first cordotomy in man was carried out by Martin at Spiller's instigation, with many technical difficulties [4]. Cordotomy operations were classically performed using the open technique through the cervical and upper thoracic region by a posterior approach.

As cordotomy patients are typically in poor health and do not tolerate open surgery well, clinicians have long sought noninvasive treatments to accommodate them. Percutaneous cordotomy (PC) is a relatively new treatment modality performed using a needle electrode system and, conventionally, X-ray guidance. This procedure was first described and performed by Mullan in 1963 using a radioactive-tipped strontium needle [5]. Thereafter, Mullan began making unipolar, anodal, electrolytic lesions in 1965 [6]. In the same year, Rosomoff described a PC technique using a radiofrequency (RF) electrode system [7], which allows the making of a small, discrete lesion in the pain-conducting system of the spinal cord. With the help of impedance measurements and stimulation, evaluation of the target's neurophysiological function became possible. The percutaneous method was performed in the lower cervical region by an anterior approach by Lin and Gildenberg in 1966 [8]. X-ray, the conventional visualization system in stereotactic pain procedures, cannot demonstrate patients' spinal cord morphology. In 1988, Kanpolat et al published the first experience with computed tomography (CT) visualization in a stereotactic pain procedure, later using CT-guidance as a visualization method in PC [9,10]. Computed tomographic visualization offers the advantage of topographic orientation. Morphological orientation and neurophysiologic evaluation of the target allowed the use of this truly stereotactic method with radiofrequency energy [11,12].

2 PERTINENT ANATOMY

The target in cordotomy is the LST (Fig. 1A), which is located in the anterolateral part of the spinal cord [13–16]. This ascending tract carries information chiefly about pain and temperature and relays some tactile information. The distribution of the pain-conducting fibers within the anterolateral spinal tract is such that the small, ventrally located fibers mainly conduct pain sensation. The organization of fibers from the outside inwards is: superficial pain, temperature, and deep pain [16]. The anterolateral sensory system has a somatotropic relationship, with fibers from higher levels laminating medially and ventrally, and fibers from lower levels laminating laterally and dorsally within the LST [14–16]. Segmentation of the fibers provides the opportunity for selective cordotomy, given that anteromedial lesions denervate the contralateral arm and upper chest region, whereas posterolateral lesions denervate the sacral and lumbar area (Fig. 1B).

Morphometric studies of the spinal cord at the level of the surgical approach have provided critical information pertaining to anatomical orientation for cordotomy. We measured the spinal cord diameters of 63 patients who underwent computed tomographic (CT) guided PC at the C1-C2 level at 7.0 to 11.4 mm (mean 8.66 ± 0.72 mm) anteroposteriorly, and 9.0 to 14.0 mm transversely (mean 10.9 ± 1.56 mm) [17].

Between the anterior extent of the pyramidal tracts and the posterior aspect of the lateral spinothalamic tracts is a narrow "safety zone" of white matter. The pyramidal tract is usually located posterior to the dentate ligament. It must be remembered, however, that in rare instances the dentate ligament is located posterior to its normal place [15]. Moreover, there is much variation in the size and location of the ventral corticospinal tract; for example, sometimes it does not decussate at all. Because motor decussation

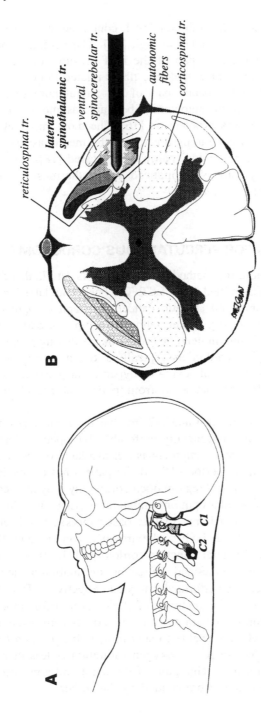

FIGURE 1 A, Schematic representation of the needle in lateral percutaneous cordotomy at the C1-C2 level. B, Ideal position of needle electrode system in the target (LST). (Copyright).

may extend from the obex to the C1 level, contralateral leg weakness may also occur if the lesion is made too high [16]. The ventral spinocerebellar tract is located in the lateral part of the LST. Lesions of this tract cause ipsilateral ataxia of the arm. Autonomic fibers related to bowel and bladder function are found in the lateral part of the lateral horn of gray matter. Immediately posterior to the autonomic fibers are vasomotor fibers, bilateral lesioning of which causes hypotension [16]. The most important region related to upper cervical cordotomy practice is the medial aspect of the LST, where the descending respiratory pathway is located [18]. Bilateral lesions of this pathway may cause sleep-induced apnea, the most important complication of bilateral cordotomy.

3   INDICATIONS FOR PERCUTANEOUS CORDOTOMY

Cordotomy is the preferred method if the surgeon is certain that the patient's intractable pain is transmitted in the LST. The best candidates for cordotomy are patients with unilateral somatic cancer pain and compression of the plexus, roots, or nerves [19]. Tasker defined two types of pain as indications for cordotomy: one is intermittent, neuralgia-like, shooting pain into the legs associated with a spinal cord injury typically at the thoracolumbar level; the other type is evoked pain—allodynia or hyperpathia—associated with neuropathic pain syndromes that arise from peripheral neurological lesions [19,20].

The indications for open and PC involve the same types of patients. Percutaneous cordotomy is generally preferable, but open cordotomy is recommended if the necessary equipment is not available or the surgeon's experience is inadequate to perform PC. If the patient has anomalies or other diseases of the upper cervical region, open cordotomy is again recommended [19,20]. Contrary to popular opinion, unilateral upper body pain (secondary to lung carcinoma, mesothelioma, or Pancoast tumors) and bilateral somatic intractable pain in the lower body and extremities can be controlled by CT-guided, unilateral, or bilateral selective cordotomy [11,12]. Nowadays, with the help of imaging techniques and the recent contribution of electrode technology, cordotomy can be performed safely and effectively. Thus, CT-guided PC should be considered the treatment of choice even before morphine therapy [11,12]. Cordotomy is contraindicated in patients with severe pulmonary dysfunction, those who are unable to stay in a supine position for 30 to 40 minutes, and those whose partial oxygen saturation is less than 80%. For patients with bilateral intractable pain of the chest and arms, bilateral high cervical cordotomy is not recommended by the author.

4 PERCUTANEOUS CORDOTOMY TECHNIQUE

Percutaneous cordotomy is routinely performed using an RF system consisting of a generator, specially designed needles, and electrodes. The diameter and length of the uninsulated tip of the electrode are critical, because the lesion size is directly related to these parameters. The author uses an electrode kit (KCTE Kanpolat CT Electrode Kit, Radionics, Inc., Burlington, MA) with 20-gauge, thin-walled needles and plastic hubs designed to avoid imaging artifact problems. Demarcations on the cannula indicate the depth of insertion (Fig. 1A). The kit also includes two open-tip thermocouple electrodes with 2-mm tips and diameters of 0.30 mm and 0.40 mm (one straight-tip electrode and one curved tip). The smaller-caliber electrode (0.30 mm) is usually used for bilateral cordotomy, whereas the larger electrode is preferred for unilateral cordotomy [21].

The patient should have been fasting for 5 hours preoperatively. In CT-guided PC, contrast material should be administered into the subarachnoid space of the spinal cord by lumbar puncture (7–8 ml of 240 mg/l Iohexol) 20 to 30 minutes before the operation. If lumbar puncture cannot be tolerated, contrast material (5 ml Iohexol) is injected at the C1-C2 level. The patient is placed in the supine position, and the upper cervical spine must be kept in a horizontal position, particularly for X-ray-guided cordotomy (Fig. 1A, B). In conventional lateral and anterior cordotomy, the head is flexed and fixed. In CT-guided cordotomy, the procedure is performed in the CT unit with the patient in the supine position. The head is placed on the head holder, flexed and fixed with a fixation band. Local anesthesia is usually adequate, but neuroleptic anesthesia may be used if necessary. General anesthesia is used by some surgeons [22], although rarely, but is not recommended by the author because of the need for communication with the patient during the procedure.

The electrode system is placed on the anterolateral aspect of the anterolateral spinal cord with the assistance of an imaging method (Fig. 2, Fig. 3). Computed tomography shows the morphology of the spinal cord segment directly, whereas X-ray allows only indirect visualization of the spinal cord without demonstration of the relationship between the spinal cord and the needle electrode.

In conventional C1-C2 lateral cordotomy, the needle is inserted perpendicularly, 1 cm below and behind the mastoid process after deep local anesthetic infiltration (Fig. 1A, B). The local anesthetic needle is used as a guide needle before the initial puncture if an X-ray or CT image is taken. As a safety precaution the author uses a cannula (Kanpolat cannula, Radionics) with demarcations demonstrating the amount penetrated.

In CT-guided cordotomy, the skin-dura distance and needle direction must be monitored. The needle is then placed 1 to 2 mm anterior to the

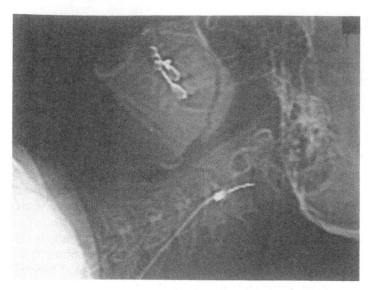

FIGURE 2   Stages of CT-guided left C1-C2 percutaneous cordotomy. Position of needle at C1-C2 level on lateral scanogram.

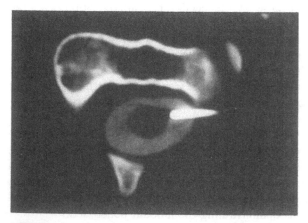

FIGURE 3   Final position of the needle on axial computed tomographic scan.

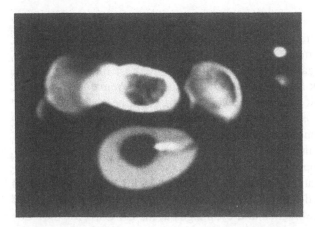

FIGURE 4   Incomplete insertion of the electrode.

dentate ligament. As lateral puncturing of the dura usually causes pain, local anesthetic infiltration is recommended. The needle position is seen at every step of manipulation on lateral scanogram and axial CT scans using a 1-mm slice thickness (Figs. 2, 3). Multiple maneuvers under CT guidance may be needed to fix the needle in this position. The active electrode is then inserted into the cannula using one insertion. The location of the electrode in the spinal cord, as well as displacement or rotation of the spinal cord, can be visualized (Figs. 1C, D; 4, 5).

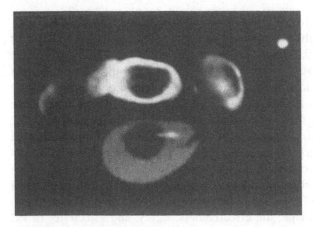

FIGURE 5   Final position of electrode in the target on axial computed tomographic scan.

If conventional cordotomy is performed using X-ray guidance, use of an image intensifier is recommended. Visualization of the dentate ligament in the lateral X-ray is mandatory. Because water-soluble dyes do not demonstrate the dentate ligament [19,20], oil-based contrast material must be used; however, the risk of arachnoiditis with such dyes remains a problem. Theoretically the anterior part of the spinal cord could be visualized by air myelogram, and the posterior part by oil-based contrast material. Anteroposterior imaging is usually used to demonstrate the position of the needle just in the lateral margin of the odontoid process.

In the anterior approach, the skin, subcutaneous tissues, and paravertebral fascia are infiltrated with local anesthetic. An 18-gauge, thin-walled spinal needle is inserted opposite the cordotomy site, medial to the carotid sheath and lateral to the trachea and esophagus at the C4-C5, C5-C6 or C6-C7 level. With the help of X-ray imaging or CT, the needle is observed as it passes through the disc space and is placed in the anterior lateral part of the spinal cord [23–25]. After reaching the subarachnoid space, only the anterior part of the spinal cord can be visualized indirectly on air myelogram [23,24].

To confirm whether the electrode is in the cerebrospinal fluid (CSF) or the spinal cord, the surgeon obtains impedance values and determines the neurophysiologic response of the compartment where the electrode is located. Impedance measurements are an important indication of passage into a new medium along the path of the electrode. Impedance values are approximately 400 Ohms in the CSF; an increase of approximately 200 Ohms is observed when there is contact between the electrode tip and the pia. The value is almost always greater than 1000 Ohms after insertion into the spinal cord.

Real neurophysiologic confirmation of the target is obtained by stimulation, necessitating that the patient be alert to cooperate. As a rule of functional neurosurgery, stimulation must be initiated at minimum voltage values: 2–5 Hz stimulation with 0.4 to 1.5 volts causes ipsilateral trapezius muscle contraction, indicating that the electrode is within or near the anterior gray matter of the LST. Ipsilateral motor responses in the arm or leg indicate that the electrode is in the corticospinal tract; 100 Hz stimulation with 0.2 to 1.5 volts causes pain, paresthesia, or warmth in the LST. Use of a curved electrode allows the surgeon to rotate the needle 0.5 mm anteriorly or posteriorly to place the electrode in a specific part of the tract in the lateral-to-medial plane. In CT-guided cordotomy, the position of the electrode must be confirmed by new CT images. The author believes that if stimulation is confirmed by the CT image, the effectiveness, safety, and selectivity of PC are gained in this golden state. This is currently only obtained with CT imaging and stimulation. The final step of the procedure is to make con-

trolled radiofrequency lesions. A test lesion should be made at 55° to 60° C
for 60 seconds before making the final lesions. The author then recommends
making two to three lesions at a temperature of 70° to 80° C for 60 seconds,
checking the patient's neurological function, particularly analgesia level and
motor function, after making each lesion.

Bilateral PC is usually performed with a 1-week interval. Bilateral
procedures may present technical difficulties, but we recommend using bilateral selective cordotomy for intractable pain in the lower Th_{10} dermatome.
If the pain is located in the upper segment, C1-C2 percutaneous lateral
cordotomy is performed on one side and percutaneous anterior cordotomy
is performed on the other [23–25]. The author prefers to use a small-caliber
electrode for CT-guided bilateral cordotomy only in cases with somatic
lower body pain. The pain-dominant side is selected for the first denervation.
After the test lesion is made, one or two lesions are made at a temperature
of 70° to 80° C.

The patient is kept in the supine position with the head elevated for 1
hour after the procedure. After an observation period of 6 hours, unilateral
cordotomy patients may go home if conditions permit, but bilateral cordotomy patients must be observed in the intensive care unit. Blood pressure
must be monitored carefully because of the risk of hypotension, especially
on the day of the procedure. Other important problems are related to lesions
of the reticulospinal tract, which controls the rhythm and depth of ventilation. Blood gases must be evaluated and sleep patterns monitored. Patients
with respiratory complications are kept in the hospital for 2 to 3 weeks. The
surgeon who performs cordotomy and controls pain successfully must remember not to stop morphine therapy suddenly. Most patients reduce their
dosages progressively and discontinue morphine use over time.

5 RESULTS AND COMPLICATIONS

Results depend on the volume of the destroyed part of the spinal cord at the
approach level, whereas complications are related to spreading of the lesion
in the area surrounding the target. With percutaneous techniques, controlled
lesions are made with the help of morphological and functional monitoring
of the target. Sindou [26] reviewed 37 series in the literature comprising
5,770 cordotomy cases. Among patients with cancer (2,022 cases), early pain
relief was achieved after open anterolateral cordotomy in 30% to 97% of
patients (mean 70.9%), and after percutaneous anterolateral cordotomy in
76% to 100% of patients (mean 88.3%). Long-term pain relief was experienced by 75% of patients at 6 months and 40% after 1 year. Among noncancer patients, Sindou reported 21.4% to 75% pain relief (mean 47%). The
best results were obtained in lower spinal cord pain or cauda equina injuries

and in painful amputation stumps or phantom limbs. Long-term results have not been described by many authors (26). Cordotomy results after 3 months to 10 years, as reported by Rosomoff, were as follows: the success rate was 84% at 3 months (495 patients), 61% between 3 months and 1 year (185 patients), 43% for years 1 to 5 (127 patients), and 37% for years 5 to 10 (32 patients) [27].

The outcome and complication rate associated with cordotomy are related to proper placement of the lesion and the lesion diameter. Lahuerta et al [30] reported that the best results were obtained by creating lesions that extended 5 mm into the cord and destroyed about 20% of the hemicord. This is a critical aspect of the success and complication rate of cordotomy. The author believes that if the location of the destruction is established through a direct imaging technique such as CT, confirmed by stimulation and destroyed with controlled lesions, the best results can be obtained with no or minimal complications. The mortality rate of cordotomy is related to the level of the procedure and whether it is unilateral or bilateral. This rate has been reported as 5.1% for open and 3% for percutaneous procedures in collected series [26]. Mortality is particularly increased in bilateral cervical cordotomy cases above the C4 level. Death occurs most commonly with destruction of a large portion of the anterolateral column of the reticulospinal tract, especially in bilateral lesions at the C1-C2 level [26–28]. This group of patients usually dies because of sleep-induced apnea. Motor weakness is another important complication and usually occurs when lesions are made in the posterior part of the target area. The complication rate is higher in the open cordotomy group, especially in bilateral cordotomy patients. The overall motor complication rate in collected percutaneous series is 3.5% [26]. Two percent of patients in Lipton's series of 710 patients, and 3% of Rosomoff's series did not recover motor function [27,28]. Ataxia usually occurs as a result of destruction of the spinocerebellar tract. In PC, ataxia usually disappears within 2 weeks. Permanent ataxia was reported at a rate of 3% by Rosomoff and 0.5% by Lipton [26,29]. Post-cordotomy dysesthesia is a real complication of cordotomy caused by sectioning of the LST, especially for patients with intractable pain in benign disorders, because of their extended life-spans. The incidence is given as 1% in large series [27,29]. Horner syndrome is frequently observed in cervical cordotomies but usually disappears in the long term [26]. Orthostatic hypotension, as well as urinary and sexual disturbances, is usually seen in bilateral lesions.

The author believes that these series and figures do not provide sufficient documentation of the real status of cordotomy, as most cordotomies were performed 30 to 40 years ago. The author thus presents his series of 169 CT-guided percutaneous lateral cordotomies performed since 1987 in 151 patients at the C1-C2 level. Of these, 144 patients had intractable pain caused by malignancy. Contrary to conventional criteria, most patients had intractable pain in the chest or arm region and were considered poor candidates for X-ray-guided PC. The majority of patients (77 cases, 53.4%) had malignancy of the chest, breast, including pulmonary carcinoma (40 cases, 27.7%), mesothelioma (18 cases, 12.5%), Pancoast tumor (13 cases, 9%), breast carcinoma (6 cases, 4.2%), and others (64 cases, 46.6%).

In the group with cancer pain, pain control was obtained in 139 patients (96.5% initial success rate). Pain relief was obtained selectively in 79.2% and nonselectively in 20.8% of cases. Bilateral selective cordotomy was performed on 10 patients with intractable pain in the lower trunk and lower extremities, with achievement of pain control in nine of them (90% initial success rate). Computed tomographic-guided PC was performed in seven patients who had some form of intractable pain originating from benign pathological states, such as painful rhizopathy after disc surgery, gunshot, sciatic nerve injury, and spinal cord injuries. Complete pain control was obtained in four patients, partial pain control in two, and the procedure was ineffective for one patient with C5 root avulsion. Overall, short-term complications included transient paresis in five cases (3.4%) and transient ataxia in five cases (3.4%). Postcordotomy hypotension was observed in three patients (two of which were bilateral), but the patients stabilized with medical treatment on the first postoperative day. In two patients who underwent bilateral cordotomy, urinary retention was observed within 2 days. The only true postcordotomy complication was dysesthesia, which was observed in four patients (2.6%).

6 CONCLUSIONS

The goal of cordotomy is to interrupt pain transmission in the LST. Conventionally, the procedure has been performed with open techniques, and some experienced surgeons continue to use these methods. If used safely and effectively, the open technique can be acceptable, but has two main disadvantages: first, open approaches, whether anterior or posterior, are not well tolerated by patients in poor health; second, this functional procedure is performed under general anesthesia. Current technology enables us to monitor some spinal cord functions but does not permit the surgeon to cooperate with the patient during the operation. The percutaneous application is performed under local anesthesia, which allows cooperation with the patient during the procedure and facilitates neurophysiological monitoring and controlled lesioning of the target. In conventional PC, the most critical problem is that the visualization system—X-ray imaging—demonstrates the spinal cord indirectly. Even with the use of contrast material, only the dentate ligament plus the anterior and posterior borders of the spinal cord are visualized, not the spinal cord segment at the approach level. With X-ray imaging, individual spinal cord diameters, which are necessary for calibration of the depth of the inserted part of the active electrode, are not measured. The needle direction cannot be superimposed on the target, which facilitates insertion of the active electrode using morphological orientation. Finally, the target-electrode relation is indirectly demonstrated.

The new version of cordotomy—CT-guided, percutaneous cordotomy —is a stereotactic, real-time, functional procedure. Three-dimensional stereotactic localization is obtained by the CT image. Each patient's spinal cord diameters are measured and used to adjust the depth of the inserted part of the active electrode for each case [18]. Direct visualization averts the need for multiple maneuvers when placing the electrode with the help of impedance measurements. Functional evaluation of the target with stimulation allows selective cordotomy to be performed unilaterally or bilaterally using controlled lesions made in close cooperation with the patient. Cordotomy is indisputably an effective procedure in neurosurgery practice and is still used by surgeons. A tremendous number of patients worldwide could benefit from PC with CT guidance. The best results are obtained in properly selected patients using the appropriate technique.

Acknowledgments

Special thanks to Helen Stevens, R.N.C., for editing, to Ahmet Sinav, M.D., for his creative drawings, and to Ali Savas, M.D., PhD, for his assistance in preparing this chapter.

REFERENCES

1. Clarke E, O'Malley CD. Function of the spinal cord. In: Clarke E, O'Malley CD (eds). The Human Brain and the Spinal Cord. San Francisco, Norman Publishing, 1996, pp 291–322.
2. Spiller WG. The location within the spinal cord of the fibers for temperature and pain sensations. J Nerv Ment Dis 32:318–320, 1905.
3. Schüller A. Über operative Durchtrennung der Rückenmarksstrange (Chordotomie). Wien Med Woch 60:2292–2295, 1910.
4. Spiller WG, Martin E. The treatment of persistent pain of organic origin in the lower part of the body by division of the anterolateral column of the spinal cord. JAMA 58:1489–1490, 1912.
5. Mullan S, Harper PV, Hekmatpanah J, Torres H, Dobbin G. Percutaneous interruption of spinal-pain tracts by means of a strontium needle. J Neurosurg 20:931–939, 1963.
6. Mullan S, Hekmatpanah J, Dobben G, Berkman F. Percutaneous, intramedullary cordotomy utilizing the unipolar anodal electrolytic lesion. J Neurosurg 22:548–555, 1965.

7. Rosomoff HL, Carroll F, Brown J, Sheptak P. Percutaneous radiofrequency cervical cordotomy: Technique. J Neurosurg 23:639–644, 1965.

8. Lin PM, Gildenberg PL, Polacoff PO. An anterior approach to percutaneous lower cervical cordotomy. J Neurosurg 25:553–560, 1966.

9. Kanpolat Y, Atalag M, Deda H, Siva A. CT-guided extralemniscal myelotomy. Acta Neurochir 91:151–152, 1988.

10. Kanpolat Y, Deda H, Akyar S, Bilgic S. CT-guided percutaneous cordotomy. Acta Neurochir (Suppl) 46:67–68, 1989.

11. Kanpolat Y, Akyar S, Caglar S, Unlu A, Bilgic S. CT-guided percutaneous selective cordotomy. Acta Neurochir 123:92–97, 1993.

12. Kanpolat Y, Savas A, Caglar S, Terniz C, Akyar S. Computerized tomography-guided percutaneous bilateral selective cordotomy. Neurosurgical Focus 2(1): Article 5, 1997.

13. Hyndman OR, Van Epps C. Possibility of differential section of the spinothalamic tract. A clinical and histological study. Arch Surg 38:1036–1053, 1939.

14. Walker EA. The spinothalamic tract in man. Arch Neurol Psychiatry 43:284–298, 1940.

15. White JC, Sweet WH. Pain and the Neurosurgeon: A Forty Year Experience. Springfield, Charles Thomas, 1969, pp 678–773.

16. Taren JA, Davis R, Crosby EC. Target physiologic corroboration in stereotaxic cervical cordotomy. J Neurosurg 30:569–584, 1969.

17. Kanpolat Y, Akyar S, Caglar S. Diametral measurements of the upper spinal cord for stereotactic pain procedures. Surg Neurol 43:478–483, 1995.

18. Nathan PW. The descending respiratory pathway in man. J Neurol Neurosurg Psychiatry 26:487–499, 1963.

19. Tasker RR. Cordotomy for pain. In: Youmans JR (ed). Neurological Surgery. Philadelphia, Saunders, 1996, pp 3463–3476.

20. Tasker RR, North R. Cordotomy and myelotomy. In: Tasker RR, North R (eds). Neurological Management of Pain. New York, Springer, 1997, pp 191–220.

21. Kanpolat Y, Cosman E. Special radiofrequency electrode system for computed tomography-guided pain-relieving procedures. Neurosurgery 38:600–603, 1996.

22. Izumi J, Hirose Y, Yazaki T. Percutaneous trigeminal rhizotomy and percutaneous cordotomy under general anesthesia. Stereotact Funct Neurosurg 59:62–68, 1992.

23. Lin MP. Percutaneous lower cervical cordotomy. In: Gildenberg PL, Tasker RR (eds). Textbook of Stereotactic and Functional Neurosurgery. New York, McGraw-Hill, 1998, pp 1403–1409.

24. Gildenberg PL. Percutaneous cervical cordotomy. Clin Neurosurg 21:246–256, 1974.

25. Fenstermaker RA, Sternau LL, Takaoka Y. CT-assisted percutaneous anterior cordotomy. Surg Neurol 43:147–150, 1995.

26. Sindou M, Daher A. Spinal cord ablation procedures for pain. In: Dubner R, Gebhart GF, Bond MR (eds). Proceedings of the Vth World Congress on Pain. Elsevier Science Publishers BV, 1988, pp 477–495.

27. Rosomoff HL, Papo I, Loeser JD. Neurosurgical operations on the spinal cord. In: Bonicca JJ (ed). The Management of Pain. Philadelphia, Lea and Febiger, 1990, pp 2067–2081.
28. Rosomoff H. Bilateral percutaneous cervical radiofrequency cordotomy. N Neurosurg 31:41–46, 1969.
29. Lipton S. Percutaneous cordotomy. In: Wall PD, Melzac R (eds). Textbook of Pain. Edinburgh, Churchill-Livingstone, 1989, pp 832–839.
30. Lahuerta J, Bowsher D, Lipton S, Buxton PH. Percutaneous cervical cordotomy: a review of 181 operations on 146 patients with a study on the location of "pain fibers" in the C-2 spinal cord segment of 29 cases. J Neurosurg 80: 975–985, 1994.

40

Dorsal Root Entry Zone (DREZ) Lesioning for Pain

Eben Alexander III
University of Massachusetts Medical School,
Worcester, Massachusetts, U.S.A.

Deepa Soni
Brigham and Women's Hospital, Children's Hospital, and
Harvard Medical School, Boston, Massachusetts, U.S.A.

1 INTRODUCTION AND BACKGROUND

The dorsal root entry zone (DREZ) operation was originally developed by Dr. Blaine S. Nashold, Jr. based on laboratory and clinical observations concerning deafferentation pain. The initial clinical indications were intractable, persistent pain resulting from plexus avulsion, for example, brachial plexus and lumbosacral plexus avulsions resulting from trauma. The first operations for DREZ lesioning were performed by Dr. Nashold on patients at Duke University Medical Center beginning in 1976 and provided substantial relief for patients with intractable pain secondary to plexus avulsions. Although Marc Sindou of Lyons had described and performed "selective posterior rhizotomy" as early as 1972, the DREZ operation was unique in that it was designed to interrupt completely the sensory pathways by destroying the second order neurons in the dorsal horn rather than preferentially destroy only the small-diameter nociceptive fibers as in Sindou's rhizotomy.

Since its introduction almost a quarter of a century ago, the indications for DREZ lesioning have expanded to include the treatment of many types of intractable pain including traumatic plexus avulsions, conus medullaris and cauda equina lesions, postherpetic pain, postamputation pain, brachial plexus radiation injuries, brachial plexus stretch injuries, cancer pain, postoperative (postrhizotomy and postthoracotomy) pain, and peripheral nerve injury pain. In addition, a specialized variation of the spinal cord DREZ lesion, the nucleus caudalis DREZ operation, was developed to treat intractable facial pain and is often indicated for other refractory cranial pain [Nashold, 1992], including trigeminal neuralgia that has failed other procedures, anesthesia dolorosa complicating prior procedures, peripheral nerve pain after infection or trauma (including dental procedures), cluster headaches, and others.

The clinical results after DREZ lesioning, in those patients who have the classic indications of traumatic plexus avulsions as well as for other pain syndromes, especially some with facial pain, continue to be substantial and durable.

2   NORMAL ANATOMY AND NEUROBIOLOGY

2.1   Spinal Cord Dorsal Horn

The dorsal root entry zone refers to the interface between the central and peripheral nervous systems in the spinal cord and specifically includes Rexed's laminae I–V, located in the posterior dorsal horn of the spinal cord. It is the pathway through which sensory afferents enter the central nervous system (CNS) during development and the area in which the first synaptic relay and integrative center for nociceptive afferents are located. Although laminae I–V each has a unique and discrete neuronal and cellular make-up, they all serve as anatomical endpoints for primary sensory afferents in which nociceptive impulses from the periphery are received, modified, and relayed by second order neurons projecting to supraspinal levels.

Nociceptors in laminae I–V can be classified as mechanical, thermal, or chemical and receive input from a number of sensory afferents, including A_α, A_β, A_δ, and C fibers. A_δ and C fibers are fine-diameter fibers that primarily terminate in laminae I, II, and V on nociceptive mechanoreceptors. The majority of unmyelinated primary afferents or C fibers that carry pain modalities pass through the first order synapse in lamina II (ie, the substantia gelatinosa).

The second order neurons also reside in this region, specifically in Rexed's lamina II for the pain pathways. Among the cell types in lamina II are Golgi type I neurons or relay neurons and Golgi type II cells, which primarily have an integrative function. Primary afferents carrying pain modalites synapse on either Golgi type I or type II cells, which in turn integrate that information and project axons that extend through the dorsal horn, cross the midline of the spinal cord over the course of two ascending segments, and then project rostrally to the thalamus by way of the ascending anterior and lateral spinothalamic pathways. Dorsal root entry zone lesioning, therefore, includes creating a lesion that extends across laminae I–V, through the entire dorsal horn.

2.2 Nucleus Caudalis

The nucleus caudalis is an elongated structure located on the dorsolateral surface of the cervicomedullary junction. It extends from the level of C2, in the upper cervical cord, rostrally to a region approximately 1 cm above the obex. It is anatomically homologous with the substantia gelatinosa in the dorsal horn of the spinal cord and harbors the second order neuronal cell bodies that project axons carrying pain and temperature sensation from facial sensory dermatomes, supplied by the branches of the trigeminal nerve, to the thalamus.

The nucleus caudalis has two main somatotopic organizations. The most fundamental organization is lateral-to-medial corresponding with trigeminal divisions V1, V2, and V3, respectively. A less obvious organization, but one that is critical to the clinical success of the nucleus caudalis DREZ operation, is a rostral-to-caudal organization with a corresponding concentric target, or so-called "reptilian" or "onion skin" dermatomal distribution. The perioral portions of V2 and V3 are found at the most rostral aspects of the nucleus, above the obex; whereas, the more peripheral facial regions away from the mouth are located progressively more caudally directed down to C2. Pain afferents from cranial nerves VII, IX, and X project to the most medial aspect of the caudalis nucleus, adjacent to the cuneate fasciculis.

3 PATHOPHYSIOLOGY OF NEUROPATHIC PAIN

Many theories have been proposed for explaining the pathophysiology of chronic pain after injury to peripheral nerves, dorsal roots, or dorsal root ganglia. The various proposed mechanisms of chronic pain production remain controversial, but it is generally accepted that hyperactivity in nociceptive pathway neurons as well as neuronal hypersensitivity to abnormal discharges from injured peripheral ganglia or neurons are involved in the pathophysiology of chronic neuropathic pain.

When a patient sustains a traumatic plexus avulsion, as in the case of a motorcyclist striking a tree impacting mainly over the lateral chest and shoulder, the sudden and forceful impact avulses some of the nerve roots directly from their attachments at the posterolateral spinal cord. The second order neuronal cell bodies in the posterior horn of the spinal cord are thus "deafferented," removing their normal input. In many cases, these deafferented cell bodies progress, over a variable period, to spontaneously fire impulses along their axons toward the third order neurons in the thalamus. A similar situation occurs after traumatic hemipelvectomy with resultant lumbosacral plexus avulsion.

The DREZ lesion was designed to coagulate and destroy these second order neuronal cell bodies in the substantia gelatinosa of the posterior horn. It, eliminates the firing of pain impulses along the spinothalamic axons and often rids the patient of pain. One typically generates a zone of hypalgesia into the previously painful region, but this is rarely cause for complaint. The exact mechanisms by which chronic pain is produced have yet to be elucidated and remain somewhat controversial; the phenomenon, however, is real and DREZ lesioning has provided effective results in eliminating chronic pain of various etiologies.

4 INDICATIONS

The DREZ lesion has been used for a wide variety of pain syndromes in addition to deafferentation pain. Dr. Nashold and several of his trainees from Duke have published their results using the spinal cord DREZ lesion to treat patients with pain of multiple etiologies, including paraplegia-associated and spinal cord injury pain, postherpetic neuralgia, phantom limb pain, reflex sympathetic dystrophy and causalgia, chronic low back pain, and various refractory peripheral nerve pains In more recent years, DREZ lesioning has shown some efficacy in the treatment of a number of other centrally mediated pain syndromes, including pain resulting from conus medullaris nerve root avulsions, pain from spinal cysts, spasticity, and hyperactive bladder.

Pain associated with syringomyelia was not originally felt to be amenable to the DREZ operation because the etiology is based in damage to the axons stretched around the syrinx rostral to the dorsal horn neurons. Recent results indicate that syrinx pain can respond well to the DREZ, presumably by eradicating the cell bodies that initiate the pain signal transmission.

The nucleus caudalis DREZ procedure is a specialized form of the operation that is used mainly for facial pain, or occasionally for other cranial discomfort [Nashold, 1992]. In general, it is not indicated for routine facial pain, or tic douloureux, unless the pain has been refractory to other procedures, such as glycerol injection, radiofrequency rhizotomy, or microvascular decompression. The nucleus caudalis DREZ operation is especially useful in these refractory cases, or in pain related to failure of these procedures (such as anesthesia dolorosa, which was the indication for DREZ in approximately half of the original series from Duke).

5 OPERATIVE NEUROANATOMICAL AND TECHNICAL DETAILS OF THE DREZ LESION

5.1 Neuroanatomical Localization of Lesion

The use of intraoperative neurophysiological measurements in neurosurgical procedures is not a new practice. In fact, a variety of neurophysiological recording techniques are commonly used to reduce the incidence of irreversible CNS damage during surgery. Less common, however, has been the use of neurophysiological intraoperative recordings for anatomical localization in the nervous system. Dorsal root entry zone lesioning has been one of the few instances when neurophysiological methods, primarily the measurement of somatosensory evoked potentials (SSEPs) and impedance, have been used to ensure correct anatomical localization of the dorsal horn and, more importantly, of the pyramidal tract so that it can be avoided. Other intraoperative techniques used to localize the dorsal horn include electromyogram (EMG) recordings peripherally while the pyramidal tract is stimulated by the DREZ electrode, myotome localization by simultaneous cord stimulation and recording over the peripheral muscle, recordings of cord dorsum potentials that have been evoked by stimulation of the dorsal roots, and spinal cord mapping with evoked responses for accurate DREZ localization.

5.2 Intraoperative Measurements of Impedance

Since its introduction into neurosurgery by Meyer in 1921, when impedance was measured while performing freehand brain biopsies in humans, impedance measurements have evolved as an invaluable intraoperative tool in many neurosurgical procedures. As defined by Ohm's Law— $Z = E/I$, ($Z =$ impedance, $E =$ electrical potential or voltage, and $I =$ electrical current)— tissue impedance is a passive electrical property that measures the resistance to electrical current through a medium. As early as 1969, the utility of impedance measurements in determining the transition zone from cerebrospinal fluid (CSF) to spinal cord parenchyma in spinal cord cordotomies was reported by both Taren et al. and Gildenberg et al. The importance of using impedance measurements was recognized early in the course of DREZ lesioning as a means of differentiating normal and damaged spinal cord tissue, thus aiding in the identification of the target dorsal root entry zone. In a repeat DREZ operation, it can also assist in localizing a region of prior DREZ lesioning.

In DREZ lesioning, the voltage required to produce a current flow between the DREZ electrode and a distant reference electrode, such as the Radionics RFG-3B RF Lesion Generator (Radionics, Inc., Burlington, MA), constitutes the impedance measurement. Before lesioning, the tissue impedance of the dorsal horn in the human has been determined to range from 900 to 1200 ohms. The impedance value decreases after a DREZ lesion. In addition, impedance values are markedly decreased in areas of spinal cord pathology and thus can provide a boundary for DREZ lesioning as impedance values decrease in the transition from normal cord to an area of damaged dorsal horn.

5.3 The Lesion: Radiofrequency versus Laser

The classic DREZ lesion operation is performed using a radiofrequency electrode to heat the target tissue to 75°C for 15 seconds. Lesions are made approximately 1 mm apart, with great care to avoid disrupting the small vessels over the surface of the spinal cord or brainstem. Earlier investigators attempting to use CO_2 lasers for DREZ lesioning found significant problems with small vessel disruption.

Different electrodes are used for the spinal cord DREZ as opposed to the nucleus caudalis DREZ. The RFG-3B lesion generator (Radionics, Inc., Burlington, MA) was the original lesioning source for the Duke series of Dr. Nashold, but has recently been replaced by the improved RFG-3C and other radiofrequency lesioning systems.

5.3.1 Spinal Cord DREZ Lesions

The standard spinal cord lesion is performed through the entire length of the affected painful dermatomes. The spinal cord DREZ electrode is inserted into the cord, at the level of the dorsal root entry zone, at a lateral to medial angle of 20 to 30 degrees off a perpendicular vertical to the cord surface.

The DREZ lesions in the spinal cord are performed using the straight Nashold DREZ electrode. One measures impedance on electrode insertion, with relatively high values indicating possible penetration into posterior columns and relatively low values suggesting possible penetration into a cyst or syrinx.

5.3.2 Nucleus Caudalis DREZ Lesions

Fortuitously, this elongated sensory relay nucleus provides the surgeon with the opportunity to preferentially limit the thermal lesion to involve primarily pain fibers, a feat that cannot be performed in the microscopic region of Rexed's lamina II in the spinal cord. This specific lesion is of great benefit for patients with facial pain, as corneal responses can be spared even if painful impulses originating from V1 and V2 dermatomal distributions are eliminated, because of preservation of light touch pathways synapsing at more rostral levels. The widespread observation that the nucleus caudalis DREZ operation is more successful at eradicating atypical types of pain may also be linked to this microscopic separation of various pain modalities and the ability to more completely lesion a broad dermatomal pain region. In contrast, the spinal cord DREZ lesion is mainly useful for true deafferentation pain, as is encountered with plexus avulsions.

For the nucleus caudalis DREZ lesion, one performs a suboccipital craniectomy biased 5 mm toward the side of the pain, approximately 3-cm wide and 2.5-cm high. The initial lesion is performed at the level of the C2 dorsal root ganglion, with mediolateral location in the root entry zone. The entry vector is in the transverse plane with approximately 20 to 30 degrees lateral-to-medial direction. From 1982, when the nucleus caudalis DREZ lesion was first introduced, the standard lesion was made for 15 seconds at a temperature of 75°C. For the first 5 years, the Nashold spinal cord DREZ electrode was used for making lesions in the nucleus caudalis. Dr. El-Naggar, working in conjunction with Dr. Nashold, redesigned the electrode to be used for the nucleus caudalis DREZ. His initial modifications called for two electrodes with different distal angles and lengths of exposed electrode tip for cord penetration. This design was the result of a careful anatomical study of the variable relationship of the shape and size of the nucleus caudalis analyzed from C2 to a centimeter above the level of the obex.

5.4 Complications

Complications related to DREZ lesioning fall into two major categories: underlesioning and overlesioning. Underlesioning is a problem that continues to be addressed and, with continued improvement in the electrodes and RF lesion generator, are decreasing in frequency.

Overlesioning, on the other hand, can have serious consequences, especially in the case of the spinal cord DREZ lesion. Complications of overlesioning range from sensory deficits to severe motor deficits, including paraplegia and death. Sensory and motor deficits are often not the result of imprecise anatomical placement of the electrode, but rather from scattering effects from the thermal injury itself. For this reason, special attention should be given to the impedance measurements intraoperatively, and the use of SSEPs during DREZ lesioning is imperative. Other common complications include infection, syrinx formation, limb ataxia, and weakness.

One reason for the failure of a DREZ lesion to be permanent may be the ability of sensory axons to regenerate after injury. The peripheral nervous system (PNS)/CNS junction, as found in the dorsal root entry zone, is especially supportive to axonal regeneration. In fact, the tendency of DREZ lesions to be temporary rather than incomplete may be the result of the temporal ability of sensory neurons to regenerate their axons and re-establish appropriate connections. In other words, DREZ lesions, when technically adequate, often produce complete relief of pain, indicating sufficient disruption of peripheral sensory input as well as the disruption of the neurons responsible for the relaying of nociceptive input to higher centers. However, with the return of pain at some later date, the regeneration of sensory axons and their subsequent re-establishment with nocieptors is likely.

6 LONG-TERM RESULTS

Spinal cord DREZ lesioning has been used to successfully treat a number of neuropathic pain syndromes refractory to conventional treatment, including deafferentation syndromes, brachial and lumbar plexus avulsions, and pain secondary to spinal cord injury. In addition, nucleus caudalis DREZ lesioning has been successful in treating facial pain. Several clinical series demonstrate the utility of DREZ lesioning in the treatment of many intractable neuropathic pain syndromes and illustrate some of the limitations of the procedure.

Bernard reviewed the records of the first 18 patients with intractable facial pain treated with nucleus caudalis dorsal root entry zone lesions at Duke. The pain etiology varied, but the largest group was that of postherpetic neuralgia. In the immediate postoperative period, 90% of patients had satisfactory pain relief in comparison to 58% on subsequent follow-up. Seventy-one percent of those with postherpetic neuralgia had satisfactory relief on subsequent follow-up. Favorable results correlated with (1) a lesser preoperative sensory deficit, (2) pain restricted to trigeminal distributions, and (3) pain of a burning or lancinating/penetrating quality [Bernard, 1987].

Bullard and Nashold have reported their results in 25 patients undergoing nucleus caudalis DREZ lesions for refractory trigeminal neuralgia, atypical headaches or facial pain, multiple sclerosis, brainstem infarction, postherpetic neuralgia, posttraumatic closed head injuries, cancer-related pain [Rossitch, 1989] and postsurgical anesthesia dolorosa. Initial postsurgery results were impressive for such usually refractory indications, with 24 of 25 patients having good to excellent pain relief at the time of discharge. Good to excellent results were maintained in 19 of 25 patients (76%) patients at 1 month and 17 of 25 patients (60%) at 3 months. Follow-up at 1 year included only 18 patients, but 12 of 18 (67%) maintained good to excellent pain relief, two reporting fair and four reporting poor pain relief. Because of disruption of the spinocerebellar pathway directly overlying the nucleus caudalis in the brainstem, 15 of 25 (60%) of patients had significant transient postoperative ataxia which resolved, in most, at 1 month. Minimal ataxia remained in three of 18 (17%) of patients at 1 year, although none of them considered it disabling. The other complications included transient diplopia in two patients and increased corneal anesthesia in 3. One general advantage of the nucleus caudalis DREZ lesion is that light touch is often preserved in the cornea so that keratitis is a very infrequent complication. Bullard and Nashold [1997] reported one case of keratitis in their 25 patients. Their manuscript confirmed prior reports indicating that the nucleus caudalis DREZ offers significant benefit in managing very difficult pain in these patients.

At a meeting commemorating the 50th anniversary of Neurosurgery in Egypt, held in Cairo in March 1999, Drs. el-Naggar and Nashold discussed their results with alterations in the maximum temperature and anatomical extent of the nucleus caudalis DREZ lesions. Specifically, a lesion temperature of 80°C was used to obtain a more complete lesion of the nucleus results in a higher initial success rate and more durable pain relief. Previously, the eradication of perioral V2 and V3 pain required the rostral-most lesion be performed 10 to 12 mm above the obex. However, by increasing the lesion temperature from 75°C to 80°C, they have obtained satisfactory relief of perioral pain without lesioning above the obex. Further clinical studies are required before this fundamental change in lesioning parameters is widely recommended. However, their early results are promising.

In general, the nucleus caudalis DREZ operation has allowed for more robust management of varied pain syndromes, including those resulting from peripheral nervous system etiologies, than has the original spinal cord DREZ. Perhaps this is because of the difference in anatomical distribution of pain pathways relative to other sensory pathways. All the sensory relay nuclei are localized in 1- to 2-mm region of the posterior horn in the spinal cord, whereas they are spread through a much larger vertical nucleus extending from the level of C2 up through the medulla, with clear anatomical separation into surgically accessible zones in the trigeminal nuclei (the nucleus caudalis being the most caudal).

7 SUMMARY

The DREZ operation has provided substantial relief of pain for thousands of patients who otherwise would have continued to suffer from their condition. Many pain syndromes previously deemed "untreatable" have become more manageable. Even anesthesia dolorosa, the dreaded complication of a minority of trigeminal neuralgia procedures, can yield to the nucleus caudalis DREZ operation in a significant number of cases. The DREZ is generally not useful for peripheral etiology pain in the spinal cord (eg, chronic back pain, postherpetic neuralgia, neuropathic pain, and causalgia), although it has a more reliable effect for such peripheral pains in the trigeminal distribution (ie, pain after dental procedures, infections, or trauma) through the nucleus caudalis.

REFERENCES

Bennett MH, Lunsford LD, Akin O, Martinez AJ. Evoked-potential monitoring during dorsal root entry zone surgery. An experimental animal model. Stereotact Funct Neurosurg 1989;53(4):247–260.

Bernard EJ Jr, Nashold BS Jr, Caputi F, Moossy JJ. Nucleus caudalis DREZ lesions for facial pain. Br J Neurosurg 1987;1(1):81–91.

Broggi G, Dones I, Ferroli P, Franzini A, Pluderi M. [Contribution of thalamotomy, cordotomy and "dorsal root entry zone" (DREZ) caudalis trigeminalis lesions in the treatment of chronic pain]. Neurochirurgie 2000;46(5):447–453. French.

Bullard DE, Nashold BS Jr. The caudalis DREZ for facial pain. Stereotact Funct Neurosurg 1997;68(1–4) Pt 1):168–174.

Campbell JN, Solomon CT, James CS. The Hopkins experience with lesions of the dorsal horn (Nashold's operation) for pain from avulsion of the brachial plexus. Appl Neurophysiol 1988;51(2–5):170–174.

Carvalho GA, Nikkhah G, Samii M. [Pain management after post-traumatic brachial plexus lesions. Conservative and surgical therapy possibilities]. Orthopade 1997; 26(7):621–625. Review. German.

Chong MS, Woolf CJ, Haque NS, Anderson PN. Axonal regeneration from injured dorsal roots into the spinal cord of adult rats. J Comp Neurol 1999;410(1):42–54.

Cosman ER, Nashold BS, Ovelman-Levitt J. Theoretical aspects of radiofrequency lesions in the dorsal root entry zone. Neurosurgery 1984;15(6):945–950.

Dreval ON. Ultrasonic DREZ-operations for treatment of pain due to brachial plexus avulsion. Acta Neurochir (Wien) 1993;122(1-2):76–81.

Edgar RE, Best LG, Quail PA, Obert AD. Computer-assisted DREZ microcoagulation: Posttraumatic spinal deafferentation pain. J Spinal Disord 1993;6(1):48–56.

Fazl M, Houlden DA, Kiss Z. Spinal cord mapping with evoked responses for accurate localization of the dorsal root entry zone. J Neurosurg 1995;82(4):587–591.

Friedman AH, Nashold BS Jr, Ovelmen-Levitt J. Dorsal root entry zone lesions for the treatment of post-herpetic neuralgia. J Neurosurg 1984;60(6):1258–1262.

Friedman AH, Nashold BS Jr. DREZ lesions for relief of pain related to spinal cord injury. J Neurosurg 1986;65(4):465–469.

Friedman AH, Nashold BS Jr. Dorsal root entry zone lesions for the treatment of postherpetic neuralgia. Neurosurgery 1984;15(6);969–970.

Friedman AH, Bullitt E. Dorsal root entry zone lesions in the treatment of pain following brachial plexus avulsion, spinal cord injury and herpes zoster. Appl Neurophysiol 1988;51(2-5):164–169.

Friedman AH, Nashold BS Jr, Bronec PR. Dorsal root entry zone lesions for the treatment of brachial plexus avulsion injuries: A follow-up study. Neurosurgery 1988;22(2):369–373.

Garcia-March G, Sanchez-Ledesma MJ, Diaz P, Yague L, Anaya J, Goncalves J, Broseta J. Dorsal root entry zone lesion versus spinal cord stimulation in the management of pain from brachial plexus avulsion. Acta Neurochir Suppl (Wien) 1987;39:155–158.

Garcia-Larrea L, Sindou M, Mauguiere F. Clinical use of nociceptive flexion reflex recording in the evaluation of functional neurosurgical procedures. Acta Neurochir Suppl (Wien) 1989;46:53–57.

Golding JP, Bird C, McMahon S, Cohen J. Behaviour of DRG sensory neurites at the intact and injured adult rat dorsal root entry zone: Postnatal neurites become paralysed, whilst injury improves the growth of embryonic neurites. Glia 1999; 26(4):309–323.

Gorecki JP, Nashold BS. The Duke experience with the nucleus caudalis DREZ operation. Acta Neurochir Suppl (Wien) 1995;64:128–131.

Gorecki JP, Burt T, Wee A. Relief from chronic pelvic pain through surgical lesions of the conus medullaris dorsal root entry zone. Stereotact Funct Neurosurg 1992; 59(1-4):69–75.

Ishijima B. [Spinal and medullary DREZ lesions for deafferentation pain]. No Shinkei Geka 1988;16(12):1331–1337. Japanese.

Ishijima B, Shimoji K, Shimizu H, Takahashi H, Suzuki I. Lesions of spinal and trigeminal dorsal root entry zone for deafferentation pain. Experience of 35 cases. Appl Neurophysiol 1988;51(2-5):175–187

Jeanmonod D, Sindou M. Somatosensory function following dorsal root entry zone lesions in patients with neurogenic pain or spasticity. J Neurosurg 1991;74(6): 916–932.

Jeanmonod D, Sindou M. Somatosensory function following dorsal root entry zone lesions in patients with neurogenic pain or spasticity. J Neurosurg 1991;74(6): 916–932.

Kumagai Y, Taga K, Hokari T, Fujioka II, Matsuki M, Shimoji K, Homma T, Tsutsui T, Takeshita H, Tsuji C. [The effect of DREZ (dorsal root entry zone) lesions on intractable pain in patients with spinal cord injury]. Masui 1990;39(5):632–638.

Kuroda R, Nakatani J, Kitano M, Yamada Y, Yorimae A. Experimental anatomical considerations of the dorsal root entry zone lesions for pain relief. Appl Neurophysiol 1987;50(1-6):420–424.

Lunsford LD, Bennett MH. Evoked-potential monitoring during dorsal root entry zone surgery. Patients with chronic pain. Stereotact Funct Neurosurg 1989;53(4): 233–246.

Makachinas T, Ovelmen-Levitt J, Nashold BS Jr. Intraoperative somatosensory evoked potentials. A localizing technique in the DREZ operation. Appl Neurophysiol 1988;51(2-5):146–153.

Mertens P, Sindou M. [Surgery in the DREZ (dorsal root entry zone) for treatment of chronic pain]. Neurochirurgie 2000;46(5):429–446.

Moossy JJ, Nashold BS Jr, Osborne D, Friedman AH. Conus medullaris nerve root avulsions. J Neurosurg 1987;66(6):835–841.

Moossy JJ, Nashold BS Jr. Dorsal root entry zone lesions for conus medullaris root avulsions. Appl Neurophysiol 1988;51(2-5):198–205.

Nashold BS Jr. Introduction to Second International Symposium on Dorsal Root Entry Zone (DREZ) lesions. Appl Neurophysiol 1988;51(2-5):76–77.

Nashold BS Jr, Ostdahl RH. Dorsal root entry zone lesions for pain relief. J Neurosurg 1979;51(1)59–69.

Nashold BS Jr, el-Naggar A, Mawaffak Abdulhak M, Ovelmen-Levitt J, Cosman E. Trigeminal nucleus caudalis dorsal root entry zone: A new surgical approach. Stereotact Funct Neurosurg 1992;59(1-4):45–51.

Nashold BS Jr, Vieira J, el-Naggar AO. Pain and spinal cysts in paraplegia: Treatment by drainage and DREZ operation. Br J Neurosurg 1990;4(4):327–335.

Nashold BS Jr, Ostdahl RH. Dorsal root entry zone lesions for pain relief. J Neurosurg 1979;51(1):59–69.

Pindzola RR, Doller C, Silver J. Putative inhibitory extracellular matrix molecules at the dorsal root entry zone of the spinal cord during development and after root and sciatic nerve lesions. Dev Biol 1993;156(1):34–48.

Powers SK, Adams JE, Edwards MS, Boggan JE, Hosobuchi Y. Pain relief from dorsal root entry zone lesions made with argon and carbon dioxide microsurgical lasers. J Neurosurg 1984;61(5):841–847.

Powers SK, Barbaro NM, Levy RM. Pain control with laser-produced dorsal root entry zone lesions. Appl Neurophysiol 1988;51(2-5):243–254.

Prestor B, Zgur T, Dolenc VV. Subpial spinal evoked potentials in patients undergoing junctional dorsal root entry zone coagulation for pain relief. Acta Neurochir (Wien) 1989;101(1-2):56–62.

Proceedings of the 2nd International Symposium on Dorsal Root Entry Zone (DREZ) Lesions. Durham, N.C., April 24–26, 1987. Appl Neurophysiol 1988;51(2-5):65–263.

Rath SA, Braun V, Soliman N, Antoniadis G, Richter HP. Results of DREZ coagulations for pain related to plexus lesions, spinal cord injuries and postherpetic neuralgia. Acta Neurochir (Wien) 1996;138(4):364–369.

Rath SA, Seitz K, Soliman N, Kahamba JF, Antoniadis G, Richter HP. DREZ coagulations for deafferentation pain related to spinal and peripheral nerve lesions: Indication and results of 79 consecutive procedures. Stereotact Funct Neurosurg 1997;68(1-4 Pt 1):161–167.

Rawlings CE III, el-Naggar AO, Nashold BS Jr. The DREZ procedure: An update on technique. Br J Neurosurg 1989;3(6):633–642. Review.

Richter HP, Schachenmayr W. Is the substantia gelatinosa the target in dorsal root entry zone lesions? An autopsy report. Neurosurgery 1984;15(6):913–916.

Richter HP, Seitz K. Dorsal root entry zone lesions for the control of deafferentation pain: Experiences in ten patients. Neurosurgery 1984;15(6):956–959.

Rossitch E Jr, Zeidman SM, Nashold BS Jr. Nucleus caudalis DREZ for facial pain due to cancer. Br J Neurosurg 1989;3(1):45–49.

Rossitch E Jr, Abdulhak M, Ovelmen-Levitt J, Levitt M, Nashold BS Jr. The expression of deafferentation dysesthesias reduced by dorsal root entry zone lesions in the rat. J Neurosurg 1993;78(4):598–602.

Sampson JH, Cashman RE, Nashold BS Jr, Friedman AH. Dorsal root entry zone lesions for intractable pain after trauma to the conus medullaris and cauda equina. J Neurosurg 1995;82(1):28–34.

Saris SC, Iacono RP, Nashold BS Jr. Dorsal root entry zone lesions for post-amputation pain. J Neurosurg 1985;62(1):72–76.

Samii M, Moringlane JR. Thermocoagulation of the dorsal root entry zone for the treatment of intractable pain. Neurosurgery 1984;15(6):953–955.

Sindou M. Laser-induced DREZ lesions. J Neurosurg 1984;60(4):870–871.

Sindou M, Turano G, Pantieri R, Mertens P, Mauguiere F. Intraoperative monitoring of spinal cord SEPs during microsurgical DREZotomy (MDT) for pain, spasticity and hyperactive bladder. Stereotact Funct Neurosurg 1994;62(1-4):164–170.

Sindou M. Drez lesions for brachial plexus injury. Neurosurgery 1988;23(4):528.

Sindou M. Microsurgical DREZotomy (MDT) for pain, spasticity, and hyperactive bladder: A 20-year experience. Acta Neurochir (Wien) 1995;137(1-2):1–5.

Singh JP, Chandy MJ, Joseph T, Chandi SM. Histopathological appraisal of carbondioxide laser dorsal root entry zone (DREZ) lesions in primates; Br J Neurosurg 1989;3(3):373–379.

Singh JP, Chandy MJ, Joseph T, Chandi SM. Histopathological appraisal of carbondioxide laser dorsal root entry zone (DREZ) lesions in primates. Br J Neurosurg 1989;3(3):373–379.

Tasker RR, DeCarvalho GT, Dolan EJ. Intractable pain of spinal cord origin: Clinical features and implications for surgery. J Neurosurg 1992;77(3):373–378.

Teixeira MJ, De Souza EC, Yeng LT, Pereira WC. [Lesion of the Lissauer tract and of the posterior horn of the gray substance of the spinal cord and the electrical stimulation of the central nervous system for the treatment of brachial plexus avulsion pain]. Arq Neuropsiquiatr 1999;57(1):56–62. Portuguese.

Thomas DG, Jones SJ. Dorsal root entry zone lesions (Nashold's procedure) in brachial plexus avulsion. Neurosurgery 1984;15(6):966–968.

Thomas DG, Kitchen ND. Long-term follow up of dorsal root entry zone lesions in brachial plexus avulsion. J Neurol Neurosurg Psychiatry 1994;57(6):737–738.

Watson CP. Postherpetic neuralgia. Neurol Clin 1989;7(2):231–248. Review.

Wang YC, Kao MC, Tao PL, Ho WL, Yang CH, Fu YM. Evaluation of laser and radiofrequency induced dorsal root entry zone lesion for pain control in rats. Chung Hua I Hsueh Tsa Chih (Taipei) 1996;58(6):421–427.

Yoshida M, Noguchi S, Kuga S, Muteki T, Kojima K, Abe T, Akeda N, Kuramoto S. MRI findings of DREZ-otomy lesions. Stereotact Funct Neurosurg 1992;59(1-4):39–44.

Young RF. Clinical experience with radiofrequency and laser DREZ lesions. J Neurosurg 1990;72(5):715–720.

Young RF. Laser versus radiofrequency lesions of the DREZ. J Neurosurg 1986;64(2):341.

Young JN, Nashold BS Jr, Cosman ER. A new insulated caudalis nucleus DREZ electrode. Technical note. J Neurosurg 1989;70(2):283–284.

Young RF. Clinical experience with radiofrequency and laser DREZ lesions. J Neurosurg 1990;72(5):715–720.

Zeidman SM, Rossitch EJ, Nashold BS Jr. Dorsal root entry zone lesions in the treatment of pain related to radiation-induced brachial plexopathy. J Spinal Disord 1993;6(1):44–47.

41

Dorsal Rhizotomy for Spasticity

**Randa Zakhary, Matthew Smyth, and
Warwick J. Peacock**
University of California at San Francisco,
San Francisco, California, U.S.A.

1 INTRODUCTION

Spasticity arises from a variety of neurologic disorders, including cerebral palsy, multiple sclerosis, cerebrovascular accidents, spinal cord injury, and head trauma.

Selective posterior rhizotomy is now an accepted procedure for relieving spasticity in carefully selected patients with spastic cerebral palsy (CP). Recent developments in electrophysiologic monitoring and refinements in surgical technique have led to a resurgence in the use of this procedure for patients with spastic cerebral palsy [1–7]. Dorsal rhizotomy is performed through bilateral L2 to S1 laminectomies or laminotomies to allow selective division of lumbosacral posterior spinal rootlets with electromyographic (EMG) guidance. In patients with cerebral palsy, judicious patient selection, intraoperative monitoring, and intensive postoperative physical and occupational therapy are essential for successful surgical outcome [1,8]. Ambulatory patients with spastic diplegia and those with pure spasticity without motor weakness or severe contractures show the greatest functional improvement [1,8,9].

2 SPASTICITY AND CEREBRAL PALSY

Spasticity in childhood is most commonly encountered as a feature of cerebral palsy, which results from an insult to the developing brain. Cerebral palsy may be classified by the type of motor involvement (spastic, dystonic, or mixed), or by the distribution of involvement (quadriplegia, diplegia, hemiplegia). Loss of fine motor control, impaired balance, weakness, and delayed motor milestones also occur. The progressive, deforming forces of spasticity can lead to secondary muscle contractures and orthopedic deformities, such as hip dislocation and scoliosis [10,11]. This disorder varies widely in severity and may be associated with other problems such as hydrocephalus, seizures, learning disabilities, language problems, or sensory processing disturbances. Developmental delay is often but not always a feature of CP. Spasticity in children is particularly problematic because of the interference with normal growth.

2.1 Patient Selection

When considering the goal of neurosurgical intervention, spastic cerebral palsy patients can be divided into two groups. The first group is composed of those patients in whom functional improvement is expected. An example would be a spastic diplegic 5 year old who walks independently with a scissoring gait, flexed hips and knees, and an equinus foot posture. There should be no evidence of dystonia and minimal fixed contractures. Although range of motion may be limited in straight leg raising because of tight hamstrings, in hip abduction because of tight adductors, and in ankle dorsiflexion because of tight gastrocnemius-soleus muscles, a large portion of the restricted movement may be caused by dynamic tightness rather than structural shortening. By reducing spasticity, range of movement and stride length should increase, posture should improve, and walking speed may be accelerated. The second group is composed of those nonfunctional, severely affected spastic quadriplegic patients in whom functional gains are unlikely, but reduction of spasticity is expected to improve patient comfort, ease patient care, and reduce the risk of developing contractures, bony deformities, and joint dislocations.

Rhizotomy is not effective in patients with severe, fixed contractures. Tendon-lengthening procedures of structurally shortened muscle groups such as hip adductors, gastrocnemius-soleus, and hamstring muscle groups by the orthopedic surgeon may be indicated. In cases in which the patient has already undergone tendon-lengthening procedures, rhizotomy is often contraindicated, as a reduction in tone may adversely affect posture.

Assessment of strength and control of voluntary movements are essential. Some patients have little voluntary control and rely on the increase in tone to maintain posture. For them, reducing spasticity may actually be detrimental. Identifying certain features can help in the difficult differentiation between spastic patterns and voluntary movement. A voluntarily controlled movement can be initiated and halted several times throughout its range, whereas spastic movements tend to occur in gross patterns that, once initiated, cannot be interrupted. If adequate voluntary power cannot be confirmed, then selective posterior rhizotomy is contraindicated.

Other factors to evaluate are truncal control, isolated muscle control and the presence of primitive reflexes. If the goal is to improve gait and truncal control is poor, then reduction of spasticity in the lower extremities is unlikely to help. In severely affected spastic, quadriplegic children, rhizotomy is unlikely to improve function, but it may help to prevent contractures or aid in positioning and posture.

The role of spasticity relative to the degree of clinical disability should be considered. If weakness is minimally present and spasticity predominates, selective dorsal rhizotomy may improve function. The procedure is contraindicated in patients with significant weakness (particularly postural muscles), extrapyramidal disorders such as dystonia, athetosis, or rigidity, poor truncal control, overlengthened tendons, severe contractures, or fixed spinal deformities.

3 OPERATIVE TECHNIQUE

Intact neuromuscular activity is essential for intraoperative monitoring; therefore, no neuromuscular blocking agents are used during the procedure after the laminectomy or laminotomy has been performed. If excessive muscular response to posterior nerve rootlet stimulation is encountered, deepening the level of anesthesia with inhaled agents decreases the abnormal excitability, preventing overt movements and facilitating the electrophysiological evaluation.

After induction of general anesthesia and placement of an indwelling Foley urinary catheter, the patient is placed prone on the operating table with bolsters under the chest and pelvis to enable the abdominal wall to move freely. This facilitates respiratory movements and prevents elevated venous pressure in the epidural veins and thus minimizes blood loss. The knees, feet, and elbows are supported and padded carefully with soft foam. The patient is positioned with the feet near the lower end of the table, with the head turned to the side on a soft circular headrest. The intercristal line between the posterior iliac crests is used as a reference to locate the level of the fourth lumbar spinous process. Alternatively, a cross-table lateral radiograph may be used for localization. Counting from the L4 spinous process, the skin is marked from L1 to S2. Local anesthetic is injected through the marked incision. After careful skin preparation, the surgical drapes are arranged over a Mayo stand positioned above the patient's feet and legs to provide access for the EMG team. A transparent drape can be used to allow visualization of the lower extremities by the surgeon. The EMG team places needle electrodes into the muscle groups of interest at this time. Standard electrode placement includes five muscle groups (hip adductors, quadriceps, tibialis anterior, hamstring, and gastrocnemius) and the external anal sphincter muscle bilaterally.

After making the midline skin incision, self-retaining retractors are placed. The lumbodorsal fascia is incised on either side of the supraspinous ligament, which is preserved. The paraspinal muscles from L1 to S1 are retracted laterally using subperiosteal dissection. The lowest mobile spinous process is identified, usually L5, but in young children may be S1. The ligamentum flavum is incised with a No. 15 blade below the laminae of L5 to expose the epidural fat. A laminectomy may be performed, but in most cases a laminotomy from L5 to L2 is preferred. The laminae from L5 to L2 are cut bilaterally with a high-speed drill with a foot-plate attachment. The facet complexes are carefully preserved and the width of the laminotomy need not exceed 10 mm. The supraspinous and interspinous ligaments are divided between L5 and S1 and the entire segment is retracted rostrally, hinged on the interspinous ligaments between L1 and L2. In similar fashion, the laminae of S1 are cut and the S1 segment is retracted and secured caudally, thereby preserving the supraspinous ligament and exposing the upper sacral dura (Figure 1). Hemostasis is achieved by applying bone wax to the bone edges and bipolar cautery to epidural veins, and the epidural fat is cleared away to expose the dura. The dura is incised using a fresh No. 15 blade, preserving the arachnoid membrane. The dural incision is extended cephalad and caudad using a grooved director and the No. 15 blade. The dural edges are tacked laterally with fine suture. The arachnoid membrane is then incised, exposing the cauda equina. Cerebrospinal fluid is aspirated through a cottonoid to protect the nerve roots.

Attention is then directed toward accurate identification of the nerve root level by stimulating the anterior roots of S1 and S2. Two specially insulated rhizotomy electrodes with blunt hooks (Aesculap Surgical Instruments, Burlingame, CA) are connected by sterile wires to the electrical stimulator. The S1 nerve root, which is usually the largest in the cauda equina, is isolated and by gentle manipulation, the cleft between its anterior and posterior roots is identified. The posterior root is broad and flat, while the anterior root is round and smaller (Figure 2). The anterior root of S1 is stimulated, and characteristic flexion at the knee and plantar-flexion at the ankle are observed. Similarly, stimulation of the anterior root of S2 should produce plantar-flexion at the ankle and flexion at the toes. At this point,

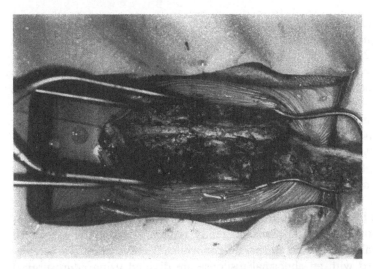

FIGURE 1 Exposure for selective posterior rhizotomy. The L5 to S1 segment has been reflected rostrally, and the S1 segment is reflected caudally. This preserves some blood flow to the posterior elements and provides for rapid and efficient bony closure. The dura mater and arachnoid membranes have been incised, revealing the cauda equina. (Printed with permission M. Smyth, Batjer, ed., Textbook of Neurological Surgery.)

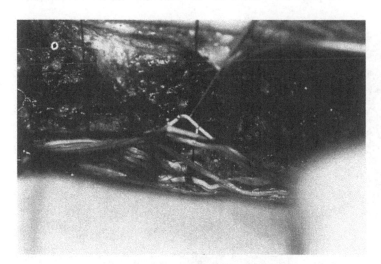

FIGURE 2 Separation of a spinal root into its round anterior root, and broad, flat posterior root. (Printed with permission M. Smyth, Batjer, ed., Textbook of Neurological Surgery.)

the anatomical levels have been identified by using (1) bony landmarks, (2) the size of the S1 root, and (3) the motor responses from the anterior roots of S1 and S2.

Counting cephalad, the L2 root is identified and separated into its anterior and posterior components. The posterior root is then picked up with the blunt hook electrodes and initially stimulated with a single 0.1 msec stimulus, which is increased incrementally until the threshold for muscular contraction is reached. The rootlets comprising the posterior root of L2 are then carefully separated and stimulated. After a threshold muscular contraction to a single-pulse stimulus is determined, each individual rootlet is stimulated with a 1-second-duration subthreshold 50 Hz tetanic stimulus, and the muscular response is monitored. The selection of rootlets for division or preservation is discussed in greater detail in the following section on intraoperative monitoring. The assistant gently retracts the rootlets associated with a normal response on a separate noninsulated nerve hook. Those rootlets associated with an abnormal response are divided using neurosurgical microscissors (Figure 3). The stimulation and recording are repeated at each level from L2 down to S2. The surgeon works with the rootlets on the contralateral side and moves to the other side of the table to repeat the procedure when the first side is completed. In a typical rhizotomy procedure, between 50 and 75 rootlets are stimulated and, depending on the degree of spasticity, between 25% and 50% are subsequently divided.

Throughout the procedure, accumulated cerebrospinal fluid is aspirated

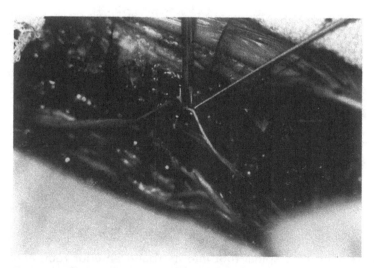

FIGURE 3 Microscissors are used to section a rootlet generating an abnormal response. (Printed with permission M. Smyth, Batjer, ed., Textbook of Neurological Surgery.)

through a small cottonoid. There are typically between two and four posterior rootlets at the L2 level, with an increasing number at each subsequent level down to S1, where there are usually between 8 and 11 rootlets. The S2 root is the first to be smaller than the preceding root and usually contains two to six very fine rootlets. When identifying the S2 root, it is important to also visualize the S3 root, which may be adherent to the S2 root and inadvertently stimulated with an S2 rootlet and divided.

After completion of the stimulation and rhizotomy stage, the dura is closed with either a continuous locking or interrupted suture. Before placement of the last stitch, sterile preservative-free saline is injected into the intrathecal space with a blunt needle. The anesthesiologist performs a Valsalva maneuver and any sites of leakage are oversewn until a watertight dural closure is confirmed. The previously rotated posterior elements are brought back into position and the medial and lateral cut edges of the ligamentum flavum are sutured at each level. Next the spinous process of S1 is sutured to that of L5 after replacing the S1 spinous process in its anatomical position. The paraspinous muscles are reapproximated through the interspinous ligament using interrupted suture. This brings the muscles into good alignment with the bone and ligaments before the supraspinous ligament is sutured to the lumbodorsal fascia. The skin is closed in two layers, the first with subcutaneous interrupted absorbable suture and the outer layer with a continuous locking nylon suture. A sterile, occlusive dressing is applied and the patient is taken to the recovery room or directly to the pediatric intensive care unit.

3 INTRAOPERATIVE MONITORING

Rootlet selection for division is based on the electromyographic response to electrical stimulation and visible muscle contraction. The overall clinical picture is considered, and sacral-level rootlets associated with anal sphincter activity are spared. Recordings from the muscles are made from 2.5 cm. stainless-steel needles, placed two each in the anal sphincter and in five muscle groups of each leg: hip adductors, quadriceps, tibialis anterior, hamstrings, and gastrocnemius. This allows bipolar recording of each muscle group, with tracings displayed on an electroencephalography chart recorder at 30 mm/sec for simultaneous viewing of activity from all 11 muscle groups.

Sterile, insulated rhizotomy electrode hooks are used to stimulate the nerve roots with an electrical stimulator that allows delivery of both single pulses and trains of stimuli. A constant-voltage electrical stimulator is used because the voltage range remains fairly constant despite rather large differences in the cross-sectional area of rootlets, whereas the amount of current required would be greater for thicker rootlets than for thin ones. The roots may then be stimulated in a bipolar manner by gently lifting the root away from the cerebrospinal fluid and applying a stimulus. The stimulating contacts are separated by 5 to 10 mm, and the voltage is varied throughout the testing procedure. Typically, between 0.2 and 5 volts are required for anterior roots and 20 to 100 volts for posterior roots. The whole posterior root at one level is first stimulated with single pulses to identify its threshold, which usually corresponds to the rootlet threshold. Next, the root is subdivided into its rootlets, which are stimulated in turn. Initial stimulation for each rootlet uses single pulses, delivered individually at gradually increasing voltages until the threshold for muscle contraction is reached. Next, 1-second trains of stimuli are applied at voltages reduced to 30% to 50% of the single pulse threshold, and gradually increased until the threshold for muscle contraction is achieved. Next, at the train threshold, several repetitions are applied to evaluate the pattern of muscle contraction and to assure reproducibility of the findings for each rootlet. Suprathreshold stimulation is avoided because diffuse spread of muscular contraction is usually produced inappropriately and may be interpreted as an abnormal response.

Several patterns of EMG response are seen during trains of stimulation (Fig. 4). "Squared" responses show a uniform amplitude of EMG across the entire 1-second interval of train stimulation. "Decremental" responses either gradually decrease in amplitude across the 1-second interval or decrease mainly in the first 100 msec and remain squared thereafter. The squared and decremental responses are considered normal. "Incremental," "multiphasic," "clonic," "sustained," "spread," and "contralateral spread" patterns are considered abnormal. The EMG amplitude of incremental responses rises abruptly or gradually during the train of stimuli. Clonic responses involve repeated bursts of EMG activity, often 5 to 12 bursts within a 1-second train. Multiphasic responses have several phases of incremental and decremental patterns within the same period of stimulation. Sustained responses show persistence of the EMG activity beyond the 1-second of 50 Hz stimulation. Equivocal responses fall outside the above categories, lying somewhere in between squared and clonic responses. Spread describes responses in which stimulation produces contraction of other muscle groups than the one being stimulated on the ipsilateral side, and contralateral spread refers to contraction of contralateral muscle groups (Figs. 5 and 6). Ongoing background muscle activity may be present and should be disregarded in the evaluation of responses. If excessive background firing is present or if higher voltages are needed to obtain responses, adjustments in the level of anesthesia may alleviate the problem.

Generally, between 25% and 50% of rootlets are cut, but slightly more may be divided in a severely affected patient. Division of all the rootlets at any level should be avoided, and a more conservative approach should be

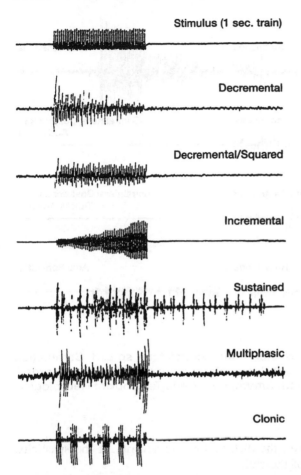

FIGURE 4 Examples of single-channel electromyogram recordings seen intraoperatively. The *decremental* and *decremental-squared* responses are considered normal, whereas the *incremental, sustained, multiphasic,* and *clonic* responses are abnormal. (Printed with permission M. Smyth, Batjer, ed., Textbook of Neurological Surgery.)

used in a root undergoing division of multiple consecutive rootlets (usually greater than three). At sacral levels, particularly S2, any activation of anal sphincter activity is a contraindication to sectioning of that rootlet, even with abnormal lower extremity responses. The decision to divide or spare a rootlet is based primarily on the EMG response pattern to trains of stimuli, but clinical judgment is also used. The behavior of the leg assessed visually or by palpation is considered, as are factors such as the number of rootlets

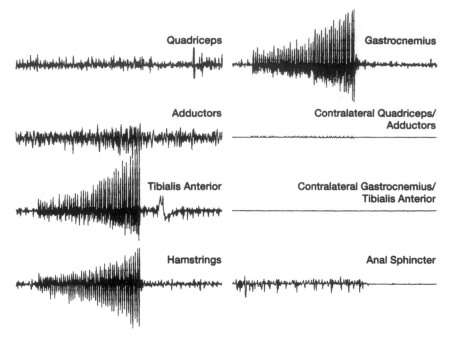

FIGURE 5 Examples of ipsilateral and contralateral spread. Stimulation of an S1 rootlet on the right demonstrating proximal ipsilateral spread. (Printed with permission M. Smyth, Batjer, ed., Textbook of Neurological Surgery.)

previously cut at that level, the distribution and severity of the spasticity, and the functional level of the child.

4 POSTOPERATIVE CARE

The patient is kept in a flat or lateral recumbent position for the first 5 postoperative days to prevent leakage of cerebrospinal fluid. Patients are logrolled without rotation of the spine to prevent strain on the incision, the lumbar muscles and the dura, and to protect the skin and mobilize respiratory secretions. Typically, intravenous narcotics are used for analgesia for the first 2 postoperative days, during which the patient remains in the pediatric intensive care unit. The Foley catheter is kept in place until at least the third postoperative day. Intra- and postoperative antibiotics are by choice of the surgeon. On postoperative day number 3, bedside physical therapy is instituted for bed mobility, range of motion, and family teaching. To avoid elevated cerebrospinal fluid pressure at the dural incision, elevation of the

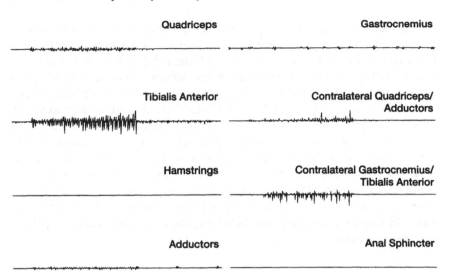

FIGURE 6 Stimulation of a right L3 rootlet demonstrating contralateral spread to the merged quadriceps/adductor and tibialis anterior/gastrocnemius channels. (Printed with permission M. Smyth, Batjer, ed., Textbook of Neurological Surgery.)

head is not allowed until the third postoperative day, whereas sitting and assisted transfers are initiated on day five. Regular, intensive physical therapy is provided on an outpatient basis after discharge to help patients regain previous strength and to improve their functional skills beyond the preoperative levels.

5 OUTCOMES

Reduction of spasticity can be appreciated on clinical examination immediately after surgery [12]. Multiple studies have documented decreased spasticity and improvements in functional ability, sitting and standing balance, and ambulation [1,2,13–22]. Assessment of function and documentation of outcome after treatment are difficult to standardize in patients with cerebral palsy because of the wide range of variability in the population as well as ongoing development and maturation. Standardized assessments, such as the Gross Motor Function Measure (GMFM), have only recently been developed [23,24] and used in evaluating treatment outcome [14]. Other measures, such as the Pediatric Evaluation of Disability Inventory [17] and the Chattecx Balance System [15] have been systematically applied to evaluation of treatment outcome, with demonstrated improvements in functional ability and sitting balance, respectively. Gait analysis has demonstrated improvements in hip and knee range of motion, stride length, and speed of ambulation [25,26], and in joint motion and foot placement [5,20,27–30]. Foot-floor contact pattern evaluation frequently demonstrates a change from primarily forefoot only at initial contact during ambulation to a heel or flatfoot position [28]. Occasionally excessive knee flexion, likely related to decreased calf muscle strength, requires orthotic intervention; however, selective posterior rhizotomy has been shown to decrease the overall rates of orthopedic procedures required in children with spastic cerebral palsy [31]. Other unexpected benefits, so-called "distant effects," such as decreased seizure frequency [32], greater bladder control [32,33], improved speech, and greater upper extremity range of movement have been observed [2,3,32]. Improvements in cognitive function [34], behavior, and emotional control [32] have also been reported.

6 COMPLICATIONS

Potential long-term neurosurgical problems include sensory loss, increased weakness, persistent spasticity, bowel or bladder dysfunction, sexual dysfunction, and spinal instability or deformity. Surgical complications such as hemorrhage, infection, or cerebrospinal fluid leakage, or anesthetic complications such as pulmonary problems are possible. The most frequent postoperative complications are fever, postcatheterization cystitis, and marginal oxygen saturation. Transient hyperesthesias are commonly noted after rhizotomy, although it has been the observation of the author that these are seen less frequently and resolve more quickly when the percentage of rootlets sectioned is kept to a minimum. After reduction in tone by rhizotomy, muscle weakness may become more apparent, either unmasked or exacerbated by the procedure. This weakness tended to improve with physiotherapy [32]. Clinically significant residual spasticity limiting improvements in functional outcome may persist. This is probably the result of an insufficient percentage of rootlets being sectioned [35,36].

Excellent outcomes and a low complication rate can be achieved through a multidisciplinary team approach combining careful patient selection, intraoperative EMG monitoring with judicious sectioning of dorsal rootlets, and intensive postoperative physical and occupational therapy. These patients should have coordinated follow-up and management with both the pediatric orthopedist, neurosurgeon, and urologist if indicated. Preexisting structural deformities are not addressed by the rhizotomy procedure, and children with neuromuscular disorders should have regular, ongoing orthopedic assessments as development progresses.

REFERENCES

1. Peacock WJ, Arens LJ, Berman B. Cerebral palsy spasticity: Selective posterior rhizotomy. Pediatr Neurosci 1987;13:61–66.
2. Fasano VA, Broggi G, Barolat-Romana G, Sguazzi A. Surgical treatment of spasticity in cerebral palsy. Childs Brain 1978;4:289–305.
3. Gros C. Spasticity. Clinical classification and surgical treatment. Adv Tech Stand Neurosurg 1979;6:55–97.
4. Albright A. Neurosurgical treatment of spasticity: Selective posterior rhizotomy and intrathecal baclofen. Sterotact Funct Neurosurg 1992;58:3–13.
5. Cahan LD, Adams JM, Perry J, Beeler LM. Instrumented gait analysis after selective dorsal rhizotomy. Dev Med Child Neurol 1990;32:1037–1043.
6. Steinbok P, Reiner A, Beauchamp RD, Cochrane DD, Keyes R. Selective functional posterior rhizotomy for treatment of spastic cerebral palsy in children: Review of 50 consecutive cases. Pediatr Neurosurg 1992;18:34–42.
7. Privat JM, Benezech J, Frerebeau P, Gros C. Sectorial posterior rhizotomy, a new technique of surgical treatment for spasticity. Acta Neurochirurg 1976;35: 181–195.
8. Peacock WJ, Staudt LA. Functional outcomes following selective posterior rhizotomy in children with cerebral palsy. J Neurosurg 1991;74:380–385.
9. Arens LJ, Peacock WJ, Peter J. Selective posterior rhizotomy: A long-term follow-up study. Childs Nerv Syst 1989;5:148–152.
10. Lance JW. Symposium synopsis. In: Feldman RG, Young RR, Koella WP, eds. Spasticity-Disordered Motor Control. St Louis: Mosby-Year Book, 1980, p. 45.
11. Samilson RL, ed. Orthopedic Aspects of Cerebral Palsy. Philadelphia, Lippincott, 1975.
12. Morin C, Perrot-Deseilligny E. Evidence for presynaptic inhibition of muscle spindle Ia afferents in man. Neurosci Lett 1984;44:137–142.
13. Foerster O. On the indications and results of the excision of posterior spinal nerve roots in man. Surg Gynecol Obstet 1913;16:463–474.
14. Yang TF, Chan RC, Wong TT, Bair WN, Kao CC, Chuang TY, Hsu TC. Quantitative measurement of improvement in sitting balance in children with spastic cerebral palsy after selective dorsal rhizotomy. Am J Phys Med Rehab 1996; 5:348–352.
15. Steinbok P, Gustavsson B, Kestle JR, Reiner A, Cochrane DD. Relationship of intraoperative electrophysiological criteria to outcome after selective functional posterior rhizotomy. J Neurosurg 1995;83(1):18–26.
16. Bloom KK, Nazar GB. Functional assessment following selective posterior rhizotomy in spastic cerebral palsy. Childs Nerv Syst 1994;10(2):84–86.
17. Peter JC, Arens LJ, Selective posterior lumbosacral rhizotomy in teenagers and young adults with spastic cerebral palsy. Br J Neurosurg 1994;8(2):135–139.
18. Engsberg JR, Olree KS, Ross SA, Park TS. Spasticity and strength changes as a function of selective dorsal rhizotomy. J Neurosurg 1998;88(6):1020–1026.
19. Subramanian N, Vaughan CL, Peter JC, Arens LJ. Gait before and 10 years after rhizotomy in children with cerebral palsy spasticity. J Neurosurg 1998; 88(6):1014–1019.
20. Wright FV, Sheil EM, Drake JM, Wedge JH, Naumann S. Evaluation of se-

lective dorsal rhizotomy for the reduction of spasticity in cerebral palsy: A randomized controlled trial. Dev Med Child Neurol 1998;40(4):239–247.

21. Buckon CE, Thomas S, Pierce R, Piatt JH Jr, Ariona MD. Developmental skills of children with spastic diplegia: Functional and qualitative changes after selective dorsal rhizotomy. Arch Phys Med Rehab 1997;78(9):946–950.

22. Park TS, Vogler GP, Phillips LH 2nd, Kaufman BA, Ortman MR, McClure SM, Gaffney PE. Effects of selective dorsal rhizotomy for spastic diplegia on hip migration in cerebral palsy. Pediatr Neurosurg 1994;20(1):43–49.

23. Russell DJ, Rosenbaum PL, Cadman DT, Gowland C, Hardy S, Jarvis S. The gross motor function measure: Validating the responsiveness of an evaluative measure. Dev Med Child Neurol 1989;31:341–352.

24. Gronley JK, and Perry J. Gait analysis techniques: Rancho Los Amigos Hospital. Phys Ther 1984;64:1831–1838.

25. Vaughan CL, Berman B, Staudt L, Peacock WJ. Gait analysis of cerebral palsied children before and after rhizotomy. Pediatr Neurosci 1989;14:297–300.

26. Boscarino LF, Ounpuu S, Davis RB 3rd, Gage JR, DeLuca PA. Effects of selective dorsal rhizotomy on gait in children with cerebral palsy. J Pediatr Orthop 1993;13:174–179.

27. Cahan LD, Kundi MS, McPherson D, Starr A, Peacock W. Electrophysiologic studies in selective dorsal rhizotomy for spasticity in children with cerebral palsy. Appl Neurophysiol 1987;50:459–460.

28. Thomas SS, Aiona MD, Buckon CE, Piatt JH Jr. Does gait continue to improve 2 years after selective dorsal rhizotomy? J Pediatr Orthop 1997;17(3):387–391.

29. Thomas SS, Aiona MD, Pierce R, Piatt JH Jr. Gait changes in children with spastic diplegia after selective dorsal rhizotomy. J Pediatr Orthop 1996;16(6):747–752.

30. Sweetser PM, Badell A, Schneider S, Badlani GH. Effects of sacral dorsal rhizotomy on bladder function in patients with spastic cerebral palsy. Neurourol Urodyn 1995;14(1):57–64.

31. Gooch JL, Walker ML. Spinal stenosis after total lumbar laminectomy for selective dorsal rhizotomy. Pediatr Neurosurg 1996;25(1):28–30.

32. Peter JC, Hoffman EB, Arens LJ, Peacock WJ. Incidence of spinal deformity in children after multiple level laminectomy for selective posterior rhizotomy. Childs Nerv Syst 1990;6:30–33.

33. Craft S, Park TS, White DA, Schatz J, Noetzel M, Arnold S. Chang cognitive performance in children with spastic diplegic cerebral palsy following selective dorsal rhizotomy. Pediatr Neurosurg 1995;23(2):68–75.

34. Steinbok P, Reiner AM, Beauchamp R, Armstrong RW, Cochrane DD. A randomized clinical trial to compare selective posterior rhizotomy plus physiotherapy with physiotherapy alone in children with spastic diplegic cerebral palsy. Dev Med Child Neurol 1997;39(3):178–184.

35. Lang FF, Deletis V, Cohen HW, Velasquez L, Abbott R. Inclusion of S2 dorsal rootlets in functional posterior rhizotomy for spasticity in children with cerebral palsy. Neurosurgery 1994;34(5):847–853.

36. Chicoine MR, Park TS, Kaufman BA. Selective dorsal rhizotomy and rates of orthopedic surgery in children with spastic cerebral palsy. J Neurosurg 1997;86(1):34–39.

42

Intrathecal Baclofen for Spasticity

Allen H. Maniker
New Jersey Medical School, Newark, New Jersey, U.S.A.

1   INTRODUCTION

The treatment of spasticity by the direct infusion of intrathecal baclofen (ITB), first proposed by Penn and Kroin in 1984, has met with significant success in treating patients with this condition [1]. To apply this therapy successfully, the surgeon must have a clear understanding of the definition of spasticity and the criteria with which to select appropriate patients. In a narrow physiological sense, spasticity may be defined as a motor disorder characterized by a velocity-dependent increase in muscle tone with exaggerated tendon jerks resulting from hyperexcitability of the stretch reflex [2]. The presence of spasticity can be thought of as pathognomonic of an upper motor lesion and is the result of both a facilitation and a disinhibition of the stretch reflex from a lack of input from descending cortical and spinal tracts [3]. The fact that it is defined as velocity dependent helps to distinguish it from other forms of rigidity, such as that caused by contractures, dystonias, or Parkinson's disease. The condition of spasticity may result from many disease states originating in either the spine or the brain. Spasticity of spinal cord origin may occur with spinal cord injury, multiple sclerosis, spinal ischemia, spinal dysraphism, degenerative myelopathy, transverse myelitis, syringomyelia, spinal tumor, cervical spondylosis, and familial spastic paraparesis. Spasticity of cerebral origin may result from cerebral palsy, traumatic brain injury, cerebrovascular accident, anoxic injury, brain tumor, and metabolic diseases of the brain [4,5]. This list is by no means complete. The end result is that spasms, rigidity, and clonus interfere with the normal initiation and completion of a smooth movement and ultimately result in weakness with a loss of mobility and dexterity.

The most effective use of oral baclofen had been in the treatment of spasticity caused by spinal cord injury or multiple sclerosis. The initial intrathecal studies were done on these patient groups after oral medications had been unsuccessful or the side effects intolerable. In these patients it was found that a small intrathecal bolus dose of baclofen was able to significantly reduce muscle tone and spasms. The effect achieved by the bolus dose could then be maintained for the long term by a continuous infusion mode. The delivery of baclofen intrathecally by a continuous infusion through a pump, in the appropriate patients, has been shown to help alleviate spasticity that may then result in improved function.

2 PATIENT SELECTION AND TEST DOSING

Baclofen, which is gamma-amino-butyric acid (GABA), acts as an agonist at the intraspinal inhibitory sites along the stretch reflex pathway, thereby effecting a decrease in the patients spasticity. Baclofen may be administered orally; however, it is water soluble and, therefore, only small amounts cross the blood-brain barrier effectively [6]. Too often maximum oral doses may not sufficiently control the patients spasticity, and patients may even experience unpleasant side effects, such as nausea, drowsiness, mental confusion, ataxia, and headache. The rationale, therefore, for administering baclofen intrathecally is that it concentrates the drug at the dorsal gray matter of the spinal cord where it is required for therapeutic effect. Furthermore, when introduced directly into the intrathecal space, effective cerebrospinal fluid (CSF) concentrations of baclofen are achieved with plasma concentrations 100 times less than those occurring with oral administration, thereby avoiding any unwanted side effects.

To assess a patient for suitability of ITB, several factors must be taken into account, including severity of spasticity, goals of the patient and family, patient responsibility to return for regular evaluations and refills, patient age, previous treatments and results, and other complicating medical conditions. Appropriate patients should be refractory to orally administered baclofen or in a situation in which their spasticity is controlled but with intolerable side effects to the drug. They should be at least 1 year posttrauma if the spasticity is of cerebral origin. A patient should initially be evaluated by the Ashworth scale (Table 1) to help quantify the severity of spasticity and for use as a baseline to determine the response to therapy. Elbow flexion and extension,

TABLE 1 Ashworth Scale

Score	Degree of Muscle Tone
1	No increase in tone (normal)
2	Slight increase in tone, giving a "catch" when affected part(s) moved in flexion or extension
3	More marked increase in tone but affected part(s) easily flexed
4	Considerable increase in tone; passive movement difficult
5	Affected part(s) rigid in flexion or extension

wrist flexion and extension, hip abduction, knee flexion and extension, and ankle dorsiflexion are all joint functions that should be evaluated and graded on the Ashworth scale. When a patient is deemed to be an appropriate candidate, as judged by the above criteria, he or she should next undergo intrathecal test dosing.

An intrathecal test dose is administered by standard lumbar puncture. Once good CSF flow is obtained through the spinal needle, a 50-microgram bolus dose is administered intrathecally. Barbitaged into the CSF over several minutes, the onset of action will generally be 30 minutes to 1 hour after administration. The peak spasmolytic effect will occur approximately 4 hours after dosing and effects may last for 4 to 8 hours. Patients are generally observed in a monitored bed setting, as adverse reactions or overdose may be life threatening. If the patient is already taking oral baclofen, this should be continued through the trial dosing, as abrupt withdrawal may result in seizures, hallucinations, and hyponatremia. If the initial dose of 50 micrograms is ineffective in alleviating spasticity (in general, at least a 2-point reduction on the Ashworth scale is considered a good response), the test dose may be repeated after 24 hours with a 75-microgram dose. If 75 micrograms is again ineffective in reducing spasticity, then a third test dose may be administered 24 hours later with 100 micrograms. If there is no response after a third test dose of 100 micrograms, then the patient should be considered a nonresponder and an inappropriate candidate for ITB.

3 OPERATIVE PROCEDURE

Once the preliminary test doses have established therapeutic efficacy, the patient may be scheduled for implantation of the pump. The patient must be free of any potential infectious sources, including urinary tract infections and open decubitus ulcers—conditions frequently found in this patient group.

Implanting a Synchromed® Infusion System (Medtronic) is a sterile surgical procedure taking approximately 2 hours (Fig. 1). It may be performed under general, regional, or local anesthetic. The patient is typically placed in the lateral decubitus position with the right flank up. Care must be taken to pad all areas well including knees, ankles, elbows, and wrists. An axillary roll is used. The sterile field must include enough room on the anterior abdominal wall over the right upper and lower quadrants to develop a subcutaneous pocket to accommodate the pump. The field must also include the area of the lumbosacral spine at the level of L3-4.

An approximately 4-cm incision should be laid out on the lumbosacral area centered over L3-4 landmarks (Fig. 2). Dissection should continue down to expose the spinous processes. With a 15-gauge Touhy needle, the thecal sac is entered. Good CSF flow is verified and sent for routine laboratory tests and cultures. The intrathecal catheter is threaded through the needle and its placement at the T10 level should be confirmed with fluoroscopy. The Touhy needle is withdrawn and the catheter clamped to prevent

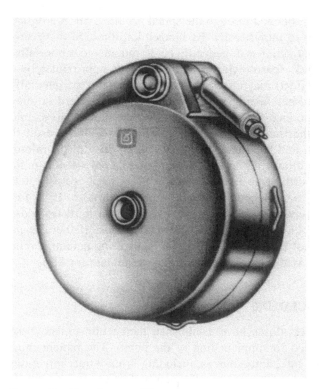

FIGURE 1 Synchromed® pump.

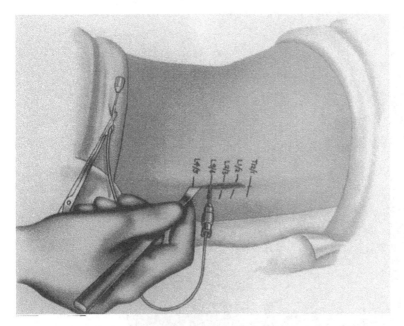

FIGURE 2   Location of lumbar incision.

additional CSF leakage. The subcutaneous pocket is developed on the anterior abdominal wall, above the rectus fascia. The pocket should be positioned sufficiently below the rib cage and above the iliac crest so that when the patient bends, the pump will not strike up against the lowest ribs or crest, causing discomfort. A larger pocket is desirable, so that the edge of the pump does not place undue pressure on the incision and precipitate an incisional dehiscence. A tunneling rod is then used to pass the proximal catheter from the pocket to the lower back incision. The catheters are then connected with the metal and Silastic connectors provided with the kit. The proximal catheter is secured to the pump, and the pump is placed within the pocket (Fig. 3). The pump may be placed in a Dacron pouch to promote fibrosis to the underlying fascia, or alternatively, newer pump series have metal loops through which the pump may be secured to the underlying fascia. One of several anchoring devices may be used to secure the distal catheter to the lumbar fascia to help prevent catheter migration. The areas are copiously irrigated with an antibiotic solution and the incisions closed in layers. Any lengths of catheter that have been trimmed away must be handed off and saved, so that the initial priming dosage may be accurately calculated. The initial dose for 24 hours is generally set at double the amount

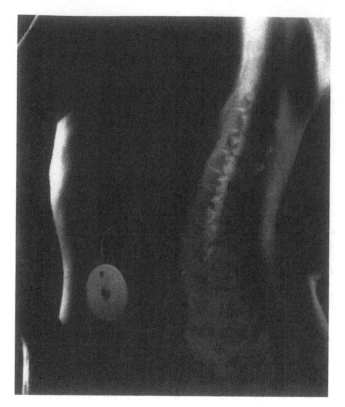

FIGURE 3 System in place.

of the bolus dose shown as effective in the testing phase. The pump is then programmed with a percutaneous wand while the patient is waking up from anesthesia. The procedure for programming takes a minute or 2 to accomplish. (Refer to company manuals for exact instructions for calculating dosage rate and programming the pump.) Once the appropriate initial dosage is calculated, it should remain at this level for at least 24 hours without further changes. Thereafter, the amount delivered may be increased by 10% to 15% every 24 hours until the desired reduction in spasticity is achieved.

4 POSTOPERATIVE CARE

The patient is generally kept in the hospital for an additional 24 hours for administration of intravenous antibiotics, and a program for tapering off any oral baclofen is begun. This taper off oral medications should be accomplished gradually as the side effects of abrupt withdrawal, as mentioned above, are severe. Sutures are removed at 10 days after operation. Depending on the amount of drug required by the patient, the pump is refilled, usually by a home nursing service, every 4 to 6 weeks. Evaluation and programming of the pump function and dosage are accomplished through a percutaneous computer system on regularly scheduled patient visits. The patient should have at least a yearly evaluation by the implanting surgeon. The pump battery is expected to last between 4 to 6 years. A low battery alarm will sound with an audible beeping noise approximately 4 to 6 weeks before battery failure. Caution should be exercised in interpreting the low battery alarm, as instillation of cold medication into the pump may also trigger its sounding. If confirmed as a true battery failure, then the patient should be scheduled for a prompt revision and replacement of the pump unit. This can usually be accomplished under local anesthetic.

5 COMPLICATIONS

5.1 Infection

Infection, as can be expected with any implanted device, can be problematic. The usual signs of redness, pain, swelling and fever should be watched for closely in the immediate postoperative period. Occasionally an infection is heralded by the development of a large amount of serous fluid build-up in the subcutaneous pocket of the pump. This may be treated with aspiration of the fluid and aggressive antibiotic therapy [7]. If headache and neck stiffness develop, this may signal meningitis, and the pump system may then require removal.

5.2 Overdosage

Overdoses of intrathecal baclofen have been reported in the literature [8]. Symptoms may include drowsiness, lightheadedness, dizziness, somnolence, respiratory depression, seizures, rostral progression of hypotonia, and loss of consciousness progressing to coma. As always, emergency procedures to maintain airway, breathing, and circulation are instituted immediately. Intubation and respirator support may be required. The pump reservoir is emptied and the pump disabled. Unless contraindicated, as in patients with heart conduction defects, physostigmine is administered intravenously. In adults, 1 to 2 mg may be administered over 5 to 10 minutes. If not contraindicated, 30 to 40 ml of CSF are also withdrawn to reduce CSF baclofen concentration. The patient should respond to the physostigmine relatively rapidly but may require additional doses if the overdose was especially large. The central effects of an overdose should clear in 24 to 48 hours; however, the patient should be observed in an intensive care setting until all vital signs and mental status return to baseline.

5.3 Tolerance

Tolerance to baclofen develops in most patients over time. Over the first 6 to 12 months, the intrathecal dose may be double that of the initial dose needed to achieve the same clinical result. However, after this period the dosage will usually stabilize [9]. In a few patients, tolerance may require a drug holiday for several weeks and may be switched to intrathecal morphine, which has some of the spasmolytic effects seen with baclofen. Abrupt withdrawal of baclofen may cause seizures and hallucinations; therefore, if a patient is begun on an intrathecal drug holiday, he or she should be restarted on an oral dosage of baclofen. Furthermore, a rebound effect may be noted in which spasticity returns to an even worse level than before the start of intrathecal therapy. This effect is, however, short lived and resolves in several days.

6 CONCLUSION

Intrathecal baclofen delivered by a subcutaneously implanted programmable pump can result in a significant improvement in spasticity, as measured by Ashworth scores, and an improved quality of life for these patients.

REFERENCES

1. Penn RD, Kroin JS. Intrathecal baclofen alleviates spinal cord spasticity. Lancet 1:1078, 1984.
2. Lance JW. Symposium synopsis. In: Feldman R, Young R, Koella W, eds. Spasticity: Disordered Motor Control. Chicago: Year Book Medical Publishers, 1980, pp. 185–203.
3. Ashby P, Verrier M, Lightfoot E. Segmental reflex pathways in spinal shock and spinal spasticity in man. J Neurol Neurosurg Psychiatry 37:1352–1360, 1974.
4. Meythaler JM, McCary A, Hadley MN. Prospective assessment of continuous intrathecal infusion of baclofen for spasticity caused by acquired brain injury: A preliminary report. J Neurosurg 87:415–419, 1997.
5. Albright AL, Barron WB, Fasick MP, Polinko P, Janosky J. Continuous intrathecal baclofen infusion for spasticity of cerebral origin. JAMA 270:2475–2477, 1993.
6. Knutsson E, Lindbloom U, Martensson A. Plasma and cerebrospinal fluid levels of baclofen (Lioresal) at optimal therapeutic responses in spastic paresis. J Neurol Sci 23:473–484, 1974.

7. Penn RD. Intrathecal baclofen for spasticity of spinal origin: Seven years of
    experience. J Neurosurg 77:236–240, 1992.
8. Krames ES. Intrathecal infusional therapies for intractable pain: Patient man-
    agement guidelines. Pain Symptom Manage 8(1):36–46, 1993.
9. Muller-Schwefe G, Penn RD. Physostigmine in the treatment of intrathecal ba-
    clofen overdose: Report of three cases. J Neurosurg 71:273–275, 1989.

43

Classification of Seizure Disorders

David A. Marks
University of Medicine and Dentistry of New Jersey,
Newark, New Jersey, U.S.A.

1 INTRODUCTION

An epileptic seizure is a behavioral event that is caused by an abnormal neuronal discharge. Epilepsy refers to the condition of recurrent seizure. Certain metabolic or medical conditions, including hypoglycemia, hyponatremia, and alcohol withdrawal may predispose an individual to a single seizure, but not recurrent seizures (epilepsy). In the United States, epilepsy affects approximately 6% of the population. Approximately 4% of individuals living to age 75 may experience a single unprovoked seizure, and if provoked seizures are included, the incidence approaches 10% [1].

It is important to classify seizure disorders. Anticonvulsant treatment differs for the various seizure types, and before initiating a treatment plan, seizure type must be classified. For example, certain generalized seizures respond best to valproate, and control may be aggravated by certain gabanergic drugs, including gabapentin. The type of seizure may influence the patient's ability to work, and different seizure types have different natural histories. Accurate classification helps with prognostication.

Currently, there is both a seizure and an epilepsy classification. In 1981, the International League Against Epilepsy (ILAE) developed a descriptive classification of seizures that used both the electroencephalogram

TABLE 1   ILAE Classification of Epileptic Seizures

I. Partial (focal) seizures.
   A. Simple partial seizures (consciousness not impaired)
      1. With motor signs (examples include a jacksonian march, loss of tone, versive movements)
      2. With sensory symptoms (examples include visual, auditory, somatosensory, olfactory, and gustatory symptoms)
      3. With psychic symptoms (involves a disturbance of higher cortical functions, eg, deja vu, hallucinations, and aphasia)
      4. With autonomic symptoms (examples include epigastric sensations, flushing, piloerection, pupillary changes)
   B. Complex partial seizures (consciousness is impaired)
      1. With simple partial onset followed by impaired consciousness
      2. With impairment of consciousness at the onset
      3. Impairment of complex partial seizures with automatisms
   C. Partial seizures evolving to secondary generalized seizures
      1. Simple partial seizures evolving to generalized seizures
      2. Complex partial seizures evolving to generalized seizures
      3. Simple partial seizures evolving to complex partial seizures evolving to generalized seizures
II. Generalized seizures (no focal onset, convulsive or nonconvulsive)
   A. Absence seizures
      1. With impaired consciousness
      2. Impaired consciousness with additional features including atonic or tonic activity, automatisms.
   B. Myoclonic seizures characterized by single or multiple jerks
   C. Tonic-clonic seizures
   D. Tonic seizures
   E. Atonic seizures
   F. Clonic seizures
III. Unclassified epileptic seizures

(EEG) and clinical symptoms to define the seizure type (Table 1) [2]. The Classification of Epilepsies and Epileptic Syndromes of the International League Against Epilepsy, developed in 1989, incorporates etiological, biological, and genetic considerations [3]. This chapter will concentrate on the former descriptive classification of epileptic seizures.

The principle feature of the seizure classification is to determine whether seizures started focally (partial seizures) or have a diffuse onset (generalized seizures). It is usually possible to make this distinction from an accurate history, but certain focal seizures spread very rapidly, and it may not be possible to make this distinction. If a focal onset is determined, the next issue is to establish whether there is an alteration in consciousness. If consciousness is not affected, seizures are classified as simple partial seizures. Conversely, if consciousness is altered, seizures are classified as complex partial seizures. Generalized seizures are divided according to their motor characteristics. It is important to determine whether the subject experienced predominantly tonic, tonic-clonic, or generalized motor activity.

Classifying seizures depends on an understanding of neuroanatomy. The initial clinical symptom, or aura, is extremely helpful to localize seizure onset. For example, visual hallucinations suggest occipital onset, whereas a deja vu feeling suggests temporal lobe onset. Patients with partial seizures may not report an aura if (1) the seizure spreads rapidly and generalizes, and consciousness is rapidly altered, (2) the individual is amnestic after the seizure (3), seizures begin in a clinically silent cortical region. Examples of "silent" areas include certain frontal and association cortical regions.

2 PARTIAL SEIZURES

When onset is focal, seizures are referred to as partial seizures, but the term focal is still used. Partial seizures occur when electrical activation begins in a localized region of one cerebral hemisphere. Partial seizures are classified primarily on the basis of whether consciousness is altered. When consciousness is preserved, seizures are referred to as simple partial seizures. When consciousness is altered or impaired, seizures are classified as complex partial seizures. If the electrical discharge spreads to involve deep subcortical structures, a partial seizure will evolve to a secondary generalized seizure.

2.1 Simple Partial Seizures

Simple partial seizures result when the ictal discharge remains localized to a restricted cortical region within one hemisphere and does not spread to the opposite hemisphere. The electrical changes may not be seen on surface EEG. Because electrical spread is limited, there is no alteration in consciousness, and the clinical manifestations will depend on the properties of the activated cortical region. Most simple partial seizures can be grouped into four clinical groups: motor, sensory psychic, and autonomic.

Simple motor seizures involve an electrical discharge activating the motor cortex. Patients will typically experience contralateral clonic activity that may be localized or spread. Focal motor seizures may be predominantly versive with contraversive head turning. When the motor activity spreads, it is referred to as a jacksonian march. Focal motor activity does not usually exceed 60 seconds. After a focal motor seizure, patients may experience transient weakness, which is referred to as a Todd's paralysis. The paralysis may lasts minutes to hours, and the clinician needs to differentiate a Todd's paralysis from a stroke. Focal motor activity may be very localized, and may persist hours to days. These seizures are referred to as epilepsia partialis continua.

Seizures occurring with activation of the sensory cortex produce somatosensory seizures. Clinical features reported include pins and needles, numbness, novocaine-type tingling, and the sensory symptoms commonly march. Involvement of the visual cortex may present with elementary or elaborate visual hallucinations. Activation of the primary visual cortex is accompanied by simple, elementary visual hallucinations, such as flashing lights, sparkles, and colors. When the association visual cortex is involved, visual symptomatology is complex, and patients may report complex shapes, illusions, and distortions. The occipital cortex has direct frontal connections, and the initial clinical manifestations may be tonic eye deviation and blinking. Involvement of the auditory cortex usually produces simple auditory hallucinations, including tinnitus and buzzing sensations. Complex auditory hallucinations, such as a fixed music tune are less common, and when patients report hearing voices, the etiology is usually psychiatric and not neurological. With activation of the temporal region, simple partial seizures may present with gustatory or olfactory sensations.

Simple partial seizures with psychic symptoms usually progress to complex partial seizures leading to impairment of consciousness. These seizures are associated with a disturbance of higher cortical function. Symptoms include aphasia, visual illusions, and complex structured hallucinations. Patients often complain of a deja vu experience. Affective symptoms include fear and anger.

Autonomic symptoms may be the most prominent seizure manifestation. A common autonomic symptom is a rising epigastric sensation and is associated with a temporal lobe seizure focus. Flushing, sweating, piloerection, pupil dilatation, and incontinence may occur as simple partial seizures.

2.2 Complex Partial Seizures

During a seizure, it is important to determine whether the subject experiences an alteration or loss of consciousness. This implies spread of the epileptic discharge across the corpus callosum to the opposite hemisphere. Patients may describe a subjective feeling or aura before losing consciousness. If the epileptic discharge does not progress, the aura constitutes the simple partial seizure. Common temporal lobe auras include a rising epigastric sensation, fear, deja vu, jamais vu, and a feeling of detachment. Alteration of consciousness has important clinical relevance, and patients should not drive, operate heavy machinery, or partake in certain sporting activities unsupervised. Complex partial seizures may be clinically bland, and it is not always possible to determine whether consciousness was impaired. At most epilepsy centers, nurses are trained to question patients during a seizure to determine whether the patient can learn and incorporate new information. Failure to follow simple instructions (ictal unresponsiveness) implies loss of consciousness. It is extremely difficult to determine whether consciousness is affected in neonates and young children. After a complex partial or generalized seizure, patients are amnestic and confused, and the postictal state may last minutes to hours. Without EEG monitoring, it is not possible to determine the transition from the ictal to the postictal state.

During a complex partial seizures, patients may carry out "automatic" behaviors or motor activities, referred to as automatisms. An automatism may be the continuation of an activity that preceded the onset of the seizure. Common automatisms include eating movements (lipsmacking, chewing, and swallowing), simple or elaborate gestures, verbal automatisms consisting of forced ictal speech, and ambulatory automatisms. Gestures include fumbling with objects and picking at one's clothes, and patients are unaware of these behaviors. Oropharyngeal and gustatory automatisms are usually associated with seizure spread to the insula and amygdala. Automatisms may occur with a prolonged generalized absence seizure, and the EEG differentiates between these two seizure types. Both simple and partial complex seizures may rapidly evolve to a generalized tonic-clonic seizure and are referred to as secondary generalized seizures. The majority (70%–80%) of partial complex seizures arise from the temporal lobe, followed by the frontal lobe.

First-line anticonvulsants for simple and complex partial seizures with or without generalization are carbamazepine, phenytoin, and valproic acid. Adjunctive agents include gabapentin, lamotrigine, tiagabine, and topiramate.

3 GENERALIZED SEIZURES

Generalized seizures are characterized by an abrupt loss of consciousness. Generalized seizures with motor activity include tonic-clonic seizures, myoclonic seizures, tonic, or clonic seizures. Generalized seizures without motor activity includes absence and atonic seizures. Generalized seizures frequently have a genetic basis, and it is important to ask about a family history. The type of generalized seizure is age dependent. Absence seizures occur in children younger than age 10, myoclonic seizures present later in the teenage years, and tonic clonic seizures typically begin in the teens. The typical EEG pattern associated with generalized seizures is a generalized spike or polyspike and slow wave discharge. In contrast, partial seizures (with or without secondary generalization) is associated with focal EEG abnormalities, including focal spike discharges, and focal slowing.

3.1 Absence Seizures

The essential feature of an absence seizure is the sudden, abrupt loss of consciousness. Seizure onset is characterized by immediate behavioral arrest, and patients are noted to have a brief motionless stare. An absence seizure typically lasts several seconds, but may last up to 30 seconds. Speech is interrupted momentarily, and the subject will then resume speaking. The attack may be influenced by sensory input, and may terminate when the individual is spoken to.

Absence seizures occur in those with a strong family history. Symptomatic children will show the classic generalized three per second spike and wave pattern, but the EEG of asymptomatic siblings may show a similar spike and wave. The course of absence seizures is variable, and absence seizures usually remit by mid-adolescence. Rarely, absence seizures will persist, and children may subsequently develop myoclonic or tonic-clonic seizures in their teenage years.

The sole manifestation of an absence seizure may be loss of consciousness with no other activity. Additional clinical features frequently accompany absence seizures. During the attack, myoclonic movements, which commonly involve eyelid fluttering or facial twitching, may occur.

Additional manifestations include atonic components. Examples are brief loss of neck and postural tone, leading to drooping of the head or slumping of the body. When diminution in tone is severe, the subject may fall. If the absence seizure is prolonged for more than 15 seconds, patients may exhibit simple or elaborate automatisms similar to the automatisms seen during complex partial seizures. An absence seizure with automatisms will have an EEG with the classic generalized spike and wave pattern. The treatment of choice for absence seizures is ethosuximide.

3.2 Myoclonic Seizures

Myoclonic seizures usually begin during the early teenage years. A myoclonic jerk is a brief shock-like contraction of an individual muscle or a muscle group. These jerks usually involve the limbs but may be confined to the face or trunk. Generalized myoclonic jerks or jerks involving the legs can be disabling, because they are associated with violent falls and frequent fractures. Myoclonic seizures have a circadian pattern and commonly occur in the morning shortly after awakening. Patients may drop or throw objects held in their hands. Myoclonic seizures are very brief, lasting approximately 1 second, and the EEG during the myoclonic jerk will show a generalized spike or polyspike and slow wave discharge. A flurry of myoclonic seizures may evolve to a generalized tonic-clonic seizure.

It is important to emphasize that not all myoclonus is epileptic. Myoclonic jerks may occur with focal spinal disease or inherited degenerative diseases. The treatment of choice for myoclonic seizures is valproate. Alternative effective anticonvulsants include lamotrigine and topirimate.

3.3 Tonic-Clonic Seizures

This is the most commonly encountered generalized seizure and is also referred to as a grand mal seizure or convulsion. Generalized seizures may occur in either childhood or adult life, and are often preceded by a flurry of myoclonic seizures. Typically, no warning precedes the seizure, although patients may complain of vague premonitions (examples include nervousness or irritability) minutes to hours before the seizure. Abrupt tonic contractions of muscles result in the patient falling to the ground in a tonic state, which may result in injury. Sustained contractions of the respiratory muscles result in stridor and a loud moan. Patients are rigid during the tonic phase, and cyanoses may occur. Patients may bite their tongue or become incontinent. The tonic phase typically lasts 30 seconds and is followed by clonic motor activity lasting 60 to 90 seconds. Shallow breathing may occur, and patients are at a risk for aspiration. The clonic phase is followed by deep sighing respiration, muscles are hypotonic, and the gag reflex is reduced, increasing the risk for aspiration. Patients may remain unresponsive for minutes to hours after a tonic-clonic seizure, and then go into a deep sleep. Patients may be amnestic for several hours after a tonic-clonic seizure (similar to the amnesia after electroconvulsive shock therapy). Sustained muscle contractions result in painful muscles and fatigue, and severe headaches are common. Patients may experience rib and vertebral fractures, and elderly women with osteoporosis are especially vulnerable. It is important to determine whether the tonic-clonic seizure was secondary generalized or occurred with no prior aura. Focal onset will suggest a structural brain lesion. Partial seizures may spread rapidly and may be difficult to distinguish from primary generalized seizures. An EEG is helpful in distinguishing between these two seizure types. Primary generalized seizures have a generalized spike and wave pattern, and they respond to valproate. Secondary generalized seizures are associated with focal interictal spikes and respond to those drugs used to treat complex partial seizures.

Absence, myoclonic, and tonic-clonic seizures are the common generalized seizure types, but generalized atonic clonic and tonic seizures do occur. Atonic seizures are very disabling, and patients experience frequent drop attacks, leading to severe injuries and bone fractures. Patients with atonic seizures need to wear a helmet to prevent severe head injuries. Atonic seizures are brief, and consciousness may be lost. Tonic seizures are also brief, and are associated with violent muscle contractions, and extensor posturing. The head and eyes may deviate, and the body may rotate. Generalized seizures may not have a tonic component, and may present as generalized clonic seizures, consisting of repetitive generalized clonic jerks. Tonic and atonic seizures do not have a familial inheritance component. These two seizure types usually occur in patients with severe underlying brain disease and are very refractory to anticonvulsants. When standard anticonvulsant therapy fails, patients may need more invasive treatments, including a corpus callosotomy or vagal nerve stimulation.

REFERENCES

1. Hauser WA, Hesdorffer DC. Epilepsy: Frequency, causes and consequences. New York: Demos, 1990.
2. The Commission on Classification and Terminology of the International League Against Epilepsy. Proposal for revised clinical and electroencephalographic classification of epileptic seizures. Epilepsia 1981;22:489–501.
3. The Commission on Classification and Terminology of the International League Against Epilepsy. Proposal for revised classification of epilepsies and epileptic syndromes. Epilepsia 1989;30:389–399.

44

Anterior Temporal Lobectomy: Indications and Technique

Thomas L. Ellis

Wake Forest University School of Medicine, Winston-Salem, North Carolina, U.S.A.

Steven N. Roper

University of Florida and Malcolm Randall VA Medical Center, Gainesville, Florida, U.S.A.

1 INTRODUCTION

Anterior temporal lobectomy (ATL) is the most commonly used and the most successful surgical treatment for intractable epilepsy. It is designed to treat a specific surgically remediable epilepsy syndrome: unilateral medial temporal lobe epilepsy. The specific characteristics of medial temporal lobe epilepsy were outlined in two papers from Yale University [1,2]. They include antecedent febrile convulsions in childhood, auras (abdominal/visceral, autonomic, emotional, and olfactory sensations are most common), partial complex seizures, characteristic memory deficits, and seizure onsets in the anterior temporal region. Hippocampal sclerosis is the pathological substrate of medial temporal lobe epilepsy and is present in about 80% of surgical specimens from ATL if foreign tissue lesions are excluded. It consists of a characteristic pattern of neuronal loss that is most severe in area CA1 with relative sparing of the dentate granule cells and area CA2. Axonal sprouting of the mossy fibers of the dentate granule cells into the dentate inner molecular layer is also seen. The etiology of hippocampal sclerosis and the exact relationship between the structural changes and seizure initiation remain to be completely understood. Other surgical resections for epilepsy may take place in the temporal lobe, such as foreign tissue lesionectomy or neocortical resections of the temporal cortex, but this chapter will describe the standard ATL for medial temporal lobectomy as modified by Spencer [3].

2 PATIENT SELECTION

Surgical success is largely dependent on proper patient selection. Intractable, disabling seizures are documented by seizure diaries and trials of antiepileptic medications. The number of antiepileptic drugs (AEDs) for partial complex seizures is growing, but a large percentage of patients remain intractable to medical therapy. Vagus nerve stimulation should not be considered an alternative to ATL, as seizure-free rates between the two procedures are not comparable. All patients undergo history and physical examination, neuropsychological testing, video-electroencephalographic (EEG) monitoring documenting seizure onsets, and magnetic resonance (MR)-imaging with special attention to the hippocampus. All patients undergo Wada testing prior to ATL to confirm language lateralization and the adequacy of the opposite temporal lobe to support memory. Additional imaging tests may also be helpful, and these include ictal single photon emission computed tomography (SPECT), interictal positron emission tomography (PET), and magnetoencephalography. To proceed directly to ATL, we require that two major tests localize to the same temporal lobe with no discordant information from any of the other tests. In the event that temporal lobe onsets have been clearly identified but the laterality is uncertain, bitemporal depth electrodes and frontotemporal subdural strip electrodes are placed for extraoperative monitoring of ictal activity. If the seizure onsets are well lateralized but frontal cannot be clearly differentiated from temporal onsets, we will place unilateral frontotemporal subdural grid and strip electrodes.

3 SURGICAL TECHNIQUE

Preoperative treatment is similar to many craniotomies. Preoperative labs are limited to a complete blood count and AED levels, unless age or other medical conditions indicate additional tests. Patients are instructed to take nothing by mouth after midnight and to take any morning AEDs when they awaken. Patients are admitted to the hospital on the day of surgery. They are given a dose of prophylactic antibiotics in the preoperative holding area. All efforts are made to maintain therapeutic AED levels throughout the surgical period. If patients are taking only oral AEDs, they are loaded with phosphenytoin intraoperatively after electrocorticography (ECoG), with the assumption that changes in gastrointestinal motility and vomiting may decrease absorption of oral medications in the early postoperative period.

At the University of Florida, a standard anesthetic regimen is given to reduce variability in intraoperative ECoG. We use a combination of isoflorane, nitrous oxide, and a narcotic agent at the beginning of the operation. Throughout the case, we hyperventilate ($PCO_2 = 30$–35 mm Hg) but do not use mannitol for nonlesional cases. After the bone work is completed, isoflorane is stopped and the rest of the surgery is carried out under nitrous/ narcotic anesthesia. We do not perform awake cortical stimulation mapping when performing standard anterior temporal lobectomies.

After induction of anesthesia and intubation, the patient's hair is clipped and shaved in the frontotemporal area. The Mayfield headholder is applied and a bump is placed beneath the contralateral shoulder. The head is turned 60 degrees from vertical with the vertex flat. Placing the vertex down is more common for craniotomies, but this angle makes the hippocampal resection slightly more difficult. The skin incision is a typical "question mark" that extends back to the level of the external auditory canal. The skin incision is marked, the area is sterilely prepared and draped, and the incision is made. We carry the scalp dissection full-thickness through the temporalis muscle and elevate the muscle with the scalp flap. The muscle dissection is extended so that 1 cm of the root of the zygoma in front of the ear and 1 cm of the zygomatic process of the frontal bone are exposed. The muscle and scalp flap are retracted using fish hooks and rubberbands after first wrapping the flap in a wet laparotomy pad to prevent an excessively acute angle of the scalp flap that could produce ischemic necrosis of the flap. The bone flap is made by placing burr holes above and below the pterion and over the posterior temporal lobe. The bone flap needs to provide very little frontal exposure but should be extended as low as possible over the middle fossa. Additional portions of the pterion and squamous temporal bone are removed with a Leksell ronguer. Mastoid air cells may be entered at this time and are filled with bone wax. The dura is opened in a C-shaped fashion based on the pterion. The dural flap is retracted and covered with moist gelatin sponge to prevent drying.

We perform intraoperative ECoG if no invasive monitoring has been performed previously. The results of the ECoG do not alter the boundaries of the standard resection, but we feel that it may provide additional information in the event that the patient is not seizure free after surgery. Two 4-contact strips are placed along the inferior surface of the temporal lobe. If placed correctly, the medial contacts of the strips will lie directly beneath the parahippocampal gyrus and give good recordings of medial temporal activity. A 9- or 20-contact grid is then placed over the lateral temporal lobe.

If interictal activity is extremely quiet, we will administer 20 mg of methohexital sodium to activate interictal spikes.

After completion of ECoG, the lateral resection margin is then measured over the middle temporal gyrus. We use 3 cm for the dominant hemisphere and 4 cm for the nondominant one (Fig. 1A). The superficial incision is then made over the lateral aspect of the temporal lobe and in the inferior aspect to the level of the collateral sulcus. We angle posteriorly as we work along the inferior surface to provide better exposure of the medial temporal structures (Fig. 1B). We then incise the pia just beneath the Sylvian fissure and coagulate and cut any anterior temporal branches of the middle cerebral artery that are confined to the area of resection. Care is taken to preserve any arteries or veins near the posterior resection margin that might be servicing tissue outside of the planned resection. The superficial Sylvian vein is also preserved as it enters the sphenoparietal sinus. The anterior portion of the superior temporal gyrus is then removed in a subpial fashion over the Sylvian fissure. Controlled, gentle suction is used so that the integrity of the pia is maintained. This dissection is continued until the lymen insulae is identified as the area of gray matter extending deep to the Sylvian fissure.

Next, the lateral cortical incision is carried out through the temporal white matter with the anterolateral temporal cortex retracted anteriorly. This dissection is extended until the temporal horn of the lateral ventricle is entered about 1 cm deep to the superior temporal sulcus. The wall of the temporal horn is heralded by the small ependymal veins running through

A

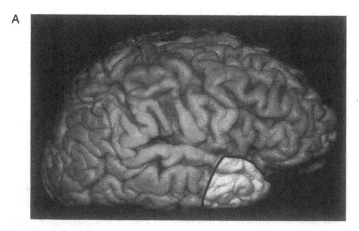

FIGURE 1   A. Photographs of a fixed brain demonstrating the extent of cortical resection in anterior temporal lobectomy. The lateral neocortical resection extends 3 cm posterior to the tip of the temporal pole in the dominant hemisphere and 4 cm in the nondominant hemisphere.

B

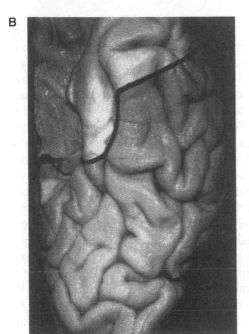

FIGURE 1   Continued. **B.** The inferior resection angles posteriorly and the medial resection (defined laterally by the collateral sulcus) is carried back to the level of the quadrigeminal plate.

the white matter in an anterior-posterior orientation. Once the temporal horn is entered, the dissection is carried anteriorly through the temporal stem to connect with the previous dissection over the Sylvian fissure. In this way the temporal horn is completely unroofed. The inferior surface of the amygdala will be appreciated forming the roof of the anterior temporal horn at this time. The anterolateral temporal specimen is then retracted laterally. The floor of the temporal horn is defined by two hemicylindrical structures running in an anterior-posterior orientation. The medial one is the dorsal aspect of the hippocampus. The lateral one is the collateral eminence. The dissection is carried through the collateral eminence to the deep surface of the collateral sulcus. The pia of the collateral sulcus is then cut, and this dissection is carried anteriorly through the rhinal sulcus. At this point, the anterolateral temporal specimen is completely separated from the brain. Any bridging veins over the surface are coagulated and cut, and the specimen is removed.

Next, the operative microscope is sterilely draped and brought into position. The Greenberg retractor system is used to retract the choroid plexus of the temporal horn superiorly and the posterior temporal cortex posteriorly. A third retractor may be used to retract the hippocampus and parahippocampal gyrus laterally as the dissection proceeds. The choroidal fissure is exposed and the fimbria is identified as a flap of white matter extending medially from the hippocampus. The fimbria is teased from the choroidal fissure with a microball dissector. Retracting the fimbria medially (or removing it) exposes the hippocampal sulcus. This sulcus is defined by two layers of pia with the hippocampal arteries running between them. The pial sleeves and the small arteries are coagulated and cut. This dissection is usually started over the body of the hippocampus. As the dissection is extended anteriorly, the pial sleeve will appear to extend laterally. At this point, the dissection is carried through the pes hippocampus and adjacent parahippocampal gyrus. Similarly, suction is used to transect the hippocampus and parahippocampal gyrus posteriorly. An effort is made to remove all the hippocampus except for the posterior tail. Next the dissection is carried in a subpial fashion over the subiculum and parahippocampal gyrus. When the dissection is lateral to the incisura, the pia over the parahippocampal gyrus is cut longitudinally. Anterior and middle temporal arteries from the posterior cerebral artery are coagulated and cut. The medial temporal specimen consisting of the hippocampus and parahippocampal gyrus is then removed. The lateral amygdala and the uncus are then removed subpially using gentle suction. During the medial resection, care is taken so that the integrity of the pia adjacent to the crural and ambient cisterns is preserved at all times. The resection bed is lined with a single layer of oxidized cellulose. Closure of the craniotomy is carried out in the usual fashion.

Postoperatively, patients are observed in the intensive care unit overnight. Decadron is started on the morning of surgery at 4 mg every 6 hours. On subsequent postoperative days it is reduced to 3, 2, and 1 mg every 4 hours, and then discontinued. Patients are continued on the usual AEDs. If intravenous phenytoin or phosphenytoin was initiated intraoperatively, it is continued until the patient demonstrates good oral intake. Patients are encouraged to get out of bed on postoperative day 1. Most patients return home on postoperative day 3 or 4.

4 OUTCOME

Many classification schemes have been proposed to assess outcome after surgery for intractable seizures. Perhaps the most popular is the four-tiered classification scheme developed by Engel [4]. The class 1 patients include those who are seizure-free for 2 years since surgery, those with occasional nondisabling simple partial seizures, and those with generalized convulsions only in the setting of antiepileptic medication withdrawal. Class II patients have rare (< 2–3 per year) disabling seizures. Those patients in class III have "worthwhile improvement," generally defined as a more than 90% reduction in seizure frequency. Lastly, patients in class IV are those with no change in seizure frequency, increased seizure frequency, or a reduction in seizure frequency without an improvement in the patient's disability. In many, the simpler scheme of seizure-free, improved, or not improved is used.

Early reports of the success of surgery in the treatment of epilepsy include those of Rasmussen in 1983 [5]. This report included 894 patients with anterior temporal lobe resections between 1928 and 1980 and documented that 37% of the patients were seizure free after 2 or more years and that 26% were improved. From the same institution, Olivier [6] more recently reported on a series of 221 patients and found that 65% were either seizure free or had a maximum of three seizures per year.

In 1989, Dasheiff [7] reviewed the available literature of reports with a minimum 2-year follow-up and found that in those reports with primarily temporal lobe resections, 40% to 62% of the patients were seizure free. An additional 21% to 35% were improved and 14% to 35% showed no improvement. In 1992, Engel [8] published the collected results of 3410 patients from 91 centers who underwent anterior temporal lobectomies and found that 67% were seizure-free, 24% were improved and 9% were not improved.

In a separate analysis, Engel [8] demonstrated the importance of following year-by-year outcomes for more than 2 years after surgery. In a group of 106 patients who underwent anterior temporal lobectomy between 1961 and 1983, only 81% of the patients who were seizure-free at 2 years remained seizure-free at 5 years, and 57% remained seizure-free at 10 years. Conversely, of those patients experiencing rare seizures after 1 year of follow-up, 57% became seizure free for at least 2 years by the end of the fifth year of follow-up. This study highlights the fact that late failures do occur and that early outcomes are not always predictive of late outcomes. Significant changes in patient outcomes continue for at least 5 to 10 years postoperatively.

Many studies have analyzed factors that may affect seizure outcomes after anterior temporal lobectomy. Dodrill et al. [9] identified patients with interictal epileptiform activity confined to the anterior temporal lobe as being likely to be seizure free. Jeong et al [10] analyzed 93 patients with mesial temporal lobe epilepsy to identify the preoperative prognostic factors that may predict good outcome after surgery. They found that 78 (84%) of the patients were seizure free at 2 years. Using multivariate analysis, they discovered that age at surgery and the presence of ipsilateral hippocampal sclerosis on MRI were the most statistically significant independent prognostic factors predictive of good outcome. This supported multiple earlier studies that identified the presence of hippocampal sclerosis, either in pathologic specimens or in preoperative MRI, as predictive of good outcome.

Foldvary et al [11] examined 79 patients who underwent anterior temporal lobectomy between 1962 and 1984. Patients were followed up for an average of 14 years, with patients having less than 2 years of follow-up being excluded from the study. Using Engel's classification, 65% of patients were class I, 15% were class II, 11% were class III, and 9% were class IV. Using Kaplan-Meier survival analysis, it was discovered that higher preoperative seizure frequency was associated with poor seizure outcome. In addition, seizure-free status at 2 years was found to be a better predictor of long-term outcome than the status at 6, 12, or 18 months.

Favorable outcomes after temporal lobectomy also have been correlated with the presence of abnormalities seen on PET scan [12], with nonspecific abnormalities of the mesial temporal lobe on MRI [13,14], and with functional deficits produced on intracarotid injection of amytal [15].

In patients with bitemporal abnormalities seen preoperatively on EEG, several factors may predict seizure-free status. Holmes et al [16] examined 44 patients with bitemporal, independent, interictal epileptiform patterns on EEG who underwent anterior temporal lobectomy. All patients underwent preoperative intracranial monitoring. Twenty-two (50%) of patients were seizure-free at 1 year, 14 (32%) had at least 75% reduction in seizures, and eight (18%) had less than a 75% reduction in seizures. A seizure-free outcome was associated with three independent factors: a history of febrile seizures, concordance of MRI abnormality and side of operation, and 100% lateralization of intracranially recorded ictal onset to the side of the operation.

Complication rates for ATL are about 5% in most series [17]. Possible complications that are relatively specific for ATL include verbal memory deficits and visual field defects. Removal of language-dominant medial temporal structures is associated with decreased verbal memory [18]. Most patients with dominant hippocampal sclerosis will demonstrate these deficits preoperatively (it is an integral part of the preoperative evaluation) so that few to no new deficits are seen after surgery. If a patient has normal preoperative verbal memory, increased verbal forgetting can be demonstrated in postoperative testing. This may show a maximal effect of a loss of about 10% to 20% of preoperative ability. Patients may notice this as increased word-finding difficulties. Testing for nondominant medial temporal deficits, both pre- and postoperatively, have been relatively unrewarding, but newer, computer-based tests of visuo-spatial memory show promise in this area. Early series reported high rates of visual field defects in the contralateral superior quadrant. The incidence of this deficit has declined with ATLs that limit the lateral temporal cortical resection, and noticeable visual field defects are now rare.

REFERENCES

1. JA French, PD Williamson, VM Thadani, TM Darcey, RH Mattson, SS Spencer, DD Spencer. Characteristics of medial temporal lobe epilepsy: I. Results of history and physical examination. Ann Neurol 34:774–780, 1993.
2. PD Williamson, JA French, VM Thadani, JH Kim, RA Novelly, SS Spencer, DD Spencer, RH Mattson. Characteristics of medial temporal lobe epilepsy: II. Interictal and ictal scalp electroencephalography, neuropsychological testing, neuroimaging, surgical results, and pathology. Ann Neurol 34:781–787, 1993.
3. DD Spencer, SS Spencer, RH Mattson, PD Williamson, RA Novelly. Access to the posterior medial temporal lobe structures in the surgical treatment of temporal lobe epilepsy. Neurosurgery 15:667–671, 1984.
4. J Engel Jr. Outcome with respect to epileptic seizures. In: Engel J Jr, ed. Surgical Treatment of the Epilepsies. New York: Raven Press, 1987, pp 553–571.
5. TB Rasmussen. Surgical treatment of the complex partial seizures: Results, lessons and problems. Epilepsia 24 (suppl 1):65–76, 1983.
6. A Olivier. Surgery of epilepsy: Overall procedure. In: MLJ Apuzzo, cd. Neurosurgical Aspects of Epilepsy. Park Ridge, IL: American Association of Neurological Surgeons, 1991, pp 117–148.
7. RM Dasheiff. Epilepsy surgery: Is it an effective treatment? Ann Neurol 25:506–510, 1989.
8. J Engel Jr, PC Van Ness, TB Rasmussen, LM Ojemann. Outcome with respect to epileptic seizures. In: J Engel Jr, ed. Surgical Treatment of the Epilepsies. 2nd ed. New York: Raven Press, 1992, pp 609–621.
9. CB Dodrill, GA Ojemann, AGA Wilkus. Multidisciplinary prediction of seizure relief from cortical resection surgery. Ann Neurol 20:2–12, 1986.
10. SW Jeong, SK Lee, KK Kim, H Kim, JY Kim, CK Chung. Prognostic factors in anterior temporal lobe resections for mesial temporal lobe epilepsy: Multivariate analysis. Epilepsia 40:1735–1739, 1999.
11. N Foldvary, B Nashold, E Mascha, EA Thompson, N Lee, JO McNamara, DV Lewis, JS Luther, AH Friedman, RA Radtke. Seizure outcome after temporal lobectomy for temporal lobe epilepsy: A Kaplan-Meier survival analysis. Neurology 54:630–634, 2000.
12. J Engel Jr. Seizures and Epilepsy. Philadelphia: Davis, 1989, pp 443–474.
13. CR Jack Jr, FW Sharbrough, CK Twomey. Temporal lobe seizures: Lateralization with MR volume measurements of the hippocampal formation. Radiology 175:423–429, 1990.
14. T Lencz, G McCarthy, R Bronen. Quantitative MRI of the hippocampus in temporal lobe epilepsy. Ann Neurol 31:629–637, 1992.
15. R Rausch, T Babb, J Engel Jr. Memory following intracarotid amobarbital injection contralateral to hippocampal damage. Arch Neurol 46:783–788, 1989.

Ellis and Roper

16. MD Holmes, CB Dodrill, GA Ojemann, AJ Wilensky, LM Ojemann. Outcome following surgery in patients with bitemporal interictal epileptiform patterns. Neurology 48:1037–1040, 1997.
17. E Behrens, J Schramm, J Zentner, R Konig. Surgical and neurological complications in a series of 708 epilepsy surgery procedures. Neurosurgery 41:1–9, 1997.
18. RJ Ivnik, FW Sharbrough, ER Laws. Anterior temporal lobectomy for the control of partial complex seizures: Information for counseling patients. Mayo Clin Proc 63:783–793, 1988.

45

Corpus Callosotomy: Indications and Technique

Theodore H. Schwartz

Weill Cornell Medical College, New York Presbyterian Hospital, New York, New York, U.S.A.

1 HISTORY

Division of the corpus callosum for the treatment of patients with seizure disorders dates back to the observations of Van Wagenen in the 1930s [1]. He noticed that patients with strokes affecting the corpus callosum often had improvement in the frequency of their attacks. Experimental evidence for the importance of commissural fibers for the spread of epilepsy was demonstrated in the primate by Erickson, lending further support for this therapeutic approach [2]. Additional reports by Bogan in adults [3] and Luessenhop in children [4] established corpus callosotomy (CC) as a standard technique in the surgical treatment of epilepsy.

2 INDICATIONS

2.1 Adults

Candidates for CC include patients with medically intractable primary generalized epilepsy or partial epilepsy with rapid secondary generalization that is either unlocalized or localized to unresectable cortex. Differentiation be-

529

tween these two groups is often difficult, although relevant, in that patients with lateralized electroencephalographic findings often have a better outcome [5,6]. The most common generalized epilepsies treated with CC are characterized by atonic or akinetic seizures, often involving sudden drop attacks. Patients with predominantly tonic or tonic-clonic seizures also respond to CC and, in fact, most patients considered for CC have multiple seizure types.

2.2 Children

In the pediatric age group, one must balance the potential disruption of cortical reorganization mediated by the intact corpus callosum with the potential excitotoxic injury of persistent frequent seizures in the developing brain [7]. The consensus is that early surgery is indicated, depending on the severity of the seizures [7]. Indications in this age group are similar to the adult, although there is a higher proportion of patients with hemispheric disease, such as infantile hemiplegia, forme-fruste infantile hemiplegia, and Rasmussen's syndrome. Although CC can be used as a substitute for hemispherectomy, if the source of the seizures can be localized and hemispherectomy can be performed, this is preferable. Corpus callosotomy to treat hemispheric disease should be reserved for children with residual neurological function in the damaged hemisphere and in whom hemispherectomy is contraindicated. Children with Lennox-Gastaut show a significant improvement in seizure control and quality of life [8,9].

2.3 Contraindications

Patients in whom a resectable focus can be identified are clearly not candidates for CC. Surgical cure after successful resective surgery is much higher than for CC. Bilateral synchronous epileptiform abnormalities do not necessarily imply a worse outcome; however, the discovery of bilateral independent foci should raise concern. Age, mixed hemisphere dominance, and mental retardation have also been considered contraindications in some series; however, many surgeons do not automatically exclude such patients, although successful outcome is less likely [10]. One third of children with severe mental retardation may benefit from CC, particularly if focal or hemispheric damage is documented [7]. Patients with multifocal, bifrontal asymmetric epilepsy may be at higher risk of developing more intense seizure foci postoperatively.

3 TECHNIQUE

Complete section is approximately twice as effective as partial section in controlling seizure frequency [6,10]. Nevertheless, most centers currently perform a partial section initially to avoid a potential acute disconnection syndrome, although even partial CC may disrupt cortical function, particularly in patients with mixed dominance (see below). Completion of CC is then performed as a second operation if seizure control is inadequate. Initial posterior CC has been described; however, anterior section with sparing of the anterior commissure and fornix is the preferred first operation unless clearly posterior epileptogenic abnormalities are documented. Preoperative evaluation for coagulopathy, including a bleeding time, is essential, as patients are generally on multiple anticonvulsants.

3.1 Anterior 2/3 Callosotomy

The surgery is performed under general anesthesia. Electroencephalogram is not necessary, but if used, requires appropriate anesthetic agents that do not interfere with the recording. Mannitol, decadron, and prophylactic antibiotics are administered intravenously. The patient is placed supine on the table with the head turned toward the nondominant hemisphere, a shoulder roll under the contralateral shoulder and the vertex elevated by 30 to 45 degrees (Fig. 1). This position permits a minimum of retraction, as the dependent hemisphere is retracted by gravity and the operating microscope retains stereoscopic vision in the horizontal plane. A partial bicoronal incision is made 2 cm in front of the coronal suture, of sufficient length to permit the craniotomy, which extends 4 cm in front of, and 2 cm behind, the coronal suture and from 1 cm over the sagittal suture to the temporal insertion of the dependent side of the cranium (Fig. 2). Reviewing the angiogram from the Wada test or obtaining a Magnetic Resonance Venogram (MRV) may be helpful in surgical planning but it is usually possible to work around any draining veins. The dura is reflected over the sinus and the interhemispheric dissection is performed using loupes or the surgical microscope (Fig. 3). If gravity alone does not supply sufficient retraction, additional force can be attained either with two rolled up cotton paddies or gentle pressure from a self-retaining retractor. The glistening white corpus callosum is identified and exposed along its length, as are the two pericallosal arteries. Division of the corpus callosum is best performed under the operating microscope by dividing a small portion of the callosum and identifying the midline cleft between the ventricles where the septum pellucidum inserts. The use of frameless stereotaxy can be helpful in distinguishing the callosum from the cingulate gyri and defining the depth of the callosum, depending on the degree of brain shift. Without entering the ventricle, this cleft is followed first anteriorly around the genu and down to the rostrum. Additional posterior division can be performed with the help of frameless stereotaxy to achieve a 2/3 division. Alternatively, a metal clip can be placed at the back of the

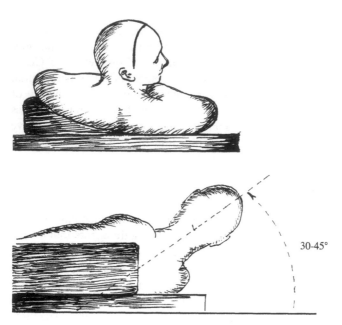

FIGURE 1 The patient is placed supine and the head is elevated to 30 to 45 degrees. The head is turned to the right so that gravity can help retract the nondominant hemisphere and the microscope can maintain stereoscopic vision.

callosal division and a lateral radiograph obtained to ensure that the callosotomy has been carried out behind the line bisecting the glabella-inion line. A final metal clip is then placed at the posterior margin of the callosotomy to demarcate the limits of the resection in case a second operation is required to complete the callosotomy. Anticonvulsants are continued postoperatively.

3.2 Posterior 1/3 Callosotomy

At least 3 months after the first procedure, decision is made regarding completion of the callosotomy. The patient is placed in a similar position with slightly more head flexion. A partial bicoronal skin incision is placed over the parietal eminence, sufficient to expose the craniotomy. The bone flap extends from 1 cm behind the lambdoid suture to 4 cm in front and from 1 cm over the sagittal suture to 4 cm lateral in the direction of the nondominant hemisphere. Division of the posterior callosum is performed down to the arachnoid to preserve the arachnoid overlying the pineal and quadrigeminal cisterns. The posterior hippocampal commissure is divided with the callosum.

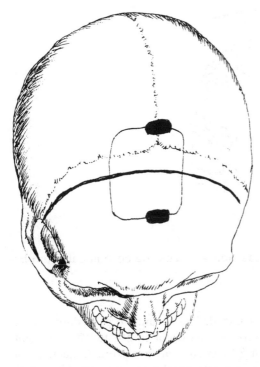

FIGURE 2   A partial bicoronal skin incision is performed and the temporalis muscle is not violated. A burr is used to drill slots over the sinus
and a craniotomy is elevated 2/3 in front and 1/3 behind the coronal
suture, extending just over the midline.

3.3 Postoperative MRI

All patients should undergo postoperative magnetic resonance imaging
(MRI), and sagittal images must be reviewed to assess the extent of the
callosal section.

4 RESULTS

4.1 Seizure Frequency and Intensity

The best results occur in patients with nonlocalizable but focal hemispheric
disease [7]. Seizure onset before age 5 has been associated with a better
outcome, and mental retardation with a worse outcome [6,9]. For all patients,
secondarily generalized seizures are controlled in 70% to 80% of patients,
whereas only 25% to 50% of patients find relief from complex-partial sei-

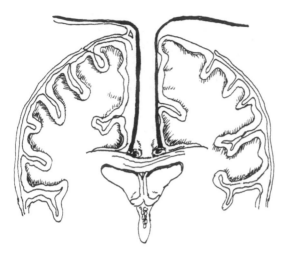

FIGURE 3 Interhemispheric dissection exposes the corpus callosum between the pericallosal arteries.

zures. Corpus callosotomy is not intended as a curative procedure, but reports of complete cessation of seizures can occur in 5% to 7% of patients [11]. In one series, greater than 80% reduction in seizure frequency was found for major seizures in 65% of patients, focal motor seizures 38%, atonic seizures in 76%, and absence in 68% [10]. For all seizures together, the percentage of patients obtaining better than 80% reduction in generalized seizures improves from 29% after anterior section to 62% after completion of callosal section [10]. Up to 30% of patients may develop more intense or newly patterned seizures postoperatively from removal of callosally mediated inhibitory interhemispheric connections, particularly in patients with bilateral independent frontal foci [12]. On the other hand, development of a lateralized focus may also occur after CC, which may be amenable to cure after further resective surgery [13,14].

4.2 Neuropsychology

Patients with early onset central nervous system (CNS) disease and signs of severe lateralized CNS dysfunction, including a structural lesion, impaired memory, neurological deficit, and contralateral speech function tend to have a good neuropsychological outcome [15]. In such patients, the preserved functions are subserved almost entirely by the intact hemisphere. In patients with mild to moderate CNS dysfunction, surgery can disrupt callosally mediated interhemispheric compensatory mechanisms causing a decrease in manual dexterity postoperatively [15]. If the speech-dominant hemisphere is contralateral to the hemisphere controlling the dominant hand, which can occur in a late-onset, left hemisphere seizure disorder, postoperative speech deterioration can occur [15]. Other forms of mixed dominance, such as memory function contralateral to speech or hemianopsia contralateral to language, may result in postoperative mutism or alexia without agraphia respectively [16]. Isolated posterior callosal section can produce a syndrome of sensory disconnection with the language-dominant hemisphere not having access to stimuli presented to the contralateral hemisphere [10]. In the pediatric age group, several authors have noticed significant improvements in behavior and attention in up to 81% of children after callosotomy [17,18].

5 COMPLICATIONS

Ventriculitis, meningitis, and death have been reported from earlier series of CC. More recent reports have noted fewer complications, including subdural hematoma, asymptomatic venous infarctions, and wound infections. Transient postoperative leg weakness and a decrease in spontaneity of speech is not uncommon after anterior 2/3 section, either from acute disconnection or retraction injury [7].

5.1 The Future of CC

The vagal nerve stimulator (VNS) has been proven efficacious at reducing seizure frequency for partial seizures [19–21] and may be useful in primarily generalized epilepsy as well [22]. Long-term results appear promising [23]. Data are lacking on the relative success of VNS compared with CC for controlling generalized epilepsy, but the advantage of the VNS is a significant reduction in operative morbidity and decreased neuropsychological sequelae. Although seizure control will probably not be as effective, the VNS may be used as a first operative intervention, before CC, for unresectable foci.

REFERENCES

1. WP Van Wagenen, RY Herren. Surgical division of the commissural pathways in the corpus callosum: Relation to spread of an epileptic attack. Arch Neurol Psychiatry 44:740–759, 1940.
2. TE Erickson. Spread of the epileptic discharge. An experimental study of the afterdischarge induced by electrical stimulation of the cerebral cortex. Arch Neurol Psychiatry 43:429–452, 1940.
3. JE Bogan, PJ Vogel. Cerebral commissurotomy in man: Preliminary case report. Bull LA Neurol Soc 27:169–172, 1962.

4. AJ Luessenhop. Interhemispheric commissurotomy: (The split brain operation) as an alternative to hemispherectomy for control of intractable seizures. Am Surg 36:265–268, 1970.

5. G Geoffrey, M Lassonde, F Delisle, M Decarie. Corpus callosotomy for control of intractable epilepsy in children. Neurology 33:891–897, 1983.

6. SS Spencer, DD Spencer, PD Williamson, K Sass, RA Novelly, RH Mattson. Corpus callosotomy for epilepsy: I. Seizure effects. Neurology 38:19–24, 1988.

7. DD Spencer, SS Spencer. Corpus callosotomy in the treatment of medically intractable secondarily generalized seizures in children. Cleveland Clin J Med 56 (Suppl):S69–S78, 1990.

8. S Collins, J Walker, N Barbaro, K Laxer. Corpus callosotomy in the treatment of Lennox-Gastaut syndrome. Epilepsia 30:670–689, 1989.

9. JM Sorenson, JW Wheless, JE Baumgartner, AB Thomas, BL Brookshire, GL Clifton, LJ Willmore. Corpus callosotomy for medically intractable seizures. Pediatr Neurosurg 27:260–267, 1997.

10. DW Roberts. Section of the corpus callosum for epilepsy. In: HH Schmidek and WH Sweet, eds. Operative Neurosurgical Techniques. Philadelphia: W.B. Saunders Co., 1995, pp 1351–1358.

11. JJ Engel, PC Van Ness, TB Rasmussen, OL M. Outcome with respect to epileptic seizures. In: JJ Engel, ed. Surgical Treatment of the Epilepsies. New York: Raven Press, 1993, pp 609–621.

12. SS Spencer, DD Spencer, GH Glaser, PD Williamson, RH Mattson. More intense focal seizure types after callosal section: The role of inhibition. Ann Neurol 16:686–693, 1984.

13. A Turmel, N Giard, G Bouvier, R Labrecque, F Veilleux, I Rouleau, JM Sainte-Hilaire. Frontal lobe seizures and epilepsy: Indications for corticectomies and callosotomies. Adv Neurol 57:689–706, 1992.

14. S Purves, J Wada, W Woodhurst, P Moyes, E Strauss, B Kosaka, D Li. Results of anterior corpus callosum section in 24 patients with medically intractable seizures. Neurology 38:1194–1201, 1988.

15. KJ Sass, DD Spender, RA Novelly, PD Williamson, RH Mattson. Corpus callosotomy for epilepsy. II. Neurologic and neuropsychological outcome. Neurology 38:24–28, 1988.

16. RA Novelly, LD Lifrak. Forebrain commissurotomy reinstates effects of preexisting hemisphere lesions: An examination of the hypothesis. In: A Reeves, ed. Epilepsy and the Corpus Callosum. New York: Plenum Press, 1984, pp 467–500.

17. F Cendes, PC Fagazzo, VL Martins. Corpus callosotomy in treatment of medically resistant epilepsy: Preliminary results in a pediatric population. Epilepsia 34:910–917, 1993.

18. R Nordgren, A Reeves, A Viguera, D Roberts. Corpus callosotomy for intractable seizures in the pediatric age group. Arch Neurol 48:364–372, 1991.

19. E Ben-Menachim, R Manon-Espaillat, R Ristanovic, RJ Wilder, H Stefan, W Mirza, WB Tarver, JF Wernicke. Vagus nerve stimulation for treatment of partial seizures. I. A controlled study of effect on seizures. First International Vagus Nerve Stimulation Group. Epilepsia 35:616–626, 1994.

20. TVNS Group. A randomized controlled trial of chronic vagus nerve stimulation for treatment of medically intractable seizures. Neurology 45:224–230, 1995.

21. A Handforth, CM DeGiorgio, SC Schachter, BM Uthman, DK Nartoku, ES Tecoma, TR Henry, SD Collins, BV Vaughn, RC Gilmartin, DR Labar, GLr Morris, MC Salinsky, I Osorio, RK Ristanovvic, DM Labiner, JC Jones, JV Murphy, OC Ney, JW Wheless. Vagus nerve stimulation therapy for partial-onset seizures: A randomized active-control trial. Neurology 51:48–55, 1998.

22. E Ben-Menachim, K Hellström, C Waldton, LE Augustinsson. Evaluation of refractory epilepsy treated with vagus nerve stimulation for up to 5 years. Neurology 52:1265–1267, 1999.

23. GL Morris, WM Mueller, TvNSSG EO1-EO5. Long-term treatment with vagus nerve stimulation in patients with refractory epilepsy. Neurology 53:1731–1735, 1999.

46

Vagal Nerve Stimulation: Indications and Technique

Arun Paul Amar and Michael L. J. Apuzzo
Keck School of Medicine, University of Southern California,
Los Angeles, California, U.S.A.

Michael L. Levy
University of California San Diego, San Diego, California, U.S.A.

1 INTRODUCTION

Vagus nerve stimulation (VNS) by the implantable neurocybernetic prosthesis (NCP) from Cyberonics, Inc. is emerging as a novel adjunct in the management of patients with medically refractory seizures. This device delivers intermittent electrical stimulation to the left cervical vagus nerve trunk, which secondarily transmits rostral impulses to exert widespread effects on neuronal excitability throughout the central nervous system (Fig. 1). We have comprehensively reviewed the theoretical rationale, practical background, and clinical application of VNS in previous publications [1–3]. The operative procedure for implanting the NCP device has also been presented in detail elsewhere [4–6]. This chapter summarizes pragmatic issues pertaining to VNS, such as patient selection and surgical technique.

2 CLINICAL UTILITY OF VNS

2.1 Review of Safety and Efficacy

Clinical experience with vagus nerve stimulation began in 1988 with the first human implantation of the NCP system. Since then, more than 1,000

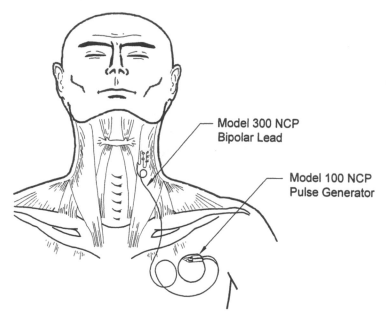

Model 300 NCP
Bipolar Lead

Model 100 NCP
Pulse Generator

FIGURE 1   Schematic representation of VNS therapy. A pulse generator
inserted in the subcutaneous tissues of the upper left chest delivers intermittent electrical stimulation to the cervical vague nerve trunk via a
bifurcated helical lead. Reproduced with permission from Cyberonics,
Inc.

patients have participated in seven clinical trials throughout 26 countries,
and more than 3000 patient-years of data have accrued. These studies confirm the long-term safety, efficacy, feasibility, and tolerability of VNS, as
well as the durability of the NCP device [1,7].

Vagus nerve stimulation gained approval by the United States Food
and Drug Administration (FDA) in 1997. Post-marketing experience with
more than 7,000 patients validates the earlier clinical trials, and in 1999, the
Therapeutics and Technology subcommittee of the American Association of
Neurology declared VNS "effective and safe, based on a preponderance of
class I evidence" [8]. Although VNS requires a large initial investment because of the price of the device itself as well as its surgical insertion, cost-
benefit analysis suggests that the expense of VNS is recovered within 2 years
of follow-up [9].

Recently, a meta-analysis was performed of the 454 patients enrolled
in one of five multicenter clinical trials conducted in the United States before
FDA approval [7]. For the study population as a whole, the median reduction

in seizure frequency was 35% at 1 year, 43% at 2 years, and 44% at 3 years. An important observation is that the response to VNS is maintained during prolonged stimulation, and unlike chronic medication therapy, seizure control actually improves with time.

The response of individual patients to VNS varies widely. Although 1% to 2% of subjects enjoy complete seizure cessation, others derive no benefit whatsoever. The remainder experience intermediate results. In the collective study experience, the proportion of patients who sustained a 50% reduction in baseline seizure frequency was approximately 23% at 3 months and 43% after 2 years. These improvements occurred in a highly refractory population of patients who typically had an average of 1.7 seizures per day despite administration of more than two antiepileptic medications.

In spite of the well-known functions of the vagus nerve as the principal efferent component of the parasympathetic nervous system, VNS has not been shown to adversely affect any aspect of physiological function, including cardiac rhythm, pulmonary function, gastrointestinal motility, and secretion. Unlike many antiepileptic medications, VNS therapy does not impair cognition, balance, or emotion. Plasma concentrations of antiepileptic medications remain unchanged.

Side effects are typically transient, mild, and limited to cycles of stimulation. Initially, patients may experience voice alteration (20%–30%), paresthesias (10%), or cough (6%), but the incidence of these adverse effects diminishes greatly over time. Surgical complications are rare, and device failures are also uncommon.

2.2 Indications and Contraindications

The selection criteria for insertion of the NCP system remain in evolution and reflect current governmental standards, as well as institutional biases and general guidelines from prior clinical trials [1,2]. Currently, the device is only approved by the FDA "as an adjunctive therapy in reducing the frequency of seizures in adults and adolescents over 12 years of age with partial onset seizures which are refractory to antiepileptic medications" [1]. However, favorable results have been obtained with off-label use among children as young as age 3 and among patients with Lennox-Gastaut or other primarily generalized seizures syndromes [10]. Preliminary experience with infantile spasms has been disappointing, however. Patients with both idiopathic epilepsy and seizures of structural etiology are considered appropriate candidates. Of note, VNS has been used successfully among patients who have failed previous surgical procedures, confirming the potential efficacy of VNS in highly refractory patient populations.

The definition of medical intractability varies from center to center. Standards from previous studies commonly required a frequency of at least six seizures per month and a seizure-free interval of no longer than 2 to 3 weeks despite therapy with multiple medications [1,2]. However, seizure frequency, seizure type, severity of attacks, drug toxicity, and overall impact on quality of life must all be considered before a patient is deemed refractory to pharmacotherapy. Adequate monitoring of patient compliance and sufficient trials of investigational drugs must also be assured.

As noted above, the response to VNS is highly variable, and previous clinical trials have failed to characterize the demographic factors that predict a favorable outcome [1,2]. Furthermore, VNS is rarely curative. Therefore, at present, we do not consider the NCP device an alternative to conventional methods of epilepsy surgery that offer a higher likelihood of seizure cessation, and we generally reserve VNS for patients in whom such operations are not indicated. These include those patients whose seizure focus is bilateral, not associated with a structural abnormality, or cannot be completely resected because of overlap with functional cortex.

The NCP system cannot be inserted in patients who have undergone a prior left cervical vagotomy. Furthermore, the safety of VNS has not been tested in several conditions in which impairment of vagus nerve function might produce deleterious effects. Thus, relative contraindications include progressive neurological or systemic diseases, pregnancy, cardiac arrhythmia, asthma, chronic obstructive pulmonary disease, active peptic ulcer disease, and insulin-dependent diabetes mellitus [1].

3   PRACTICAL BACKGROUND

3.1   Anatomy and Physiology of the Vagus Nerve

The vagus nerve is generally regarded as an efferent projection that innervates the larynx and provides parasympathetic control of the body; however, the majority of its fibers are special visceral and general somatic afferents leading towards the brain [1]. The latter originate from receptors in the viscera and terminate in diffuse areas of the central nervous system, many of which are potential sites of epileptogenesis. These include the cerebellum, diencephalon, amygdala, hippocampus, insular cortex, and multiple brainstem centers. Some of these projections relay through the nucleus tractus solitarius, whereas others form direct, monosynaptic connections with their targets. It remains unclear which of these pathways underlies the mechanism of VNS action, but the locus coeruleus and raphe nucleus appear to be key intermediaries, as bilateral lesions of these centers abolish the seizure-suppressing effects of VNS therapy in animal models [2].

Several branches of the vagus nerve arise cephalad to the midcervical trunk, where the VNS electrodes are applied [5]. These include projections to the pharynx and carotid sinus, as well as superior and inferior cervical cardiac branches leading to the cardiac plexus. Both the right and left vagus nerves carry cardiac efferent fibers, but anatomical studies in dogs suggest that those on the right side preferentially supply the SA node of the heart, whereas those on the left side preferentially innervate the AV node. For this reason, the NCP system is generally inserted on the left side. Nevertheless, stimulation of the left vagus nerve rarely may cause bradycardia or asystole, even at FDA-approved settings.

As mentioned, the NCP device is generally applied to the midcervical portion of the vagus nerve trunk, distal to the origin of the superior and inferior cervical cardiac branches; this may represent another reason why the incidence of bradycardia is low [5]. Nonetheless, the diameter, appearance, and location of the cardiac branches may approximate those of the nerve trunk itself, and care must be taken to avoid mistaking the two. If the cardiac branches are stimulated directly, small currents as low as 0.8 mA may produce significant bradycardia [5].

The midcervical portion of the vagus nerve is relatively free of branches [5]. The superior laryngeal nerve arises rostral to the carotid bifurcation before descending toward the larynx, and high currents applied to the midcervical nerve trunk may recruit these fibers, leading to tightness or pain in the pharynx or larynx. The recurrent laryngeal nerve travels with the main trunk and branches caudally at the level of the aortic arch before ascending in the tracheo-esophageal groove. As a result, hoarseness is a common occurrence during periods of stimulation or after VNS implantation.

3.2 Regional Anatomy of the Carotid Sheath

In addition to branches of the vagus nerve trunk, several other nerves in the vicinity of the carotid sheath risk hazard from the implantation procedure itself or from subsequent stimulation. The hypoglossal nerve arises cephalad to the midcervical region, making unilateral tongue weakness an infrequent complication of VNS implantation. The phrenic nerve lies deep to a fascial plane beneath the carotid sheath, and hemiparalysis of the diaphragm has been reported with stimulation at high output currents, although not as an operative complication.

The sympathetic trunk lies deep and medial to the common carotid artery. It gives off fibers that ascend with the internal carotid artery (ICA) toward the intracranial contents. We are aware of one case of Horner's syndrome after insertion of the VNS device, caused either by manipulation of the sympathetic plexus itself or by traction on the sympathetic fibers around the ICA.

Weakness in the muscles of the lower face may result from injury to branches of the facial nerve, which ramify through the caudal aspect of the parotid gland. In general, hypoglossal and facial nerve injury are more common sequelae of carotid endarterectomy incisions, which tend to be higher than those used for placement of the VNS device.

4 NCP DEVICE COMPONENTS

Figure 1 depicts a schematic representation of VNS therapy. A pulse generator inserted in the subcutaneous tissues of the upper left side of the chest delivers intermittent electrical stimulation to the cervical vagus nerve trunk through a bifurcated helical lead.

In addition to the implantable lead and pulse generator, the NCP system includes a number of peripheral components, such as a telemetry wand that interrogates and programs the pulse generator noninvasively. This programming wand is powered by two 9V batteries and is interfaced with an IBM-compatible computer that runs a menu-based software package furnished by Cyberonics. The system also includes a hand-held magnet that patients may carry with them to alter the character of stimulation that the generator delivers.

The pulse generator has approximately the same size and shape as a cardiac pacemaker. It contains an epoxy resin header with receptacles that accept the connector pins extending from the bifurcated lead. The generator is powered by a single lithium battery encased in a hermetically sealed titanium module. Under normal conditions, the generator has a projected battery life of approximately 6 to 8 years. Once it has expired, the generator can be replaced with the patient under local anesthesia during a simple outpatient procedure.

The generator contains an internal antenna that receives radiofrequency signals emitted from the telemetry wand and transfers them to a microprocessor that regulates the electrical output of the pulse generator. The generator delivers a charge-balanced waveform characterized by five programmable parameters: output current, signal frequency, pulse width, signal on-time, and signal off-time. These variables are titrated empirically in the outpatient setting, according to individual patient tolerance and seizure frequency. Altering the parameters of stimulation will have various consequences on VNS efficacy, side effects, and battery life.

The generator has two accessories. One is a hairpin-shaped resistor used during preliminary electrodiagnostic testing before implantation, to test the internal impedance of the generator. The other is a hexagonal torque wrench used to tighten the set screws that secure the lead connector pins to the epoxy resin header of the generator.

The generator is still contained within its package, but it can be interrogated by the telemetry wand. The generator must pass this system check before it is opened onto the sterile field. The failure rate of the generator is extremely low, but it is recommended that a backup generator be available in the operating room at all times.

The bipolar lead is insulated by a silicone elastomer, and can thus be safely implanted in patients with latex allergies. One end of the lead contains a pair of connector pins that inserts directly into the generator, whereas the opposite end contains an electrode array consisting of three discrete helical coils that wrap around the vagus nerve. The middle and distal coils represent the positive and negative electrodes, respectively, whereas the most proximal one serves as an integral anchoring tether that prevents excessive force from being transmitted to the electrodes when the patient turns his neck. The leads come in two sizes, measured by the internal diameter of each helix. The majority of patients can be fitted with the 2-mm coil; however, it is desirable to have the 3 mm one available in the operating room as well.

Each electrode helix contains three loops. Embedded inside the middle turn is a platinum ribbon coil that is welded to the lead wire. This shape permits the platinum ribbon to maintain optimum mechanical contact with the nerve. Suture tails extending from either end of the helix permit manipulation of the coils without injuring these platinum contacts. Damage to the vagus nerve itself is greatly reduced by the self-sizing, open helical design of the NCP electrode array, which permits body fluid interchange with the nerve. Thus, compared with cuff electrodes, mechanical trauma and ischemia to the nerve are minimized. The electrode is intended to fit snugly around the nerve while avoiding compression, thus allowing the electrode to move with the nerve and minimizing abrasion from relative movement of the nerve against the electrode.

The hand-held magnet performs several functions. When briefly passed across the chest pocket where the generator resides, it manually triggers a train of stimulation superimposed on the baseline output. Such on-demand stimulation can be initiated by the patient or a companion at the onset of an aura, in an effort to diminish or even abort an impending seizure. The parameters of this magnet-induced stimulation may differ from those of the prescheduled activation. Alternatively, if the device appears to be malfunctioning, or if the patient wishes to terminate all stimulation for any other reason, the system can be indefinitely inactivated by applying the magnet over the generator site continuously. Finally, patients are instructed to test the function of their device periodically by performing magnet-induced activation and verifying that stimulation occurs. Most patients can perceive the stimulation as a slight tingling sensation in the throat.

5   SURGICAL CONSIDERATIONS

5.1   Operative Procedure

Insertion of the NCP device takes less than 2 hours and is typically performed under general anesthesia, thus minimizing the possibility that an intraoperative seizure might compromise the surgery. However, regional cervical blocks have also been used in awake patients. It can be performed as an outpatient procedure, but it may be desirable to observe patients overnight for vocal cord dysfunction, dysphagia, respiratory compromise, or seizures induced by anesthesia, even though these complications are rare. Prophylactic antibiotics are administered preoperatively and maintained for 24 hours postoperatively.

The patient is positioned supine with a shoulder roll beneath the scapulae to provide mild neck extension. This facilitates passage of the tunneling tool that connects separate incisions in the neck and chest. The head is rotated 30 to 45 degrees toward the right, bringing the left sternocleidomastoid muscle into prominence.

Many options exist for placement of the skin incisions. Often, a 5-cm transverse chest incision is made approximately 8 cm below the clavicle, centered above the nipple. The underlying fat is dissected to the level of the pectoralis fascia, and a subcutaneous pocket is fashioned superiorly. Others have suggested a deltopectoral incision with inferior dissection to create the pocket, but we believe that the scar tissue formed beneath the pectoral incision helps prevent caudal migration of the generator. Recently, we have been using a lateral incision along the anterior fold of the axilla, which affords better cosmetic results, especially among women.

Next, a 5-cm longitudinal incision is made along the anterior border of the sternocleidomastoid muscle, centered over its midpoint. Generally, this incision is a little lower than that for an endarterectomy. Alternatively, a transverse skin incision at C5-6, similar to the approach for an anterior cervical discectomy, can be made. For the inexperienced surgeon, the longitudinal incision permits a wider exposure, which facilitates electrode placement through this aperture.

The platysma muscle is divided vertically, and the investing layer of deep cervical fascia is opened along the anterior border of the sternocleidomastoid, allowing it to be mobilized laterally. After palpation of the carotid pulse, the neurovascular bundle is identified and sharply incised to reveal its contents. Self-retaining retractors with blunt blades expedite this stage of the procedure. Care is taken to limit the exposure between the omohyoid muscle and the common facial vein complex, thus minimizing potential hazard to adjacent neurovascular structures.

Within the carotid sheath at the level of the thyroid cartilage, the vagus nerve is generally encountered deep and medial to the internal jugular vein, encased in firm areolar tissue lateral to the common carotid artery. Great variability exists in the relative position of these structures, however, and the strategy by which the nerve is isolated from the remainder of the neurovascular bundle must account for such individual diversity. We attempt to minimize direct manipulation of the nerve itself. Instead, we prefer to mobilize the vessels away from the nerve. Dissection generally commences with isolation and retraction of the internal jugular vein using vessel loops.

Next, the nerve trunk is identified and dissected with the aid of the operating microscope or surgical loupes. At least 3 to 4 cm of the nerve must be completely freed from its surrounding tissues. At this stage, we have found that the insertion of a blue background plastic sheet between the nerve and the underlying vessels greatly facilitates the subsequent steps of the procedure. The technique of mobilizing the vessels away from the nerve usually preserves the vasa nervosum. This nuance may reduce the incidence of postoperative complications, such as hoarseness.

A tunneling tool is then used to create a subcutaneous tract between the two incisions. The tool is directed from the cervical to pectoral sites, to minimize potential injury to the vascular structures of the neck.

Depending on the relative size of the exposed nerve, either a small or large helical electrode is then selected for insertion. The lead connector pins are passed through the tunnel and emerge from the chest incision, whereas the helical electrodes remain exposed in the cervical region. Before applying the electrodes, the lead wire should be directed parallel and lateral to the nerve, with the coils occupying the gap between them.

Each coil is applied by grasping the suture tail at either end and stretching the coil until its convolutions are eliminated. The central turn of this unfurled coil is applied either obliquely or perpendicularly across or beneath the vagus trunk and wrapped around the surface of the nerve. The coil is then redirected parallel to the nerve as the remainder of its loops are applied proximal and distal to this midpoint (Fig. 2). The memory within the elongated coil will cause it to reassume its helical configuration and conform to the nerve snugly.

While all these maneuvers are taking place, additional electrodiagnostic testing of the generator is simultaneously carried out between the neurology team and the scrub technician. With the hairpin resistor inserted into the receptacles for the lead connector pins, the telemetry wand interrogates the device from within a sterile sheath to measure its internal impedance. Once the generator passes this preimplant diagnostic test, it is ready for insertion.

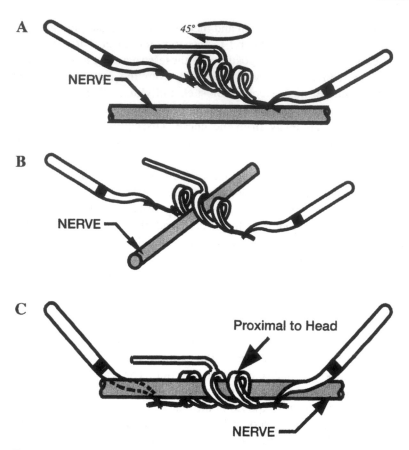

FIGURE 2 Technique of helical electrode placement. **A**, Each coil is applied by grasping the suture tail at either end and stretching the coil until its convolutions are eliminated. **B**, The central turn of this unfurled coil is applied either obliquely or perpendicularly across or beneath the vagus trunk and wrapped around the surface of the nerve. **C**, The coil is then redirected parallel to the nerve as the remainder of its loops are applied proximal and distal to this midpoint. Modified with permission from Cyberonics, Inc.

The lead connector pins are connected to the pulse generator and secured to their receptacles with set screws, using the hexagonal torque wrench. It is important to completely insert the hex wrench into its socket in the epoxy header, to decompress the backpressure that builds up as the connector pins enter the receptacles. This step is essential to form a good contact between the lead and the generator. If the connector pins fail to make such contact, the generator may attempt to overcome the resulting increased impedance by augmenting the output current, leading to intermittent symptoms of overstimulation.

Additional electrodiagnostic examination is then performed to appraise the coupling of all connections and to verify the integrity of the overall system. Then, a 1-minute lead test is performed at a frequency of 20 Hz with an output current of 1 mA and a pulse width of 500 microseconds. During this test stimulation, the responses of the patient's vital signs and electrocardiogram are monitored. Rarely, profound bradycardia will result, necessitating the use of atropine. The incidence of this event is thought to be less than 1 in 1000 [11]. If it occurs, attention should be directed to the lead to assure that the electrodes encircle the vagus nerve trunk itself, rather than one of its cardiac branches [5]. After the test stimulation, the generator is restored to its inactive status until 1 to 2 weeks postoperatively. This waiting period allows for resolution of postoperative edema and proper fixation of the electrode to the nerve.

The redundant portion of the lead between the generator and electrode is secured to several areas of the cervical fascia with Silastic tie-downs. The objective is to form superficial and deep-restraint configurations that help prevent excessive traction from being transmitted to the electrodes during repetitive neck motion. First, a U-shaped strain relief bend is made inferior to the anchoring tether, and the distal lead is secured to the fascia of the carotid sheath. Next, a strain relief loop is established by securing the lead to the superficial cervical fascia between the sternocleidomastoid and platysma muscles. Care is taken not to sew the lead directly to the muscle.

Finally, the generator is retracted into the subcutaneous pocket and secured to the pectoralis fascia with O-Prolene or similar nonabsorbable suture, using the suture hole contained within the epoxy resin header. Any excess lead is positioned in a separate pocket at the side of the generator. To prevent abrasion of the lead, however, it should not be placed behind the pulse generator. Wound closure then proceeds in standard multilayer fashion, using a subcuticular stitch for the skin. The cosmetic results are generally very good.

5.2 Lead Removal or Revision

In some circumstances, it may become necessary to remove or replace the electrodes that encircle the vagus nerve trunk. Fibrosis and adhesions may develop in the vicinity of the vagus nerve; however, Espinosa [12] has demonstrated that the spiral electrodes may be safely removed from the nerve, even years after they were implanted.

5.3 Complication Avoidance and Management

In the meta-analysis mentioned above [7], the most commonly observed surgical complication was infection of either the generator site or lead implantation site. The overall infection rate was 2.86%, but more than half these patients were successfully treated with antibiotic therapy alone, whereas only about 1.1% required explantation of the device.

Transient vocal cord paralysis is the second most common surgical complication of VNS implantation. The incidence of this event in the collective study experience was only 0.7%. However, because video stroboscopy and formal swallowing assessments are rarely performed after surgery, it is possible that more cases went undetected, and the true prevalence of vocal cord paresis is poorly understood [5]. Fortunately, most reported cases resolve clinically.

Temporary lower facial hypesthesia or paralysis occurred in another 0.7% of patients in the meta-analysis. As stated above, excessively high surgical incisions could have been a cause.

To date, of more than 7,000 implantation procedures, only four cases of intraoperative bradycardia or asystole have been reported during the lead test, accounting for an incidence of less than 0.1%. Asconape [11] has analyzed the factors that potentially contribute to this event and the means of their prevention. As mentioned, the superior or inferior cervical cardiac branches might be mistaken for the vagus trunk itself, and correct positioning of the electrodes on the intended nerve must be verified. Proper placement of the skin incision, centered over the midcervical portion of the nerve, will also help avert this complication. Current spread to the cardiac nerves can be minimized by measures that insulate them from the midcervical trunk during the lead test, such as placement of a Silastic dam beneath the nerve trunk and removal of pooled blood or saline from the vicinity. Finally, the current should be ramped up in small increments during the lead test, starting with 0.25 mA.

As stated above, we have found it preferable to mobilize the vascular structures away from the nerve trunk, thus minimizing direct manipulation of the nerve itself. We believe that this practice may improve the efficacy of subsequent stimulation and diminish the incidence of surgical complications, such as hoarseness. Other precepts of good surgical technique, gained from experience and familiarity with the implantation procedure, will also contribute to improved outcomes.

REFERENCES

1. Amar AP, Heck CN, Levy ML, Smith T, DeGiorgio CM, Oviedo S, Apuzzo MLJ. An institutional experience with cervical vagus nerve trunk stimulation

for medically refractory epilepsy: Rationale, technique, and outcome. Neurosurgery 43:1265–1280, 1998.

2. Amar AP, Heck CN, DeGiorgio CM, Apuzzo MLJ. Experience with vagus nerve stimulation for intractable epilepsy: Some questions and answers. Neurologia medicochirurgica 39:489–495, 1999.

3. Amar AP, DeGiorgio CM, Tarver WB, Apuzzo MLJ, E05 Study Group. Long-term multicenter experience with vagus nerve stimulation for intractable partial seizures: Results of the XE5 trial. Stereotact Funct Neurosurg. In press.

4. Amar AP, Levy ML, Apuzzo MLJ. Vagus nerve stimulation for intractable epilepsy. In: S Rengechary, ed. Neurosurgical operative atlas, Volume 9. Chicago: American Association of Neurological Surgeons, 2000, pp 179–188.

5. DeGiorgio CM, Amar AP, Apuzzo MLJ. Vagus nerve stimulation: Surgical anatomy, technique, and operative complications. In: S Schachter and Schmidt D, eds. Vagal Nerve Stimulation: A manual. In press.

6. Amar AP, Levy ML, Apuzzo MLJ. Vagus nerve stimulation for intractable epilepsy. In: R Winn, ed. Youmans Neurological Surgery. 5th ed. In press.

7. Morris GL, Mueller WM, Vagus Nerve Stimulation Study Group. Long-term treatment with vagus nerve stimulation in patients with refractory epilepsy. Neurology 53:1731–1735, 1999.

8. Fisher RS, Handforth A. Reassessment: Vagus nerve stimulation for epilepsy. Neurology 53:666–669, 1999.

9. Boon P, Vonck K, Vandekerckhove T, D'have M, Nieuwenhuis L, Michielsen G, Vanbelleghem H, Goethals I, Caemaert J, Calliauw L, DeReuck J. Vagus nerve stimulation for medically refractory epilepsy: Efficacy and cost-benefit analysis. Acta Neurochir 141:447–453, 1999.

10. Amar AP, Levy ML, Apuzzo MLJ. Vagus nerve stimulation for control of intractable seizures in childhood. Child's Nerv Syst. In press.

11. Asconape JJ, Moore DD, Zipes DP, Hartman LM, Duffell WH. Bradycardia and asystole with the use of vagus nerve stimulation for the treatment of epilepsy: A rare complication of intraoperative device testing. Epilepsia 40:1452–1454, 1999.

12. Espinosa J, Aiello MT, Naritoku DK. Revision and removal of stimulating electrodes following long term therapy with the vagus nerve stimulator. Surg Neurol 51:659–664, 1999.

47

A Note on Intraoperative Imaging

Michael Schulder and Danny Liang
New Jersey Medical School, Newark, New Jersey, U.S.A.

1 INTRODUCTION

Imaging is the cornerstone of stereotactic surgery. With the advent of digital sectional imaging and its integration with stereotactic devices, imaging has come to mean computed tomography (CT) or magnetic resonance imaging (MRI) (described extensively in this book). Specifically, it means preoperative scanning and use of a stereotactic frame or "frameless system." Imaging technology has become increasingly sophisticated—new frames, faster computers, more versatile software, fancier graphics, and Ethernet connections are all means of improving the manipulation of preoperative images. A scan(s) is obtained before surgery, image fusion is done as needed, the plan is made, and surgery completed. Then, the surgeon waits until a postoperative scan confirms that the surgical goals were obtained.

This paradigm is about to change. The ability to acquire high quality neuroimaging in the OR exists, and is becoming increasingly available. Neurosurgeons may resist this technology, citing the supposed expense, the lack of significant added value, etc. But we are not strangers to intraoperative imaging. Stereotactic surgery was first done with this technology, in the form of ventriculography. Now that we can perform modern neuroimaging in the OR there seems little reason not to fashion stereotaxis around this capability.

553

Of course, disagreement exists regarding intraoperative imaging technology, as is expected with the introduction of any new technology.

2 INTRAOPERATIVE MRI

Intraoperative imaging with MRI (iMRI) is being accomplished with systems that meet the needs of the neurosurgical OR in different ways. The ideal iMRI will provide the best possible images, create the least amount of interference with the OR as possible, include a means of stereotactic navigation, and be as versatile as possible.

The first iMRI was built at the Brigham and Women's Hospital in Boston as a collaborative effort between the Neurosurgery and Radiology departments and General Electric Medical Systems [1]. This system, the Signa SP, employs two vertically oriented magnet poles in a 0.5 T superconducting magnet. The patient is always positioned within the magnet and stereotactic space is defined as such. The Signa SP includes an integrated infrared-based navigational device. A full set of MRI compatible OR equipment was designed for use with this system, which is installed in a specially constructed suite. Other services may use the Signa for such procedures as nasal sinus surgery, breast biopsy and hyperthermic treatments, and prostate implants.

The Siemens corporation developed a 0.2 T iMRI known as the Magnetom Open [2]. It has 2 horizontally oriented poles with a 25 cm gap and using the "fringe field" concept regular OR instrumentation can be used, with the patient rotated into the magnet for imaging [3]. Positioning options are limited and navigation is not available. Siemens has developed a newer system, with a 1.5 T magnet, that will allow for any patient position and includes an infrared navigational tool (Falhbusch, personal communication, 2002). The fringe field concept will be used and the OR table, mounted on a special pedestal, will be rotated towards the gantry for imaging.

Other investigators have developed 1.5 T iMRI units that have been in use for several years. Sutherland spearheaded a project in Calgary whereby a ceiling mounted device is stored in an alcove adjacent to the OR and moved in on a track for imaging [4,5]. The patient and table are enclosed in a copper shield during image acquisition, so the Calgary system allows for the use of regular OR equipment. It also has an integrated IR navigational tool. Hall and Truwit, at the University of Minnesota, adapted a Philips 1.5 T MRI for shared use—on one side of the bore is an OR, and on the other side patients can be brought in for the full gamut of image acquisitions [6]. On the OR side, most of the surgery can be done far enough from the magnet to allow for the use of regular instrumentation; still, there are limits to positioning and navigation is not available. The authors have developed a very useful skull-mounted device (Navigus, Image-Guided Neurologics, Melbourne, Florida) for stereotactic targeting using MR images acquired at the time of surgery [7].

The shared use concept was also employed at the University of Cincinnati, where a 0.2 T Hitachi MRI with a horizontal magnet gap was adapted for OR use and at other times for diagnostic imaging [8]. Despite the low magnet field strength, routine brain and spine imaging can be done with this system. However, navigation is not integrated and patients must be transported from the main OR to the MR suite for imaging.

A lower magnetic field was employed in the development of the Odin PoleStar iMRI. Hadani and collaborators designed a system using a 0.12 T magnet, built from scratch primarily to enhance intracranial neurosurgery [9]. This device is meant to function in a regular OR; radiofrequency interference is eliminated by shielding the room or more recently, by using a "local shield" that surrounds the patient during imaging. Scanning and other functions are controlled by the surgeon or the OR staff. The field of view is 16 cm by 11 cm, more than enough to image most intracranial lesions. The magnet poles typically sit under the OR table and are raised when imaging is done. A navigational probe using passive infrared reflecting spheres is integrated in this system, and updating stereotactic accuracy is done simply by acquiring a new scan.

These systems represent the various approaches to iMRI that are available today and whose uses are being investigated. Clearly, there are major conceptual differences between these devices, which also range widely in price from about $750,000 to $4,000,000. A neurosurgical department contemplating implementing iMRI will need to examine carefully what its needs are and, how much they want to spend on installing a new technology. There is some new data that suggest that iMRI guidance yields shorter stays in the ICU and the hospital, which may help to justify purchase prices to some extent [10].

3   INTRAOPERATIVE CT

Digital imaging in the neurosurgical OR was first done using CT, where a dedicated unit was installed at the University of Pittsburgh [11]. In general, CT scanners are less expensive than MRI units, but acceptance of this technology has been limited by several factors. These include the lower soft tissue contrast compared to MRI, bone hardening artifact in the posterior fossa, the use of ionizing radiation, and likely need for a dedicated technologist to operate the system. Nonetheless, the rapid scan times and the potential applications for spine surgery make iCT potentially useful, and investigators have continued to evaluate its use [12].

4 ULTRASOUND

Ultrasound (US) has been used in neurosurgery for over 20 years [13]. Its major limitation has been image quality and the need to image through the open skull. Neurosurgeons accustomed to interpreting CT and MR images may not readily understand the US images that reflect echogenicity, and items such as cottonoids that have an echo must be removed before imaging. Interpreting the two dimensional images in a 3D manner may also pose problems.

Still, a useful iUS system is attractive because it has a lower price tag than iMRI or iCT. Also, ionizing radiation would not be used, and room shielding or instrument modification would not be needed. As a result, investigation of iUS imaging and navigation technology continues [14].

5 CONCLUSION

It is natural to question the utility of intraoperative imaging, especially as the available methods range considerably in price. Some cost benefit needs to be demonstrated, keeping in mind that much of contemporary neurosurgical technology has become part of the routine without demonstrating cost benefit (the operating microscope, deep brain stimulation, intensive care, and stereotactic frames and frameless systems, for instance).

The logic of imaging in the OR is unavoidable. It is another step towards eliminating guesswork in neurosurgery, the process that began with neurological localization 150 years ago, and that is represented by the concept of stereotaxis itself. Debate regarding the best technology and device is healthy. It is unlikely that one single solution will be found as "best" for intraoperative imaging. As the methods and devices mature, neurosurgeons will be able to choose which system best suits their needs. It is hard to imagine that in the near future stereotactic surgery will be done without the ability to plan, adjust, and confirm based on images acquired in the operating room.

REFERENCES

1. Black P, Moriarty T, Alexander E, 3rd, et al. Development and implementation of intraoperative magnetic resonance imaging and its neurosurgical applications. Neurosurgery 41:831–42; discussion 842–5, 1997.
2. Fahlbusch R, Ganslandt O, Nimsky C. Intraoperative imaging with open magnetic resonance imaging and neuronavigation. Childs Nerv Syst 16:829–31, 2000.
3. Rubino G, Farahani K, McGill D, Van De Wiele B, Villablanca J, Wang-Mathieson A. Magnetic resonance imaging-guided neurosurgery in the mag-

netic fringe fields: the next step in neuronavigation. Neurosurgery 46:643–53; discussion 653–4, 2000.

4. Sutherland G, Kaibara T, Louw D, Hoult D, Tomanek B, Saunders J. A mobile high-field magnetic resonance system for neurosurgery. J Neurosurg 91:804–13, 1999.

5. Kaibara T, Saunders J, Sutherland GR. Advances in mobile intraoperative magnetic resonance imaging. Neurosurgery 47:131–138, 2000.

6. Hall W, Liu H, Martin A, Pozza C, Maxwell R, Truwit C. Safety, efficacy, and functionality of high-field strength interventional magnetic resonance imaging for neurosurgery. Neurosurgery 46:632–41; discussion 641–2, 2000.

7. Hall W, Liu H, Martin A, Truwit C. Comparison of stereotactic brain biopsy to interventional magnetic–resonance–imaging–guided brain biopsy. Stereotact Funct Neurosurg 73:148–153, 2000.

8. Bohinski R, Kokkino A, Warnick R, et al. Glioma resection in a shared-resource magnetic resonance operating room after optimal image-guided frameless stereotactic resection. Neurosurgery 48:731–742, 2001.

9. Hadani M, Spiegelman R, Feldman Z, Berkenstadt H, Ram Z. Novel, compact, intraoperative magnetic resonance imaging–guided system for conventional neurosurgical operating rooms. Neurosurgery 48:799–807; discussion 807–9, 2001.

10. Schulder M, Thosani A. Intraoperative magnetic resonance imaging: impact on length of stay and hospital charges. Neurosurgery 51:595, 2002.

11. Lunsford L, Parrish R, Albright L. Intraoperative imaging with a therapeutic computed tomographic scanner. Neurosurgery 15:559–61, 1984.

12. Hum B, Feigenbaum F, Cleary K, Henderson F. Intraoperative computed tomography for complex craniocervical operations and spinal tumor resections. Neurosurgery 47:374–381, 2000.

13. Chandler W, Knake J, McGillicudy J, Lillehei K, Silver T. Intraoperative use of real–time ultrasonography in neurosurgery. J Neurosurg 57:157–163, 1982.

14. Unsgaard G, Gronningsaeter A, Ommedal S, Hernes T. Brain operations guided by real–time two–dimensional ultrasound: new possibilities as a result of improved image quality. Neurosurgery 51:402–412, 2002.

Index

About the Editor

MICHAEL SCHULDER is Associate Professor of Neurological Surgery and Director of Image-Guided Neurosurgery at New Jersey Medical School/University of Medicine and Dentistry of New Jersey, Newark. The author or coauthor of numerous professional papers, lectures, book chapters, and books, he is a member of the American Association of Neurological Surgeons, the Congress of Neurological Surgeons, the International Stereotactic Radiosurgery Society, and the American Society of Stereotactic and Functional Neurosurgery, among other organizations. He completed his undergraduate and medical education at Columbia University, New York, and his residency in neurosurgery at the Albert Einstein College of Medicine, New York.

Milton Keynes UK
Ingram Content Group UK Ltd.
UKHW020004071024
449327UK00031B/2650